The Advanced Practitioner in Mental Health

The Advanced Practitioner in Mental Health

Edited by

Clare Allabyrne

College of Health and Life Sciences
London Southbank University
London, UK

WILEY

This edition first published 2026
© 2026 John Wiley & Sons Ltd

All rights reserved, including rights for text and data mining and training of artificial intelligence technologies or similar technologies. No part of this publication may be reproduced, stored in a retrieval system, or transmitted, in any form or by any means, electronic, mechanical, photocopying, recording or otherwise, except as permitted by law. Advice on how to obtain permission to reuse material from this title is available at http://www.wiley.com/go/permissions.

The right of Clare Allabyrne to be identified as the author of the editorial material in this work has been asserted in accordance with law.

Registered Office(s)
John Wiley & Sons, Inc., 111 River Street, Hoboken, NJ 07030, USA
John Wiley & Sons Ltd, New Era House, 8 Oldlands Way, Bognor Regis, West Sussex, PO22 9NQ, UK

For details of our global editorial offices, customer services, and more information about Wiley products visit us at www.wiley.com.

The manufacturer's authorized representative according to the EU General Product Safety Regulation is Wiley-VCH GmbH, Boschstr. 12, 69469 Weinheim, Germany, e-mail: Product_Safety@wiley.com.

Wiley also publishes its books in a variety of electronic formats and by print-on-demand. Some content that appears in standard print versions of this book may not be available in other formats.

Trademarks: Wiley and the Wiley logo are trademarks or registered trademarks of John Wiley & Sons, Inc. and/or its affiliates in the United States and other countries and may not be used without written permission. All other trademarks are the property of their respective owners. John Wiley & Sons, Inc. is not associated with any product or vendor mentioned in this book.

Limit of Liability/Disclaimer of Warranty
The contents of this work are intended to further general scientific research, understanding, and discussion only and are not intended and should not be relied upon as recommending or promoting scientific method, diagnosis, or treatment by physicians for any particular patient. In view of ongoing research, equipment modifications, changes in governmental regulations, and the constant flow of information relating to the use of medicines, equipment, and devices, the reader is urged to review and evaluate the information provided in the package insert or instructions for each medicine, equipment, or device for, among other things, any changes in the instructions or indication of usage and for added warnings and precautions. While the publisher and the authors have used their best efforts in preparing this work, including a review of the content of the work, neither the publisher nor the authors make any representations or warranties with respect to the accuracy or completeness of the contents of this work and specifically disclaim all warranties, including without limitation any implied warranties of merchantability or fitness for a particular purpose. No warranty may be created or extended by sales representatives, written sales materials or promotional statements for this work. The fact that an organization, website, or product is referred to in this work as a citation and/or potential source of further information does not mean that the publisher and authors endorse the information or services the organization, website, or product may provide or recommendations it may make. This work is sold with the understanding that the publisher is not engaged in rendering professional services. The advice and strategies contained herein may not be suitable for your situation. You should consult with a specialist where appropriate. Further, readers should be aware that websites listed in this work may have changed or disappeared between when this work was written and when it is read. Neither the publisher nor authors shall be liable for any loss of profit or any other commercial damages, including but not limited to special, incidental, consequential, or other damages.

Library of Congress Cataloging-in-Publication Data Applied for:
Paperback ISBN: 9781394232673

Cover Design: Wiley
Cover Images: © anand purohit/Getty Images, © Péter Mocsonoky/Getty Images, © creative/stock.adobe.com

Set in 10.5/13pt STIXTwoText by Straive, Pondicherry, India
Printed and bound by CPI Group (UK) Ltd, Croydon, CR0 4YY
C9781394232673_110326

Dedication

This book is dedicated with love to my parents Charlie and Carmel; my children Kerry and Conor; my grandson Rory and my sister and brothers Carmel, Colin and John.

Contents

	Contributors	ix
	Foreword	xi
	Acknowledgements	xii

PART 1 Advanced Practice in Mental Health: An Overview — 1

CHAPTER 1	Introduction to Advanced Practice in Mental Health *Clare Allabyrne and Wendy York*	3
CHAPTER 2	Implementing and Governing Advanced Practice in Mental Health *Katie Cooper and Rebecca Burgess-Dawson*	10

PART 2 Advanced Practice in Mental Health: Guiding Principles — 25

CHAPTER 3	Holistic Care and the Biopsychosocial Framework *Stuart Maddock*	27
CHAPTER 4	Physical Health and Integrated Care *Kirstie Tomlinson*	48
CHAPTER 5	Clinical Reasoning and Complexity: An Overview *James Tighe*	63
CHAPTER 6	Cognitive Bias and Heuristics *Steve Bown*	89
CHAPTER 7	Advanced Practice in Mental Health and Trauma-Informed Care *Rachael Smith, Alicia Bailey and Elizabeth Hearn*	107
CHAPTER 8	Psychopharmacology for Advanced Practice *Diksha Kara and Masuma Tashnim Hussain*	130
CHAPTER 9	Mental Health and Legal Issues *Christine Hutchinson and Steve Hardy*	150

CHAPTER 10	Collaborative Care Planning and Shared Decision-Making Ann Cox and Jan McAdam	166
CHAPTER 11	Digital Technology in Advanced Practice: Mental Health Emma Taylor	181
CHAPTER 12	The Role of Experts by Experience (Including Co-production and Co-creation) in Advanced Practice in Mental Health Narenza Dhanasar	197

PART 3 Advanced Practice in Mental Health and Specific Populations — 221

CHAPTER 13	Perinatal Mental Health Claire Hargrave	223
CHAPTER 14	Child and Adolescent Mental Health Services (CAMHS) Ann Cox and Narenza Dhanasar	244
CHAPTER 15	Mental Health in Older People and the Advanced Practitioner Kirstie Tomlinson	266
CHAPTER 16	Supporting People with Learning Disabilities and Autistic People Jo Delrée and Sue Bridges	284
CHAPTER 17	Advanced Risk Assessment and Forensic Mental Health Elizabeth Hearn	301
CHAPTER 18	Substance Use – Including Co-occurring Mental Health and Drugs and Alcohol (COMHAD) Lois Dugmore	326

PART 4 The Role of the Advanced Practitioner in Mental Health — 351

CHAPTER 19	Mapping the Role to the Four Pillars of Advanced Practice Chloe Parkin	353
CHAPTER 20	Advanced Practice in Mental Health: Personal and Professional Growth Kayleigh Brown and Stephanie Tempest	380
	Index	397

Contributors

Clare Allabyrne
Division of Advanced Clinical Practice
and Non Medical Prescribing
School of Nursing and Midwifery
Institute of Health and Social Care
London Southbank University
London, UK

Alicia Bailey
Alder Hey Children's Hospital Trust
Liverpool, Merseyside, UK

Steve Bown
Sheffield Hallam University
Sheffield, UK

Sue Bridges
Norfolk and Suffolk NHS Foundation Trust
Norwich, UK

Kayleigh Brown
Mental Health Division
Humber Teaching NHS Foundation Trust
Hull, UK

Rebecca Burgess-Dawson
Workforce, Training and Education
NHS, England, UK

Katie Cooper
Workforce, Training and Education
NHS, England, UK

Dr Ann Cox
Derbyshire Healthcare NHS Foundation Trust
Derby, UK

Jo Delrée
Delree Training and Consultancy
London, UK

Narenza Dhanasar
East London NHS Foundation Trust
London, UK

Dr Lois Dugmore
Leicestershire Partnership NHS Trust
Leicester, UK

Steve Hardy
Oxleas NHS Foundation Trust
London, Kent and the South West of England
UK

Claire Hargrave
Central and North West London
Foundation Trust
London, UK

Elizabeth Hearn
St George's, Epsom, and St Helier University
Hospitals and Health Group
London, UK

Masuma Tashnim Hussain
Southwest London and St George's Mental
Health NHS Trust
London, UK

Christine Hutchinson
School of Nursing and Midwifery
Faculty of Health, Social Care and Medicine
Edge Hill University
Ormskirk, Lancashire, UK

Diksha Kara
East London NHS Foundation Trust
London, UK

Stuart Maddock
Norfolk and Suffolk Foundation Trust
Norfolk, UK

University of East Anglia
Norwich, UK

Jan McAdam
Tees, Esk and Wear Valleys NHS Trust
North Yorkshire, UK

Chloe Parkin
Cornwall Partnership NHS Foundation Trust
Cornwall, UK

South West Clinical School
University of Plymouth
Plymouth, UK

Rachael Smith
Essex Partnership Foundation Trust
Essex, UK

Emma Taylor
Digital Mentality
London, UK

Stephanie Tempest
Stephanie Tempest Consultancy Ltd.
London, UK

James Tighe
Royal Marsden Hospital
London, UK

Kirstie Tomlinson
Nottinghamshire Healthcare NHS Trust
Nottingham, UK

Wendy York
Division of Advanced Clinical Practice
and Non Medical Prescribing
School of Nursing and Midwifery
Institute of Health and Social Care
London Southbank University
London, UK

Foreword

It is with great pride that we introduce *The Advanced Practitioner in Mental Health*, the first book of its kind dedicated to advanced practice in the mental health field.

As clinicians and strategic leaders, we have had the privilege of working alongside colleagues who, over many years, have helped to shape and grow the role of the advanced practitioner. What began as a vision to recognise and harness advanced clinical expertise within mental health is now taking form as a defined and expanding field of practice. This book marks an important milestone in that journey.

What makes this volume unique is both its scope and its voice. It brings together contributions from established clinicians, academics, and experts by experience, each offering perspectives that reflect the true breadth and depth of advanced practice. From clinical reasoning and trauma-informed care to digital technology, perinatal mental health and forensic settings, the chapters set out not only the principles but also the realities of advanced practice in diverse contexts.

We hope this book will serve as both a starting point and a touchstone: a resource for aspiring and current advanced practitioners, a reference for leaders and educators and a statement of intent for the future development of services; supporting a culture where advanced practitioners' experience, expertise and professionalism is recognised and valued across the multidisciplinary team.

At its heart, advanced practice is about improving outcomes for people, families and communities. By developing, supporting and embedding these roles, we strengthen patient safety, enhance quality of care and build more resilient services. This book is a significant step in making that vision a reality.

Rebecca Burgess-Dawson
National Specialist Education Advisor (Mental Health) (WT&E)
NHS England

Katie Cooper
National Head of Multi-professional Advanced Practice
NHS England Workforce, Training & Education

Acknowledgements

Thank you to Katrina Maclaine and Sally Hardy without whose innovation and expertise this book would not have been possible.

The biggest thank you of all must go to Gemma Ford who worked so hard with me on the origin of the book, recruiting authors alongside me, assisting in the editing of some of the chapters and supporting me throughout the whole process. She has been both inspirational and instrumental in getting this book to publication.

Contributions

Chapter 19

Gemma Morshead, Linda Rowse, Sam Pearce, Lucy Bentley, Jodie Ley, Lauren Oliver, Fiona Ramsay, Dr Daniel Smith, Alison Bartlett, Dr Amber Simler, Lindsay Parkin, Joby Plant, Toby Parkin

PART 1

ADVANCED PRACTICE IN MENTAL HEALTH: AN OVERVIEW

CHAPTER 1

Introduction to Advanced Practice in Mental Health

Clare Allabyrne and Wendy York

Division of Advanced Clinical Practice and Non Medical Prescribing, School of Nursing and Midwifery, Institute of Health and Social Care, London Southbank University, London, UK

Aim

This brief chapter is intended to set a context and remind the reader of the origins, underpinning principles, education, some of the current positioning and potential next steps for advanced practice in mental health. It is significantly expanded on and developed in both the second and final chapter of the book.

INTRODUCTION

Mental health issues continue to be a neglected, yet highly essential, element of global health and well-being. The aims of global mental health are to promote mental health and well-being, provide access to treatment for populations across the world and combine transdisciplinary approaches to enable mental health equity and attention to human rights [1, 2].

Advanced practice in healthcare has emerged in response to the ever-changing societal needs, continually evolving healthcare systems and the growing complexity of patient care.

Understanding how advanced practice in mental health has evolved from and in parallel to advanced practice in physical health internationally and within the United Kingdom provides context for its current and future role in mental healthcare.

This chapter briefly explores that journey incorporating some of the drivers including parity of esteem, diagnostic overshadowing and education.

The Advanced Practitioner in Mental Health, First Edition. Edited by Clare Allabyrne.
© 2026 John Wiley & Sons Ltd. All rights reserved, including rights for text and data mining and training of artificial intelligence technologies or similar technologies. Published 2026 by John Wiley & Sons Ltd.

Definition of Advanced Practice

For the purposes of this text, we will use the definition provided by NHS England (NHSE) in their Multi-professional framework for advanced practice in England 2025. It should be noted that 'advanced practice' is now more commonly used than 'advanced clinical practice' as an overall term to avoid over-emphasis on the clinical pillar.

> 'Advanced practice is delivered by accomplished registered health and care professionals. It is a level of practice characterised by a high degree of autonomy and designated responsibility for complex decision making. This is underpinned by a post-registration master's level award or equivalent undertaken by an experienced practitioner that encompasses all four pillars of clinical practice, leadership and management, education, and research. Advanced practice embodies the ability to manage care in partnership with individuals, families, and carers. It includes the analysis and synthesis of complex problems, and management of clinical risk and uncertainty across a range of settings, enabling innovative solutions to expedite access to care, optimise people's experiences, and improve outcomes'. [3]

History

We began to see the emergence of advanced practice in healthcare in the 1960s. This was initially in response to an increasing demand for healthcare services, the need to expand access to care and medical workforce shortages. The original professional focus was on nursing. The first Nurse Practitioner (NP) programme at the University of Colorado was developed in 1965 focusing on paediatric care and aiming to extend the reach of healthcare services, particularly in areas where there were scant healthcare resources [4]. Psychiatric and mental health nursing embraced advanced roles early on, with a recognition of the potential for nurses to function as therapeutic agents in complex mental health systems [5].

Across Canada, Australia and parts of Europe, shaped by local healthcare needs similar developments unfolded. For example, Australia formally recognised the nurse practitioner role in the 1990s with mental health identified as a priority area. The Nurses Amendment (Nurse Practitioners) Act 1998 in New South Wales then allowed nurse practitioners to address mental health service gaps, especially in rural and underserved communities [6]. While the structure and titles varied globally, what became apparent was the need for healthcare professionals who could deliver high-level clinical expertise autonomously, particularly in complex fields like mental health.

Advanced practice roles in mental health have evolved internationally along similar lines to that of physical health but with additional pressures, particularly in relation to deinstitutionalisation and the inherent rise in demand for community-based mental health services with Psychiatric-Mental Health Nurse Practitioners (PMHNPs) in the United States gaining prominence in the 1990s as one response to these issues [7].

The Australian framework for mental health nurse practitioners who assess, diagnose, treat and manage mental illnesses across the lifespan emphasises collaborative, consumer-led care, aligning with contemporary mental health service delivery models [8], which is increasingly reflected in other countries.

The progression of advanced practice in the United Kingdom has been shaped by the ever-changing landscape and policy reforms in healthcare delivery. In 1966, The Salmon Report [9] laid the groundwork by proposing a new clinical nursing structure, recognising the need for senior clinical roles within nursing. These specialist nursing roles emerged throughout the 1970s and 1980s, although definitions and scopes of practice remained inconsistent.

It was not until the publication of the Multi-professional Framework for Advanced Clinical Practice in England by Health Education England (HEE) in 2017 [10] (recently updated in 2025 [3]) that a standardised definition and framework for advanced practice was established which was not nurse-centric and incorporated other professions. The framework delineated four pillars of advanced practice:

1. Clinical practice
2. Leadership and management
3. Education
4. Research [10]

In the United Kingdom, the shift from custodial care models to community-based mental health services during the 1980s and 1990s drove the need for new competencies and roles for mental health nurses. This transition then led to the gradual emergence of advanced practice roles in mental health, although there was initially little to no consistency in education, titles or expectations [11].

Then in 2020, HEE published the Advanced Practice Mental Health Curriculum and Capabilities Framework [12]. This framework outlines the capabilities required to achieve advanced practitioner-level practice in mental health and emphasises the importance of clinical competencies, supervision and support, as well as the assessment of competencies. The framework also serves as a guide for the collaborative development of advanced practice roles between providers and higher education institutions. The framework was further endorsed/credentialled by NHS England in 2022 [13].

PARITY OF ESTEEM

Central to advancing practice in the United Kingdom has been the concept of parity of esteem. Parity of esteem refers to valuing mental health equally with physical health. The term came into being to recognise the disparity in healthcare provision for mental health clients when compared with physical health clients. It means that whether due to stigma or resource/commissioning issues, mental health clients should not face inequality in treatment and their physical health issues should not be overshadowed by their mental health presentation, also known as diagnostic overshadowing [14]. This is discussed in more detail further in the chapter.

Parity of esteem was formally described in the No Health Without Mental Health strategy published in 2011 [14]. The Health and Social Care Act 2012 then enshrined the principle in legislation [15], and the need for parity of esteem was further recognised in 2014 in the NHS England Five Year Forward View [16].

Progress on this is difficult to measure, though there are three common concepts recognised as indicators of parity:

1. Excess mortality – the negative impact mental health has on life expectancy.
2. Burden of disease – measuring the impact of a disease. Mental health is one of the leading causes of ill health and disability in the world.
3. Treatment gap – the difference between the number of people thought to have a particular condition and those receiving treatment for it [17].

Advanced Practitioners in Mental Health (APMH) are uniquely suited to progressing the parity of esteem agenda in a climate of workforce and economic paucity by shaping delivery models, meeting ever-changing demands in clinical practice and leading innovative transformational change in safe, cost-efficient, quality-assured, person-focused services.

DIAGNOSTIC OVERSHADOWING

Diagnostic overshadowing is a term first used in conjunction with learning disabilities [18], in recognition that physical symptoms and/or behaviours are often overlooked and attributed to the individual's cognitive deficits. This has been widened out to encompass those with mental health difficulties, with physical health complaints being ascribed to psychiatric symptomatology [19]. Diagnostic overshadowing can be seen as partly responsible for the 15–20-year mortality gap between those with serious mental illness (SMI) and the general population. This delay in treatment can contribute to the development of further acuity and clinical complexity, adding to a decrease in the quality of life, poorer outcomes and an increase in cost to healthcare providers [20–22].

Factors that can be involved in practitioners' sometimes faulty clinical decision-making can include the severity of the mental illness, stigma, cognitive bias (addressed in detail in Chapter 6), staff attitudes, a lack of training in mental health/ill health or a lack of confidence in physical health symptom recognition [20, 23].

Strategies to minimise diagnostic overshadowing can include enhancing skills in complex thinking, diagnostic formulation and diagnostic differentials; considering the case from multiple perspectives and developing high levels of self-awareness with continuous reflection on practice, attitudes and training needs.

Specialist APMH programmes attempt to mitigate diagnostic overshadowing and address parity of esteem. The combination of skills in advanced physical health assessments, an elevated level of knowledge and skills in mental health assessment and therapeutic interventions, being able to autonomously manage clinical complexity and an episode of care from referral through to discharge go some way to address these issues which in turn make these roles attractive to employers when fully understood how they can be utilised [3, 12].

EDUCATION

Having been involved in creating and then running the first Royal College of Nursing (RCN) accredited specialist Advanced Practice MSc in Mental Health in England (at the time RCN accreditation was the only gold standard quality marker for these courses) since 2016 [22], we have both seen and been part of the emergence of a tripartite infrastructure supporting this specialist education work, including an APMH national steering group, an education forum and an Advanced Mental Health Community of Practice (AMHCoP) [23], as well as five early adopter sites in higher education institutions, a portfolio route to the qualification and the development of a Centre for Advancing Practice.

POSTIONING

The role of the APMH lends itself well to acute mental health services such as inpatient, home treatment teams and psychiatric liaison. Forensic mental health services are also seeing the benefit of the APMH role, meaning with the combination of advanced physical health and mental health knowledge and skills, service users are able to have the continuity of care and a more holistic approach in one place. The autonomous role has also seen APMHs joining doctors' rotas and clerking in at admission. There are, however, new and emerging roles. Primary care, for example, is an area in which the APMH role is being utilised to good effect. APMHs are being employed in GP surgeries offering mental health assessments, consultations, signposting and making referrals to other services. Close collaboration with secondary and tertiary mental health services is also part of the role.

In terms of service delivery, there has been a definite shift. Some of the professions that would traditionally have undertaken the generic physical health programme, for example paramedics, are now undertaking the mental health programme. The announcement [24] that the police would be responding to less mental health call outs will undoubtedly put more pressure on first responders such as paramedics to meet this need. Paramedic mental health units are being set up to address this, and there is a clear recognition of the training requirements needed to be able to deliver this service effectively and competently. The NHS Long Term Plan [25] also recognises the need to develop the mental health competency of ambulance staff. It cites several studies where the inclusion of mental health professionals in paramedic teams has reduced the number of attendances to the emergency department and hospital admissions.

The NHS Long Term Plan [25] also recognises the role that Advanced Practitioners (AP) in mental health settings can play, being strategically placed to manage some of the current workforce challenges. This is very much in line with the workforce transformation long-term plan [26] with an emphasis on train, retain and reform. New ways of working have to be implemented to meet the challenges of a stretched health service.

Advanced practice in mental health can potentially meet the needs of the mental health population where there are significant staff shortages and is intrinsic to workforce planning. Retention of the current workforce is key, and helping staff plan their career trajectory is important. Those working at an enhanced level of practice may find the dynamic APMH roles attractive, allowing the individual to stay clinical without having to move into management to progress. An expansion of consultant roles is also being further explored, which potentially can offer the APMH future development [26].

Currently, there is a limited amount of research about the APMH role and more research into the effectiveness of the APMH role is imperative. Whilst only a very small sample size, there is some evidence to show that APMHs who have undertaken the physical health advanced practice programme with a specialist mental health module have greatly benefited from this additional knowledge, arguably offering a more holistic approach to their patients [26, 27].

The recent Nuffield Trust report [28] has highlighted that the AP role in nursing and midwifery is not fully understood by colleagues as well as the public with a call for regulation by the Nursing Midwifery Council. This finding is supported [29] more specifically about the AP in mental health services. Clarification about roles, expectations and responsibilities is still a work in progress.

CONCLUSION

As the number of professionals who move through the various accredited courses in Advanced Practice in Mental Health grows and there is a more visible presence, public understanding should also increase. Utilising the four pillars and ensuring that the roles are not just clinical is imperative to the quality-of-service provision and the future workforce development. APMHs are in a prime position to be researching their own roles and the impact of said roles, as well as educating fellow healthcare professionals and the public about these roles, as their value continues to grow and there is increasing recognition of their importance in the ever-changing landscape of healthcare delivery.

REFERENCES

1. Collins, P.Y. (2020). What is global mental health? *World Psychiatry* 19: 265.
2. Bass, J., Chibanda, D., Petersen, I. et al. (2023). Introducing Cambridge prisms: global mental health. *Global Mental Health* 10: e7.
3. NHS England (2025). Multi-professional framework for advanced practice. MPF 2025 – Advanced Practice. https://advanced-practice.hee.nhs.uk/mpf2025/ (accessed 14 June 2025).
4. Ford, L.C. and Silver, H.K. (1965). Expanding the role of the nurse. *The American Journal of Nursing* 65 (12): 66–69.
5. Haber, J. (1999). Hildegard Peplau: the mother of psychiatric nursing. *Nursing and Health Care Perspectives* 20 (4): 228.
6. Driscoll, A., Worrall-Carter, L., O'Reilly, J., and Stewart, S. (2005). A historical review of the nurse practitioner role in Australia. *The Australian Journal of Advanced Nursing* 23 (1): 6–11.
7. Delaney, K.R. and Vanderhoef, D. (2019). Advanced practice psychiatric nursing: a core resource. *Journal of the American Psychiatric Nurses Association* 25 (1): 5–15.
8. Wand, T., White, K., and Patching, J. (2011). Realistic evaluation of an emergency department-based mental health nurse practitioner outpatient service in Australia. *Nursing & Health Sciences* 13 (2): 199–206.
9. Ministry of Health (1966). *Report of the Committee on Senior Nursing Staff Structure (The Salmon Report)*. London: HMSO.
10. Health Education England (2017). Multi professional framework for advanced clinical practice in England. https://www.hee.nhs.uk/sites/default/files/documents/Multi-professional%20framework%20for%20advanced%20clinical%20practice%20in%20England.pdf
11. Department of Health (1999). National service framework for mental health: modern standards and service models. London: Department of Health.
12. Health Education England (2020). Advanced practice mental health curriculum and capabilities framework. London: Health Education England.
13. NHS England (2022). Mental Health Advanced Practice area specific capability and curriculum framework. https://advanced-practice.hee.nhs.uk/wp-content/uploads/sites/28/2025/01/Mental-health-advanced-practice-area-specific-capability-and-curriculum-framework-NHSE.pdf
14. HM Government (2011). No health without mental health: a cross-government mental health outcomes strategy for people of all ages. London: HM Government.
15. Health and Social Care Act (2012). Health and Social Care Act 2012. London: The Stationery Office.
16. NHS England (2015). The five year forward view for mental health. A report from the independent Mental Health Taskforce to the NHS in England. London: NHS England.
17. Baker, C., Gheera M. Mental health: achieving 'parity of esteem'. https://commonslibrary.parliament.uk/mental-health-achieving-parity-of-esteem/ (accessed 2 May 2025).
18. Reiss, S., Levitan, G., and Szyszko, J. (1982). Emotional disturbance and mental retardation: diagnostic overshadowing. *American Journal of Mental Deficiency* 86: 567–574.
19. Jones, S., Howard, L., and Thornicroft, G. (2008). Diagnostic overshadowing: worse physical health care for people with mental illness. *Acta Psychiatrica Scandinavica* 118: 169–171.
20. Nash, M. (2013). Diagnostic overshadowing: a potential barrier to physical health care for mental health service users. *Mental Health Practice* 17 (4): 22–26.

21. Shefer, G., Henderson, C., Howard, L.M. et al. (2014). Diagnostic overshadowing and other challenges involved in the diagnostic process of patients with mental illness who present at emergency departments with physical symptoms – a qualitative study. *PLoS One* 9 (11): e111682. https://doi.org/10.1371/journal.pone.0111682.
22. Allabyrne, C., Chaplin, E., and Hardy, S. (2020). Advanced nursing practice in mental health: towards parity of esteem. *Nursing Times* 16 (12): 21–23.
23. NHS England (2022). Advanced practice in mental health implementation guide - Advanced Practice. https://advanced-practice.hee.nhs.uk/advanced-practice-in-mental-health-implementation-guide/
24. BBC (2023). Police in England to attend fewer mental health calls - BBC News. https://www.bbc.co.uk/news/uk-66304472
25. NHS (2019). Long term plan. [ARCHIVED CONTENT] The NHS Long Term Plan. https://webarchive.nationalarchives.gov.uk/ukgwa/20250707103655/https://www.longtermplan.nhs.uk/wp-content/uploads/2019/08/nhs-long-term-plan-version-1.2.pdf
26. NHS (2023). Long term workforce plan. https://www.england.nhs.uk/publication/nhs-long-term-workforce-plan/.
27. Chadwick, A. and Murphy, N. (2019). An exploration of providing mental health skills in a generic advanced clinical practice programme. *British Journal of Nursing* 28 (13): 842–847.
28. Palmer, W., Julian, S., and Vaughan, L. (2023). Independent report on the regulation of advanced practice in nursing and midwifery. London: Nuffield Trust.
29. Brimblecombe, N. and Nolan, F. (2021). A qualitative study of perceptions of senior health service staff as to factors influencing the development of advanced clinical practice roles in mental health services. *Journal of Psychiatric and Mental Health Nursing* 28: 829–837.

CHAPTER 2

Implementing and Governing Advanced Practice in Mental Health

Katie Cooper and Rebecca Burgess-Dawson
Workforce, Training and Education, NHS, England, UK

> **Aim**
>
> This chapter will critically examine the role of advanced practice in mental health within UK health policy and workforce transformation, evaluating governance. It will then consider the development and application of the NHS England capabilities framework, describing the alignment of practice with the four pillars to support safe, effective service redesign.

LEARNING OUTCOMES

- Critically analyse the role of advanced practice in mental health within the context of UK health policy and workforce transformation.
- Evaluate governance frameworks that underpin safe and effective implementation of advanced practice roles.
- Apply the HEE (now NHS England) Advanced Practice Mental Health Curriculum and Capabilities Framework to real-world service redesign.
- Examine and apply strategies for ensuring scope of practice, education and clinical governance align with the four pillars of Advanced Practice in Mental Health (APMH).
- Identify risks, safeguarding considerations and red flags in the development and delivery of advanced practice roles in mental health.

INTRODUCTION

The development of advanced roles within UK mental health services has been characterised by an iterative and often organic process, reflecting both the evolving complexity of care and the necessity for workforce innovation. Historically, many roles incorporating the title 'advanced' emerged in response to local service pressures without the benefit of a standardised national framework or clearly defined competency expectations. This lack of uniformity created challenges in assuring public confidence, as titles did not consistently equate to a predictable or verifiable level of skill, autonomy or clinical accountability across organisations and regions [1, 2].

At the same time, the trajectory of mental health workforce development has required the creation of a more nuanced and flexible skill mix. Key disciplines, including nursing, occupational therapy, psychology and social work, have long been broadening their scope of practice and enhancing their competencies in response to increasingly complex population needs. The drive towards a multi-professional advanced practice workforce has therefore been less about adding a new layer of hierarchy and more about maximising the existing potential of experienced practitioners to deliver holistic, safe and high-quality care within integrated service models [3, 4]. Establishing rigorous education standards, competency-based assessment and robust governance frameworks has been critical in transforming these organically developed roles into a coherent and credible national workforce, capable of inspiring confidence among patients, the public and professional peers alike.

In 2024, the Secretary of State for Health and Social Care commissioned Lord Darzi to conduct an immediate and wide-ranging independent investigation into the NHS. The Lord Darzi report [3] clearly sets out the current challenges faced, in terms of resources available to deliver safe, high-quality, effective care and the patient and public demands and expectations in the way services are commissioned in the future. It signalled how the health service needs to change, arguing for a more engaged relationship with people and communities to promote well-being and prevent ill health. This requires workforce transformation and a consistent approach to the expansion of new roles and new ways of working, which includes the further development and implementation of advanced practitioner roles as set out in the NHS Long Term Workforce Plan [5].

The NHS Long Term Workforce Plan [5] and later 'Fit for the Future', the NHS 10 Year Health Plan for England [6], clearly articulate the continued drive to develop the advancing practice workforce as part of the multidisciplinary team, recognising the impact these roles can have not only on improving patient care but also on increasing the number of senior clinical decision-makers within the NHS to improve productivity and increase capacity.

Also, in the new 10 year plan is an acknowledgement that in order to have long and successful careers in health and social care, the importance of retaining experienced senior staff is vital. Advanced practice and the identification of that development is one of the ways in which staff feel valued, entrusted and recognised as having highly developed knowledge and skills and the ability to provide high-quality, safe, effective care to patients and their families.

Overall, there now seems to be relatively routine acknowledgement that advanced practitioners have an established role in supporting and driving service transformation [7]. Fundamentally, they are well placed to provide supportive clinical leadership to the UK government's three key shifts to modernise the NHS [6]:

1. **From Hospital to Community**
   Emphasis on delivering more care outside hospital settings by expanding neighbourhood health centres and enhancing primary, community, mental health and home-based care services. The goal is to reduce reliance on acute hospital infrastructure and bring proactive, personalised care closer to patients' homes.

2. **From Analogue to Digital**
   A comprehensive digital transformation including expansion of the NHS App, creation of a unified patient record and deployment of artificial intelligence and telehealth solutions. This shift aims to empower patients, streamline administrative burdens and enhance access to care through technology by 2028.
3. **From Sickness to Prevention**
   Moving the focus from treating illness to preventing it through public health interventions, lifestyle support, regulation (e.g. obesity management, tobacco control) and early detection measures –shaping a future where the NHS proactively keeps people healthy.

WHAT IS ADVANCED PRACTICE?

Advanced practitioners have been introduced successfully across multiple healthcare sectors, and the numbers continue to grow due to service needs and drivers. Historically, however, these roles had often been implemented as a reactive service response, rather than with a planned and coordinated approach which led to large variations in how organisations had deployed these roles and their scope and level of practice.

To remove these inconsistencies and to support the ability to develop a sustainable and transferable advanced practice workforce, the Multi-professional framework for advanced clinical practice in England, 2017 [1], was published. For the first time, this provided a clear definition and consistent approach to advanced practice in the United Kingdom.

This was the first time that advanced practice had been formally aggregated into four overarching and interdependent pillars: clinical practice, education, leadership and management and research. This structural consolidation was significant because it provided a unified, cross-professional language and set of capabilities that could be applied consistently across diverse disciplines and care contexts. The introduction of the four pillars created a national benchmark for competence, emphasising that advanced practice is not defined by job title or profession but by a level of capability underpinned by breadth across all domains. In doing so, it established a critical foundation for assuring public confidence, supporting workforce mobility and enabling organisations to evaluate and develop roles against shared standards [1, 2]. For mental health services in particular, the four pillar model was transformative in validating the complex mix of clinical expertise, therapeutic alliance, leadership in service redesign and commitment to evidence-informed practice required to deliver safe, holistic and person-centred care.

The Framework has recently been updated; however, the core competencies and capabilities across the four pillars of advanced practice remain unchanged [2].

Although the initial work to formalise multi-professional advanced practice in this way was done in England, similar frameworks exist for healthcare professionals in the other UK countries:

- In **Scotland**, this is the 'Nursing, Midwifery, and Allied Health Professionals (NMAHP) development framework – post-reg framework' NHS Education for Scotland 2024 [8].
- In **Wales**, the 'Professional Framework for Enhanced, Advanced, and Consultant Clinical Practice', Health Education and Improvement Wales 2023 [9].
- In **Northern Ireland**, the 'Advanced Allied Health Professionals (AHP) practice framework', Department of Health 2019 [10].

As each country has published its own framework(s), some of the definitions, language and professional capabilities do vary. However, the approach of each of these countries, including the basic structure of career frameworks, definitions of advanced practice and the pillars of clinical practice, is in fact very similar.

Overall, the central paradigm remains the same. Being an advanced practitioner is to demonstrate the delivery of care with a greater degree of expertise.

The following definition of advanced practice is taken from the *Multi-professional Framework for Advanced Practice in England* [2]:

'Advanced practice is delivered by accomplished registered health and care professionals. It is a level of practice characterised by a high degree of autonomy and designated responsibility for complex decision making. This is underpinned by a post-registration master's level award or equivalent undertaken by an experienced practitioner that encompasses all four pillars of clinical practice, leadership and management, education, and research.

Advanced practice embodies the ability to manage care in partnership with individuals, families, and carers. It includes the analysis and synthesis of complex problems and management of clinical risk and uncertainty across a range of settings, enabling innovative solutions to expedite access to care, optimise people's experiences and improve outcomes'

Of course, this expertise must be contextualised to the individual's scope of practice – the area, environment and role that the person is in.

For this reason, the Framework articulates the capabilities that underpin advanced practice across all the four pillars of practice. They remain generic rather than profession-specific. It is then incumbent upon the individual health and care professional working at this level of practice to demonstrate the capabilities in relation to their profession, job role and area of practice.

All registered health and care professionals working at the level of advanced practice within the mental health workforce can then demonstrate that they have developed their skills and knowledge to enable them to meet the minimum capabilities and competencies as outlined by their regulator, national frameworks and any professional bodies guidance across all the four pillars of advanced practice (see Figure 2.1).

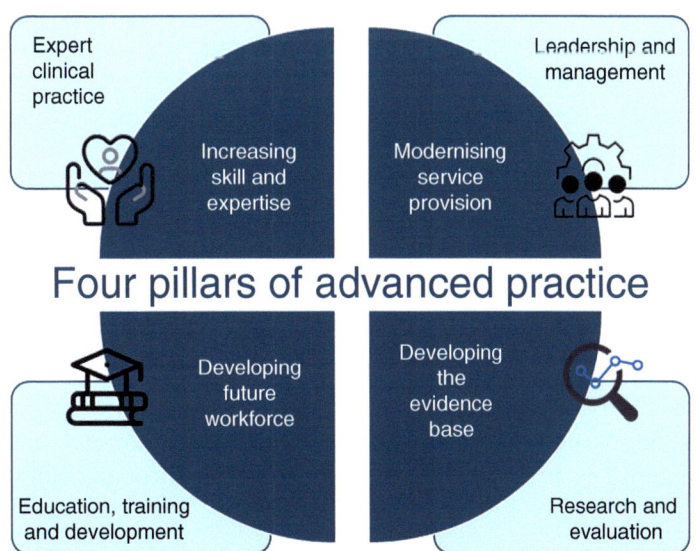

FIGURE 2.1 The four pillars of advanced practice.

IMPACT OF ADVANCED PRACTICE ROLES ON WORKFORCE AND SERVICE TRANSFORMATION

The NHS Long-term Workforce Plan [5] acknowledged the importance of optimising the workforce and the impact advance practice roles can have on workforce and service transformation, as outlined next.

- Ability to retain valued, experienced staff and realise the full scope of practice within and across each profession.
- Support teams to increase multidisciplinary team senior clinical decision-making capability and capacity.
- Release time for more experienced clinical professionals to provide training and care delivery only they can do.
- Increase person-centred care, focusing on self-care, pre- and re-habilitation with the aim of keeping people at home and as independent as possible.
- Optimise access to services and reduce waiting times.
- Support early intervention and diagnosis.
- Support workforce and service redesign and transformation.
- Increase capacity to supervise and develop multi-professional workforce.

A central driver underpinning the implementation of advanced practitioner roles is the imperative to enable experienced clinicians to operate at the highest level of their professional scope, thereby realising their full potential and optimising their contribution to the delivery of care across the continuum – from individuals, families and carers to the health and well-being of entire populations [11].

In the context of a post-Covid, resource-constrained health system, the principle of working at the 'top of one's licence' has, at times, been misinterpreted as being synonymous with achieving more with fewer resources. This interpretation diverges from the strategic intent of advanced practice, which is not to fill systemic gaps through role substitution but to formalise and elevate expertise, ensuring that complex decision-making, leadership and holistic, person-centred care are delivered by clinicians with the requisite knowledge, skill and accountability [12].

In mental health in particular, where therapeutic alliance, nuanced clinical judgement and integrated biopsychosocial approaches are critical, maximising the capabilities of advanced practitioners ensures the delivery of care at a formally recognised expert level. This enables services to embed safe, evidence-based and innovative interventions; strengthen multidisciplinary collaboration; and ultimately achieve improved outcomes for service users and populations while maintaining professional credibility and public trust [13].

IMPLEMENTING ADVANCED PRACTICE

The development of an advanced practitioner role should initially be driven by an analysis of service need and scrutiny of the capabilities and capacity of the existing and available workforce. It should always be inextricably linked to workforce development plans, which identify where advanced practice will have the greatest benefit and maximise positive impact in a person's journey through health and care pathways.

To establish advanced practice roles, organisations will need to articulate a clear business case. This is a significant investment in the workforce, including those individuals and their career development. In collaboration with the advanced practice and relevant multi-professional leads, NHS England Southwest Faculty for Advancing Practice has developed an 'Emerging Areas in Advanced Practice Workforce Transformation Resource' [14] that is designed to support and standardised the approach to workforce transformation for advanced practice.

Key principles for developing an advanced practice role would mean that the organisation or service has:

1. Reached a shared understanding of advanced practice.
2. Defined the pathway/service under consideration.
3. Defined the problem within and across the pathway – ensuring that there is a clearly demonstrated need for the service and workforce transformation.
4. Designed the role(s) to address local need – ensuring that there is a clearly demonstrated need for the role at an advanced level of practice working across all four pillars and identifying the impact on the problem(s).
5. Defined the knowledge, skills and competencies and capabilities required for the specific scope of practice.
6. Operationalised – exploring the readiness for advanced practice, considering system priorities, team engagement and the workforce.

It should be noted that there are additional specialist roles and statutory responsibilities within mental health services that clinicians may undertake following further post-qualification training and assessment. These roles, while often held by experienced practitioners, sit outside the scope of advanced practitioner education and capability frameworks, as they are governed by distinct legislative and regulatory requirements.

Examples include the **Approved Clinician (AC)** and **Responsible Clinician (RC)** roles, which carry specific legal powers and duties under the Mental Health Act 1983 [15] (as amended). These roles require additional formal training, approval by the Secretary of State and ongoing revalidation to ensure compliance with statutory responsibilities for patient assessment, treatment planning and review under compulsory care.

Similarly, the role of **Approved Mental Health Professional (AMHP)**, which may be undertaken by a range of registered professionals including social workers, nurses and occupational therapists, requires completion of a nationally accredited programme and local authority approval to exercise legal functions relating to the assessment, application and safeguarding processes under the Mental Health Act [15].

These statutory roles are complementary to, but distinct from, advanced practice in mental health. While advanced practitioners frequently work alongside ACs, RCs and AMHPs – and may themselves hold such positions concurrently with their advanced practice role – it is essential to differentiate between clinical advancement grounded in the four pillars of practice and the legal authority conferred by these statutory designations. The ability to integrate advanced clinical expertise with statutory functions can significantly enhance service delivery; however, both domains require robust governance, role clarity and ongoing professional development to ensure safe and effective care.

Finally and not exclusively to mental health facing roles, advanced practitioners in mental health from multi-professional backgrounds with **prescribing rights** under the Human Medicines Act [16] can address medicines-related issues and support people with the supply, administration and management of medicines, within their existing scope of practice. This may be via an independent or supplementary prescribing route or by using the mechanisms where available for Patient-Specific Direction (PSD) and Patient Group Direction (PGD).

It is not a pre-requisite or a mandatory requirement for all advanced practitioners in mental health to prescribe medicines. Being a prescribing practitioner is only one of the ways that some professional groups extend their skills and advance their practice but certainly not in all cases. Other core professions without legal prescribing rights and even some that have them already have identified many other ways in which to enhance their knowledge, skills and expertise to a recognised advanced level. Employers and workforce planners are encouraged to consider the needs of the specific population they serve when designing the requirements of individual posts.

More recently, as practice roles and responsibilities at an advanced level are becoming more established across health and social care, NHS Employers, the organisation representing NHS employers in England, provides advice, support and resources to help workforce leaders consider the benefits of advanced practice roles in all sectors, including mental health [17].

GOVERNANCE OF ADVANCED PRACTICE ROLES

All advanced practice is delivered by health and care professionals who are already registered by a statutory regulatory body. Each of their regulators, such as the Health and Care Professions Council (HCPC) [18] and Nursing and Midwifery Council (NMC) [19], publish standards which its registrants, including those working at an advanced level, are required to meet. Advanced practitioners have a responsibility to ensure that they have the underpinning education and training and that competencies are maintained to work safely and effectively within their scope of practice [20].

Robust, credible organisational governance is also central to the safe, effective and successful employment and deployment of the multi-professional advanced practitioner workforce.

Deployment of Advanced Practitioners within Organisations

As a minimum, any organisation which already employs or is considering implementing advanced practice roles should have an advanced roles governance framework that can evidence and provide guidance on the following and which should be agreed and supported at board level:

- There must be a named person(s) with lead responsibility for the advanced practice workforce that has a reporting line at senior board level.
- The advanced practice leads should have a job description and allocated time for their leadership role within their job plans, enabling effective partnership working with professional leads such as Chief Nurse, Chief AHP, Medical Director and Chief Pharmacist.
- There must be clear and consistent reporting and accountability lines, which include professional leads.

- Organisations must have clear oversight of all practitioners working at an advanced level, including up-to-date and accurate staff records, ensuring that regulatory standards, national frameworks and professional guidance(s) are followed.
- Advanced practice roles must be integrated into organisational workforce planning at all levels, with clarity about the roles in team structures and by the public.
- There must be inclusive recruitment processes that do not disadvantage people from underrepresented groups from applying for or being recruited to positions.
- Organisations should have consistent job description templates, job plans, appraisals and scope of practice documents that are representative of clinical responsibility and inclusive of the four pillars of practice.
- There must be processes in place to identify and agree advanced practitioner competencies and capabilities that will support service needs and for specific service settings, with reference to applicable frameworks.
- Practitioners should be supported to maintain a portfolio of competence, which is maintained and reviewed annually. Including all underpinning education and training and relevant scope of practice documents.
- There must be robust arrangements in place for workplace supervision and assessment of trainee advanced practitioners and ongoing supervision for qualified practitioners.

Meeting the aforementioned requirements will support organisations in meeting their responsibilities in relation to The Health and Social Care Act 2008 (Regulated Activities) Regulations 2014, particularly in relation to:

Regulation 12(1) and 12(2)(c) [13]
'Care and treatment must be provided in a safe way for service users ... ensuring that persons providing care or treatment to service users have the qualifications, competence, skills and experience to do so safely'.

Regulation 18(2)(a) [21]
'Persons employed by the service provider in the provision of a regulated activity must ... receive such appropriate support, training, professional development, supervision and appraisal as is necessary to enable them to carry out the duties they are employed to perform'.

SCOPE OF PRACTICE

For an advanced practitioner in mental health, the scope of practice is the defined range of complex, autonomous clinical, educational, leadership and research activities that they are educated, trained and competent to deliver safely and effectively within their professional regulation and organisational governance, tailored to the needs of individuals, families and populations.

Establishing and maintaining this scope of practice is a dynamic process that requires alignment between organisational priorities, national standards, regulatory frameworks and individual professional development. As described at the organisational level, defining the scope of a role begins with analysing population health needs, service pathways and workforce capacity. Through this lens, organisations identify the knowledge, skills and capabilities required to meet demand and articulate these in a role-specific scope of practice. This provides the structural foundation for governance, ensuring safe, effective and sustainable delivery of advanced practice roles.

Once the role is defined, the individual practitioner's scope is shaped by their regulated professional skillset and the education, training and supervised experience they undertake. Many advanced practitioners will deepen their expertise within the primary scope of their originating profession, while others will expand into adjacent or cross-disciplinary areas. Such expansion must be deliberate, underpinned by structured education, supervised practice and robust competency assessment to ensure safe and effective care. This iterative process enables clinicians to evolve their practice beyond the baseline of initial registration, while always maintaining alignment with professional standards and organisational governance.

Outside of a regulatory agency, there are other national bodies, such as Royal Colleges, professional associations and NHS England, that further influence scope of practice by publishing frameworks and capability standards grounded in evidence and professional consensus. The Multi-Professional Framework for Advanced Practice in England [2] and the Advanced Practice Mental Health Curriculum and Capabilities Framework [4] provide national benchmarks that allow local roles to be mapped to consistent expectations.

In this way, regulatory authorities such as the NMC and HCPC do not prescribe detailed scope for advanced practitioners but establish the overarching duty to practise safely and effectively within the bounds of education, training and competence. Their standards create the legal and ethical parameters within which scope is developed and extended. Legislation further defines specific tasks reserved for regulated professions, such as prescribing under the Human Medicines Regulations 2012 [16], ensuring that any extension of scope is consistent with statutory protections and public safety.

Organisations carry responsibility for ensuring these layers align in practice. This includes using learning needs analyses, reviewing professional portfolios and implementing structured supervision to bridge any gaps between role expectations and individual competence. Ongoing governance through appraisal, annual portfolio review and audit of practice provide assurance that scope remains current and responsive to evolving service demands.

In mental health, this alignment is particularly critical. The complex, relational nature of care requires a balance between role-level clarity and individual capability development. By integrating organisational role design, national frameworks, regulatory standards and personalised professional growth, advanced practice in mental health achieves both workforce transformation and the assurance of safe, holistic and expert-level care (see Figure 2.2).

Organisations will need to ensure that they have suitable arrangements for agreeing to or changing the scope of practice of advanced practitioners.

To do this, the following points should be considered:

- Fully understand what the practitioner is able to do – both legally and as a result of their previous education, training and experience. This should be led by the relevant professional lead(s) and achieved by reviewing the individual's professional portfolio.

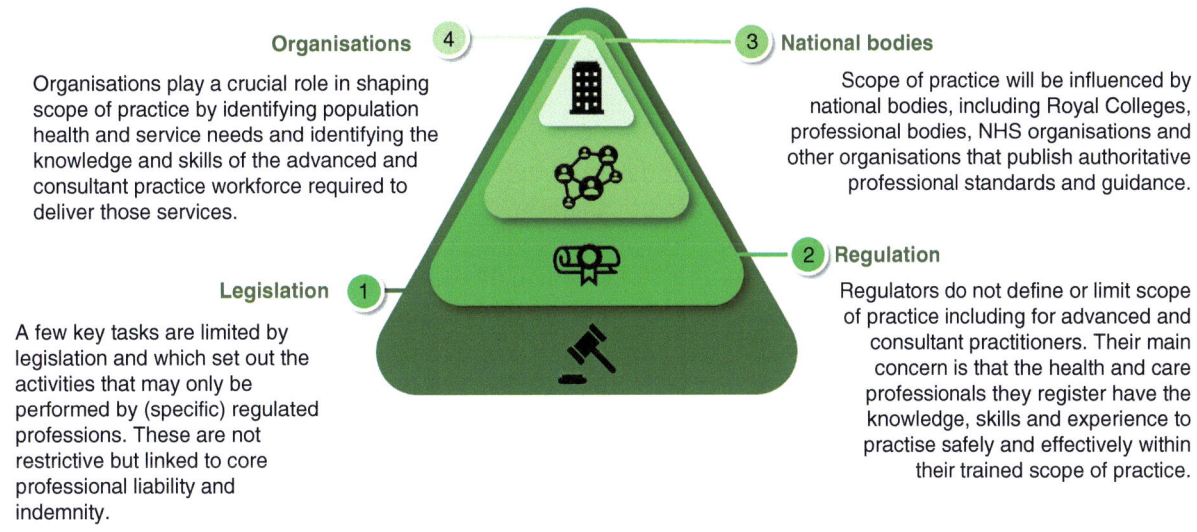

FIGURE 2.2 Factors influencing scope of practice.

- Undertake a learning needs analysis to assess how far the individual's education, training and experience meet the required competencies and capabilities for the role and to identify any gaps which need to be addressed.
- Understand that prior education and training may have been undertaken whilst working at a different level of practice or whilst working in a different area of speciality. Additional education and training may therefore be required to support the practitioner to meet the required competencies and capabilities to ensure safe, effective care for patients and their families.
- As a result of the learning needs analysis, put in place an appropriate package of training, supervision and support for the advanced or consultant practitioner in the early stages of their employment, including arrangements for sign-off of the required capabilities.
- Once the advanced practitioner has demonstrated the required capabilities, ensure that they have access to ongoing training, supervision and support, underpinned by an annual appraisal that includes a review of capabilities.

DEVELOPMENT OF MENTAL HEALTH FOCUSED ADVANCED TRAINING

The development of education and training for advanced practitioners across the United Kingdom's four nations has been shaped by a shared commitment to standardise capability while accommodating distinct policy and service contexts.

Key to upskilling the workforce is ensuring robust training and education underpins the accelerated development of practitioners' clinical decision-making skills, supports the education of the multi-professional workforce, builds productive teams and provides effective leadership and quality management that is progressive and supports workforce, digital and service transformation ability.

ADVANCED PRACTICE MENTAL HEALTH CURRICULUM AND CAPABILITIES FRAMEWORK (NHSE CENTRE FOR ADVANCING PRACTICE-ENDORSED AREA-SPECIFIC CAPABILITY)

A key element of the preparation for individuals to practice at the level of advanced practice will be a formal assessment of achievement of the capabilities, specific to the context of their practice. It is critical to the implementation, acceptance and sustainability of advanced practice that health and care professionals working at this level are widely recognised as having a consistent level of competence [20]. They must also be equally capable of fulfilling the specialist requirements of functioning at this level.

Most core advanced practice learning programmes to date have centred on developing the physical health assessment and intervention skillset typical of general practice and acute care settings. This emphasis, even when helpful in raising parity of esteem for mental health practitioners, often resulted in insufficient provision for the teaching and assessment of specialist mental health interventions. Moreover, these broadly framed curricula frequently failed to meet the educational needs of multi-professional mental health therapy roles, where specialist physiological assessment or physical health monitoring is not part of their core professional discipline.

To address this gap, in England a dedicated Advanced Practice Mental Health Curriculum and Capabilities Framework was launched in 2022 [4] under the auspices of Health Education England. This was the first nationwide master's level curriculum devoted wholly to advanced mental health practice, aligned with the four pillar Advanced Practice framework (clinical practice, leadership/management, education, research) [2]. It has been made available via a growing number of specialist Higher Education Institutions (HEIs) and endorsed by the Centre for Advancing Practice as an area-specific capability framework recognised across professions and service contexts [20]. Early adopters found it well suited both to clinicians in core mental health roles and to practitioners in broader mental health facing roles seeking structured advanced learning. However, rollout has been constrained by the fact that not all HEIs possess the specialist faculty required to deliver the curriculum and cohort sizes remain relatively small – limiting scale and pace of workforce transformation.

Nonetheless, the number of HEIs offering the mental health specific programme is growing and more information can be obtained in England from the learner's own regional advanced practice faculty [22].

The Advanced Practice Mental Health Framework has six domains (see Figure 2.3) recognising, primarily, the importance of the person-centred therapeutic alliance. The broad overarching learning outcomes must be applied to the individual's sphere of practice to ensure relevance and safe and effective practice. The programme is delivered at academic level 7 master's level and incorporates academic and experiential learning. It is anticipated to take a minimum of two years to complete (based on whole-time equivalence), although it will normally be completed in three to five years for individuals in a full-time trainee role.

There are two main audiences for the Framework: the first is as described earlier and for people who identify the need to undertake the whole programme as stand-alone learning. The second audience is for experienced advanced practitioners in mental health who can use the capabilities as a framework to map their existing experience and academic study in part to support recognition of their level of practice via the NHS England ePortfolio (Supported) route.

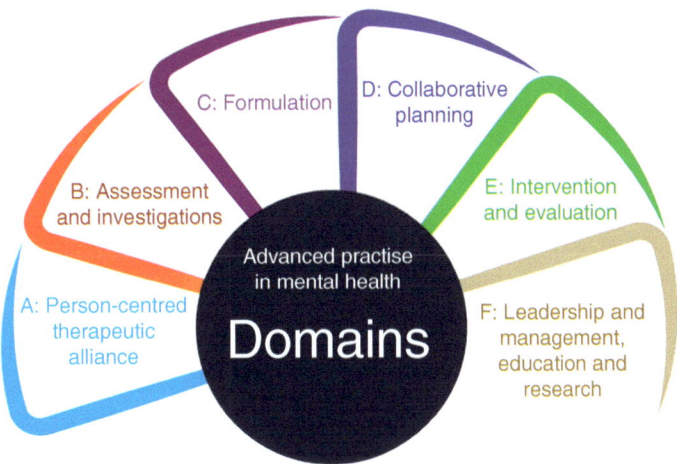

FIGURE 2.3 The Advanced Practice in Mental Health curriculum domains.

Given the increased interest in specific mental health focused learning programmes and a growing number of advanced practitioners in mental health, the developmental infrastructure within NHS England continues to form to support this work. There is an Advanced Practice in Mental Health Network (APMHN), begun in England but welcoming voices from all the four nations of the United Kingdom, to support the advanced practice mental health workforce and ensure that forums exist for all voices to be represented as this work is embedded into the system (see Figure 2.4).

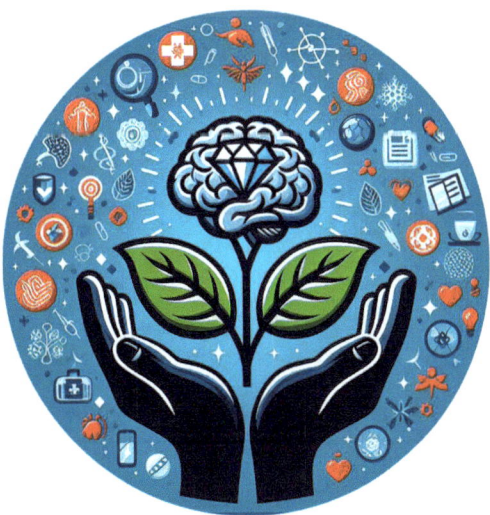

FIGURE 2.4 The logo for the Advanced Practice in Mental Health Network.

CONCLUSION

Advanced practice in mental health has emerged as a pivotal component of modern service delivery, bridging policy ambition with the realities of complex, person-centred care. This chapter has demonstrated that the shift from locally defined, ad hoc roles to nationally governed, competency-based frameworks is essential to sustaining public confidence and ensuring safe and effective practice. By embedding the four pillars of clinical practice, leadership, education and research within robust governance structures, advanced practitioners can drive workforce transformation, enhance multidisciplinary decision-making and deliver care that is both holistic and evidence-informed.

The implementation of the Advanced Practice Mental Health Curriculum and Capabilities Framework marks a critical step in standardising education, assuring consistent competence and strengthening the professional identity of advanced practitioners across diverse settings. Central to this endeavour is the alignment of individual scope of practice with organisational priorities, national standards and regulatory expectations.

As the NHS continues to navigate increasing demand, digital transformation and the shift towards prevention and community-based care, advanced practitioners are uniquely positioned to provide the expertise and leadership required. In mental health, their role is not simply an extension of existing practice but a transformative force that embeds high-level clinical judgement, therapeutic alliance and integrated service redesign at the heart of care.

REFERENCES

1. Health Education England (2017). Multi-professional framework for advanced clinical practice in England. London: HEE.
2. NHS England (2025). Multi-professional framework for advanced practice in England. London: NHS England.
3. Darzi A. (2024). Independent review of the NHS. London: Department of Health and Social Care.
4. NHS England Centre for Advancing Practice (2023). Credential specification: advanced practice mental health curriculum and capabilities framework. London: NHS England.
5. NHS England (2023). NHS Long Term Workforce Plan. London: NHS England.
6. Gov.UK (2025). Fit for the future, 10 year health plan for England. https://assets.publishing.service.gov.uk/media/6866387fe6557c544db7a/fit-for-the-future-10-year-health-plan-for-england
7. Mahoney, M.R. (2021). The key role of advanced practice providers in today's new normal. *Physician Leadership Journal* 8 (2): 89–93.
8. NHS Education for Scotland (2024). Nursing, midwifery and allied health professionals (NMAHP) development framework – post-registration framework. Edinburgh: NHS Education for Scotland.
9. Health Education and Improvement Wales (2023). Professional framework for enhanced, advanced and consultant clinical practice. Cardiff: HEIW.
10. Department of Health Northern Ireland (2019). Advanced AHP practice framework. Belfast: DoHNI.
11. Evans, C., Poku, B., Pearce, R. et al. (2021). Characterising the outcomes, impacts and implementation challenges of advanced clinical practice roles in the UK: a scoping review. *BMJ Open.* 11 (8): e048171.

12. Unsworth, J., Greene, K., Ali, P. et al. (2024). Advanced practice nurse roles in Europe: implementation challenges, progress and lessons learnt. *International Nursing Review* 71 (2): 299–308.
13. The Health and Social Care Act 2008 (Regulated Activities) Regulations 2014 | UK Statutory Instruments 2014 No. 2936 PART 3 SECTION 2 Regulation 12. https://www.legislation.gov.uk/uksi/2014/2936/regulation/12/made
14. NHS England Southwest Faculty for Advancing Practice (2025). Advancing practice in emerging areas: workforce transformation resource. NHS England. https://advanced-practice.hee.nhs.uk/regional-faculty-for-advancing-practice (accessed 28 July 2025).
15. United Kingdom (1983). Mental Health Act 1983, c.20. London: The Stationery Office. https://www.legislation.gov.uk/ukpga/1983/20/content (updated 3 August 2025; accessed 15 August 2025).
16. UK Government (2012). The Human Medicines Regulations 2012. London. https://www.legislation.gov.uk/uksi/2012/1916/contents
17. NHS Employers (2023). Advanced practice. London: NHS Employers. https://www.nhsemployers.org/articles/advanced-practice (accessed 15 August 2025).
18. Health and Care Professions Council (2024). Standards of conduct, performance and ethics. https://www.hcpc-uk.org/standards/standards-of-conduct-performance-and-ethics/
19. Nursing and Midwifery Council (2018). The Code: Professional standards of practice and behaviour for nurses, midwives and nursing associates. https://www.nmc.org.uk/standards/code/
20. NHS England (2022). Advanced practice mental health curriculum and capabilities framework. London: NHS England.
21. The Health and Social Care Act 2008 (Regulated Activities) Regulations 2014 | UK Statutory Instruments 2014 No. 2936 PART 3 SECTION 2 Regulation 18. https://www.legislation.gov.uk/uksi/2014/2936/regulation/18/made
22. NHS England (2025). Regional faculties for advancing practice. London: Health Education England. https://advanced-practice.hee.nhs.uk/regional-faculty-for-advancing-practice (accessed 28 July 2025).

PART 2

ADVANCED PRACTICE IN MENTAL HEALTH: GUIDING PRINCIPLES

CHAPTER 3

Holistic Care and the Biopsychosocial Framework

Stuart Maddock[1,2]

[1] Norfolk and Suffolk Foundation Trust, Norfolk, UK
[2] University of East Anglia, Norwich, UK

> **Aim**
>
> The aim of this chapter is to be aware of the evolution and current context of holism, the evolution of the biopsychosocial framework, its relation to integrated care and its application to advanced practice in mental health.

LEARNING OUTCOMES

After reading this chapter, the reader will:

1. Be aware of the history and philosophies in relation to holism and the connection to the biopsychosocial model.
2. Understand the evolution of the biopsychosocial model and its relevance to healthcare today in clinical practice.
3. Understand the role of the advanced practitioner in mental health (APMH) in providing holistic care that is person-centred and delivered via an integrated approach.
4. Be able to clinically apply the biopsychosocial model in advanced practice in mental health.

The Advanced Practitioner in Mental Health, First Edition. Edited by Clare Allabyrne.
© 2026 John Wiley & Sons Ltd. All rights reserved, including rights for text and data mining and training of artificial intelligence technologies or similar technologies. Published 2026 by John Wiley & Sons Ltd.

INTRODUCTION

To be able to fully understand and evaluate the biopsychosocial model and its evolution, a thorough appraisal of philosophical approaches within healthcare is first required. These are the ways in which the human organism is interpreted and approaches to healthcare are subsequently formulated, whether this takes a reductionist, materialist, behaviouralist or holistic approach. These historical developments will be discussed within the chapter to highlight the debates that have taken place throughout time and their relevance to how modern healthcare is delivered. It will be argued that as the nature of the biopsychosocial model encompasses biological, psychological and social approaches that the driving philosophy is holism.

DEFINITIONS

Holism/Holistic Care

For the purposes of this chapter, the definition of holistic care has been synthesised from a review of the literature including the American Holistic Nurses Association [1, 2] and with consideration of literature from the Allied Healthcare [3, 4] and Pharmacy professions [5] and is defined as follows:

Holism in healthcare is the philosophical approach that views individuals synergistically, as integrated wholes, greater than the mere sum of their biological, psychological, social, cultural and spiritual components. It necessitates an understanding of the intricate interplay and mutual influence among all these dimensions in shaping a person's overall well-being and lived experience.

Biopsychosocial Model

The biopsychosocial model is a comprehensive framework that views health and illness as the result of complex interacting biological, psychological and social processes. It emphasises that to understand and treat individuals effectively, healthcare providers must consider not only physiological processes but also a person's thoughts, emotions, behaviours and social environment. This approach lends itself to holistic assessment and treatment strategies across healthcare disciplines and can be applied generally both to healthcare structure and design and to individualised conditions when utilised with more specific clinical guidance [6] (see Figure 3.1).

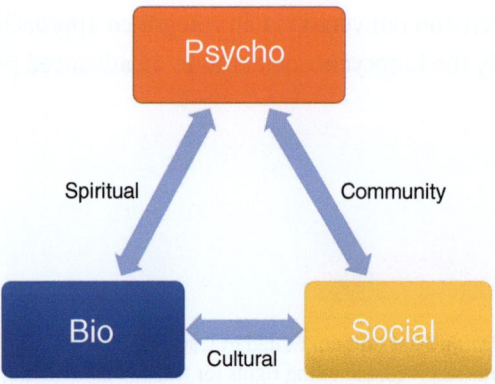

FIGURE 3.1 The interconnected nature of biopsychosocial aspects adapted from Engle's model [6], with the addition of cultural, spiritual and community aspects for a further holistic approach.

HISTORICAL INFLUENCES

Prior to examining holism and the biopsychosocial model and its applicability to advanced practice in mental health, it is important to consider historical philosophical perspectives that influenced this work.

Aristotle (384–322 BC), an ancient Greek philosopher and scientist who made major contributions in many areas, including biology and psychology, adopted a holistic approach in relation to understanding the human organism, emphasising the unity between 'soul', which included aspects of mind, with perception and cognition, and the body [7]. Socrates, (c. 470–399 BC) who has been credited with pioneering Western medicine, is also said to have taken a holistic stance when teaching medicine [1].

Holistic care can also be traced back to Florence Nightingale, a pioneering nurse, who differentiated the different aspects of care involved in the healing process, including medical, surgical and the significance of the environment for healing [8].

While holism remains an important philosophical underpinning for healthcare, particularly within advanced practice [9, 10], person-centred care has now emerged as the primary philosophical orientation guiding practice across a range of professions. This approach is central to nursing [11], allied health professions [12] and pharmacy [5]. Developed by Carl Rogers in the 1940s and 1950s, person-centred care represents a significant shift away from the traditional medical model. Rogers, an influential psychologist, emphasised the inherent capacity of individuals (whom he termed clients) to find solutions to their own challenges [13]. This philosophy continues to be promoted by the World Health Organization (WHO) as a fundamental approach to healthcare delivery [14].

Other philosophical schools of thought also emerged and need to be examined in relation to holism and the further evaluation of the biopsychosocial model as applied to advanced practice in mental health. Whilst holism seems logical, established, accepted and sensible, initially supported in healthcare, there was a time when the dominant outlook was reductionist both in medicine and in the understanding of the human [15]. This reductionist approach focused on understanding illness by attributing it to a single, purely biological cause within the body and treating mental processes as separate issues [16]. This was referred to as 'dualism' and associated with Descartes (1596–1650), a father of modern philosophy. Descartes proposed that the biological aspects of the body were more worthy of scientific investigation than the mind. The reductionist approach remained dominant for many years with further contributions that built on Descartes existing work by Locke and Hume [17] who were classic empiricist philosophers of the early modern era. However, there was a shift away from dualism in the mid-20th century. This shift was informed by materialism, which asserts that in order to exist, everything must be physical and therefore tangible, which became the more dominant viewpoint serving to reduce the dualistic movement and leading to a move towards behaviouralism, whereby mental state is understood through observation [18]. Notably, Gilbert Ryle, a philosophical behaviouralist/phenomenologist from Oxford, famously critiqued dualism in his book *The Concept of Mind* where he introduces the phrase 'the ghost in the machine' to mock the dualist perspective that a non-physical mind could somehow be housed separately within the physical machine of the body [19].

The biopsychosocial model arose in contrast to the dualist separation of mind and body and the reductionist focus on biological factors in illness and health. It aimed to provide a more holistic framework integrating biological, psychological and social factors to ensure that the person was treated as a whole, rather than with a focus on specific symptoms or aspects of disease.

It is often misreported that Engle coined the term *biopsychosocial model* whilst these developments had in fact already been underway. Roy Grinker was a psychiatrist with an interest in psychiatry training following the Second World War. He first utilised the term *biopsychosocial* in 1954 [20]. His driver for this was to extend Freud's psychoanalytical theory which was the most prevalent approach and treatment for

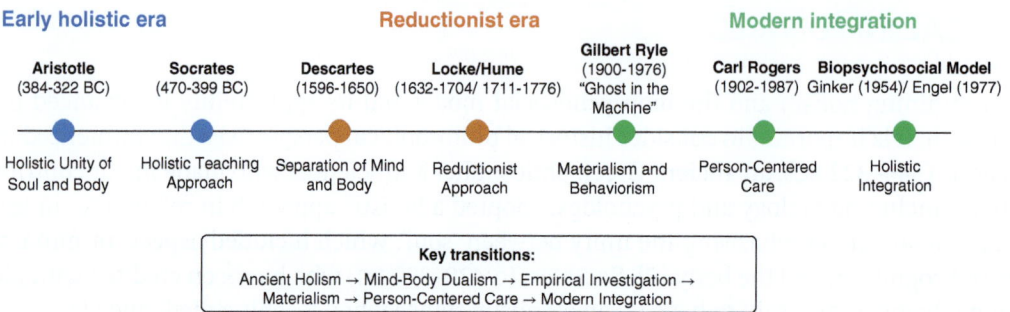

FIGURE 3.2 Historic timeline.

mental health problems at this time [21]. Grinker expressed that he wanted 'to add to the sum total of knowledge' and proposed that this would be possible through incorporating a biological approach which would include genetics and social psychiatry, to create psychoanalytic psychiatry. Grinker went on to describe this philosophical approach as 'eclecticism' [20, p. 452] which can be defined as a conceptual approach drawing from multiple theories rather than a single paradigm [22] and would continue to be debated and criticised in later years [23]. See Figure 3.2 for a historic timeline.

The Influence of History on Contemporary Issues in Practice

As has already been discussed, the concept of holistic care in healthcare has deep historical roots. Florence Nightingale's approach to holistic care emphasised the importance of the environment. This included the presence of light in the healing process. Today, this has been validated evidentially with light therapy being proven to be as beneficial as fluoxetine in treating depressive disorders, with improvements seen as early as the first week of treatment [24].

However, the landscape of healthcare began to shift in the 1900s. Priorities moved away from holistic care centred on patient connection, particularly in America, where the focus increasingly turned to profit. Arguably this led to a return to a biological and disease focused approach to increase turnaround times and therefore profit [25]. This shift set the stage for future challenges in healthcare delivery.

The increasing focus on the biological aspects of disease, often at the expense of psychological factors, prompted George Engel to develop the biopsychosocial model. Expanding on Grinker's earlier work, Engel sought to address what he perceived as a crisis in medicine, particularly psychiatry, caused by this overemphasis on biology [6]. His experience in psychosomatic medicine led him to create a model applicable to both physical conditions, such as diabetes, and mental health disorders like schizophrenia, which frequently co-occur [26]. This underscored the need to integrate psychological and social dimensions into medical understanding [27].

The biopsychosocial model represented a significant paradigm shift, aiming to balance psychological and biological approaches to mental health treatment. Engel formally introduced the model to the mental health community in 1980, using a case of ischemic heart disease as an illustrative example [28]. However, the model has not been without its critics. Ghaemi, for instance, argued that its broad scope rendered it insufficiently specific [27], while proponents suggested its application should be guided by condition-specific guidelines to enhance clinical utility [29].

These debates have spanned a range of perspectives. Some praised the model for empowering healthcare professionals to integrate effective approaches in care delivery [30], while others expressed concerns that this freedom bordered on unscientific 'anarchy' [28, p. 3]. While Grinker and Engle viewed this integrative potential positively [20], Ghaemi argued that this very eclecticism fostered dogmatism by lacking clear parameters [27]. This ongoing tension between psychological and biological perspectives continues to fuel academic debate, hindering the widespread implementation of the biopsychosocial model.

The discussion of the evolutional uses of the biopsychosocial model begins to illustrate how the model can be applied to advanced practice in mental health to further enhance these roles and define scope of practice and training requirements. The biopsychosocial model can be viewed as a framework for providing holistic care, providing advanced practitioners in mental health (APMHs) with the required autonomy to drive forward comprehensive treatment approaches [10].

Historically, healthcare education has always tended to prioritise biological factors over psychological and social ones [29]. This may be due to greater scientific understanding of biological processes, easier quantification/measurement of biological factors or cultural perceptions of mind-body dualism and how this had led to positivism and empirical investigation [31]. Within the context of medicine in Britain, more humanistic elements were not added to the curriculum until much later which were described as embryonic in the late 1970s and driven forward by students within the field of general practice [32]. This is useful to consider in terms of a paradigm shift in the National Health Service (NHS), as psychologists began teaching in medical education at this time and the shape of healthcare services was evolving and becoming more integrated. As these changes continued to progress, in later years there would be the development of health psychology roles within health services, evidencing this shift and integration towards a biopsychosocial approach in service delivery [33].

To appreciate this focus on biological approaches further and how it has remained through history, it is useful to examine it philosophically. Doing so through the lens of physicalism, it can be argued that without biology and chemistry, psychological factors of an organism cannot exist [29]. Further to this, to start to investigate something, a reductionist approach is required to look at the components to first learn how each work, prior to then looking at how they interact. It has been stated that now that we have achieved knowledge and understanding of biological factors, a more integrative approach makes sense [34].

It could, however, be argued that dualism remains when examining the development of more recent advanced-level clinical education programs including physician associate (PA) and advanced practice. The Physician Associate Curriculum whilst containing consideration of humanistic and holistic approaches is generalist and medically focused with an absence of explicit capabilities focusing on psychological or mental health domains [35]. Yet, it is of note that there is further guidance supplied by the Royal College of Psychiatry with suggestion for further competencies that are required to work in the field of mental health, including completion of a biopsychosocial assessment [36]. However, this was developed some years after the first formal PA program developed in the United Kingdom in 2008 [37] with remaining scope for its evolution. This is relevant to advanced practice as a similar pattern of development has taken place, with the establishment of a generalist-based competencies framework developed in 2017, which acknowledged that there was a requirement for more 'speciality-specific competencies' to be incorporated alongside these [10]. This was some years prior to the development of the Health Education England (HEE) Advanced Practice Mental Health Curriculum and Capabilities Framework [9]. This delay in the evolution of mental health specific capabilities is further highlighted when seen in contrast to the development of advanced practice in emergency medicine which developed a speciality-specific set of capabilities specific to its field supported by the Royal College of Emergency Medicine in 2015 [38] many years ahead of mental health.

Whilst it can be stated that development of advanced practice is driven by public demand, where there is greatest need [39], in America the first advanced practice program that was developed was actually in mental health in 1954 [40]. To further demonstrate the lack of parity between biological and physical domains within healthcare, it may be useful to highlight that whilst the Royal College of Nursing adopted the American National Organization of Nurse Practitioner Faculties Competencies in 2002 [41], it was considerable years later that we have seen the creation of the advanced practice in mental health curriculum and capabilities framework in 2020 [9].

THE BIOPSYCHOSOCIAL MODEL AND THE CONTEXT AND CONNECTION TO ADVANCED PRACTICE IN MENTAL HEALTH

The biopsychosocial model has been described as holistic, which has benefits over the reductionist approach of the prior biomedical model [6] with an increasing emphasis on integrative care [42, 43]. Bolton and Gillett view the biopsychosocial model as both functioning in a general sense to conceptualise health and disease and at a clinical level to understand specific disorders and presentations. They state that as a general model it can be applied to healthcare to inform estimates on population health, planning and prioritising healthcare services, research funding and planning syllabuses for health education. This highlights the model's merit to both mental health services and the advanced practitioner.

They go on to state that the biopsychosocial model can have multiple applications and can inform clinical care. However, this must be done by incorporating clinical guidance relevant to specific conditions [29]. This may include guidance such as The National Institute for Health and Care Excellence (NICE), British Association of Psychopharmacology (BAP), the Maudsley Prescribing Guidelines, or BMJ Best Practice. It is of note that this directly addresses Ghaemi's criticism of the biopsychosocial model in that it is unspecific and eclectic [44] and highlights its continued relevance at multiple layers and across the healthcare system. This evidences the model's ability to be both holistic and specific and that it remains current and sustainable in application to APMH roles, including examination of these roles, training, governance, implementation and continued professional development therein.

Whilst it is of note that much of the discussion so far has been around the development of the biopsychosocial model within the context of medical education and how this has impacted healthcare in England, further consideration will now be paid to how this relates to advanced practice in mental health. There has been much debate around the loss of identity of roles within mental health in England and how this links to the parity of esteem agenda in this case in education [45]. There is a lack of clear identification for the mental health model and a move to increasing genericism in care that cannot be met by reductionist generic approaches [46], and as such it is positive to see mental health specific advanced practice capabilities [9].

There is a call for mental healthcare to move away from the biomedical approach to understanding psychological distress with further claims of widespread acknowledgement stating that current classification systems such as the Diagnostic Statistical Manual (DSM) and International Classification of Diseases (ICD) are no longer fit for purpose and a requirement to move towards more psychological-based care [47]. With these changes in the paradigm of mental healthcare, the biopsychosocial model remains relevant in maintaining a sense of identity in mental health through holism, enabling consideration of the unique contributions of roles within services. However, just as Jull argues that the relative contributions of each of the three domains of the biopsychosocial model must be shifted for individual patient presentations [48], this can also be applied to a generic shift in the model throughout time to reflect increasingly less weight applied to the biological sphere. Advanced practice in mental health capabilities addresses this well with the capabilities covering all three domains of the biopsychosocial model [9] to ensure that the training and roles will be fit for purpose in a modern healthcare system [49, 50].

A key challenge in implementing advanced practice in mental health has been a lack of clarity regarding role definitions and the necessary balance of physical and mental health education [51, 52]. This lack of role clarity hinders both operational and clinical understanding of these roles, impacting their effective implementation. While national policies have aimed to define advanced practice [9], these efforts have not fully resolved the issue [53]. However, the biopsychosocial model, in conjunction with team-specific drivers and the Advanced Practice Mental Health Curriculum and Capabilities Framework [9, 10], offers a potential solution. By providing a holistic framework that considers biological, psychological and social factors, the biopsychosocial model can help define the scope and focus of advanced practice roles within specific team contexts. This holistic approach, combined with clear competencies outlined in the Capabilities Framework, can provide the necessary clarity for advanced practice roles, addressing the current barriers to their successful implementation within England's healthcare services in particular [54].

Towards the Future

As we look to the future, the integration of the biopsychosocial model with specific frameworks and team-driven approaches may offer a path forward. By combining this holistic perspective with clear role definitions and specific clinical guidelines, advanced practice in mental health can potentially address the longstanding issues of staff retention, role clarity and comprehensive patient care, as, despite current efforts, significant challenges persist in healthcare. Staffing shortages in the NHS, coupled with increasing service demands and the need for improved recruitment and retention, remain pressing issues [55, 56]. As had occurred earlier in the 1900s, many staff continue to cite the move away from holistic care as a primary reason for leaving the NHS [25, 57].

While the biopsychosocial model emerged as a call for a more holistic approach in contrast to purely biomedical models, the biological realm remains valuable. For example, neuroscience can inform clinical care through advancements in diagnostic classification systems. These include hierarchical family tree frameworks for grouping-related conditions and incorporating dimensional approaches to diagnosis, as well as network analyses that map symptoms, causes and reinforcing symptoms, resembling a spider web analogy [58]. Furthermore, epigenetics demonstrates the bidirectional interaction between environment and biology, linking social determinants with behaviour and psychological factors. This has broad implications for understanding people's needs and service provision [59, 60] and more specific applications for issues like depression, informing both assessment and interventions [60].

Although the role of genetics in mental health has been discussed for over sixty years [20], genetic testing is only now beginning to emerge in the field [61], with some attributing the delay to DSM's insufficient focus on biological/genetic factors [62]. Future directions in mental health may include blood and urine tests for neurotransmitter and immune factors, measurement of brain electrical activity to refine diagnoses and predict treatment response, and the use of technology to analyse variations in the P450 cytochrome system to inform drug metabolism [62].

The NHS England Advanced Practice Mental Health Curriculum and Capabilities Framework acknowledges the importance of biological aspects in advanced practitioner assessment, but its phrasing – 'psychological, biological, and social' – may suggest a greater emphasis on the psychological domain [9, p. 9]. This contrasts with the traditionally more biologically focused training of core psychiatry trainees, even while acknowledging their inclusion of trauma and psychological aspects [63]. However, the core psychiatry curriculum has recently shifted towards a more person-centred and holistic model, also emphasising the psychological aspects of the biopsychosocial model [64]. This illustrates that while biological aspects of mental health care continue to evolve, there is a concurrent shift towards a more psychological approach, aligning with Engel's 1977 proposal [6]. The biopsychosocial model provides a framework for analysing these developments, facilitating discussions on integrative working between roles [65] and informing healthcare design and service provision [60] to ensure the complementary nature of the APMH role.

While some might argue that a focus on biological aspects of mental health persists, including investigations into genetic and structural brain trends to explain personality [66]; whilst contemporary research acknowledges the interaction of genetics and environment [67], effectively moving beyond the 'nature versus nurture' debate. Biological predispositions to mental health problems are recognised as a significant component of the stress-vulnerability model [68]. This helps explain the high rates of mental health comorbidities observed in conditions with strong biological underpinnings, such as attention deficit hyperactivity disorder (ADHD) [69], Prader–Willi syndrome (which has a significant genetic component) [70] and bipolar disorder (which exhibits high heritability) [71]. Similarly, Paediatric Autoimmune Neuropsychiatric Disorders Associated with Streptococcal Infections (PANDAS), typically presenting with sudden onset of obsessive-compulsive symptoms and/or tics following streptococcal infection, also highlights the role of biology [72]. Other biological factors, such as diabetes and cardiovascular problems, are also known to increase the risk of developing mental health problems [29].

These examples underscore the validity of considering biological factors in mental healthcare and justify their inclusion in advanced practitioner training [9]. However, as Ghaemi points out, the presence of a biological aetiology does not necessitate a biological treatment; a genetic cause, for instance, may be effectively addressed through environmental interventions [73]. This reinforces the value of a holistic approach for advanced mental health practitioners.

Psychology and Technology Advances Which Connect Biology to Psychology

At the opposite extreme to biological dogma lies psychological dogma, which discredits diagnostic classification systems [47], suggesting that promised gains from biological advances like biomarkers may never materialise, arguing that diagnosis itself can be harmful and contending that we are incorrectly formulating human distress and natural responses to trauma [74]. However, the field of psychology has seen numerous advancements, including increased availability and accessibility of psychological treatments through the digitalisation of healthcare, such as chatbot-delivered therapies [65]. Chatbots have proven immensely popular, particularly among younger generations, due to their accessibility and cost-effectiveness [75]. While these technologies have primarily been developed outside the NHS by commercially driven entities [60], this is expected to change [65]. Technology will further bridge the biological and psychological domains through wearable devices that monitor physiological responses like heart rate variability and smartphone apps that support mental health treatment goals [76]. Chapter 11 speaks in more detail to digital technology in this field.

The existence of these opposing dogmas – biological and psychological – suggests that balance is achieved through exploring these extremes. Following the early influence of figures like Descartes and Freud, a call for a more integrative approach within healthcare has been growing for many years [65, 77]. Mental health nursing, often described as a blend of psychiatry (which shares common ground with psychology) and traditional nursing practice [78], exemplifies this holistic approach. This shared space extends to allied healthcare professionals and pharmacists, who bring their unique professional backgrounds to collaborative advanced practice. Advanced practice in mental health, therefore, increasingly involves integrating the core principles of psychology and psychiatry while retaining the distinct contributions of the practitioner's background discipline (e.g. nursing or allied health).

The biopsychosocial model provides a framework for understanding this balance, bridging the perceived dogmas of purely biological or psychological approaches. It offers a unique contribution by promoting integrative practice, clarifying the complex interplay between these perspectives.

Social Determinants for Mental Health and Their Role in the Biopsychosocial Model

The WHO states that the social determinants of health refer to the environments and situations people encounter throughout their lives that affect their well-being. These social determinants, shaped by the distribution of money, power and resources at global, national and local levels, include the circumstances around one's birth, upbringing, residence, occupation and aging [79, 80]. There is growing recognition that such life conditions influence mental health in addition to physical health, creating disparities in outcomes between different societies and communities. Recent studies highlight how factors like socioeconomic status can determine mental health trajectories and lead to inequities [81]. The social determinants that may impact mental health include social status, nutrition, housing, patterns of interaction, finances, debt and education [82]. Though originally conceptualised in terms of physical health, researchers now appreciate that social determinants have profound impacts on mental health over the life course as well. This also includes adverse childhood experiences (ACEs) [29], which are discussed in more detail in Chapters 7 and 14. Other factors may include racial discrimination, social exclusion, unemployment or social norms that disadvantage certain groups [58].

> **Case Study – Assessment with Specific Consideration of a Social Determinant View Point for Person Presenting with Depression and Diabetes**
>
> To illustrate how social determinants can impact someone with both mental health problems and a history of diabetes, consider the following:
>
> Limited resources can negatively affect diet, access to healthcare, time for stress management and self-education, the ability to purchase exercise equipment or books and awareness of the benefits of exercise – all of which increase the risk of physical, mental and emotional health problems. This highlights the holistic nature of healthcare; for example, a poor diet stemming from limited education and a social environment that normalises unhealthy eating and inactivity, perhaps learned during childhood, can significantly impact both physical and mental well-being. This underscores the need for APMHs to conduct thorough, holistic assessments using the biopsychosocial model before formulating, diagnosing, prescribing medication or planning treatment.
>
> A holistic approach is essential for advanced practitioners assessing these social, lifestyle and health factors alongside psychological elements. In this example, the individual presents with low mood, reporting depression, alongside a pre-existing diagnosis of type 2 diabetes mellitus. A comprehensive depression assessment should explore symptom onset, duration, severity and patterns, as well as lifestyle factors, coexisting conditions, family history, environmental and social contributors and risk factors such as self-harm or suicidal ideation and medication history. Validated questionnaires can formally evaluate symptom severity, functioning and treatment response. Assessing mental state, cognitive status and conducting a physical examination or further biological investigations where indicated are also crucial. This multifaceted evaluation, encompassing symptoms, history, risk factors and overall health, allows for a comprehensive understanding of contributing factors and guides individualised diagnosis and treatment [83, 84].

Considering the biopsychosocial model and a holistic assessment approach, the comorbidity of depression and diabetes is particularly relevant. Depression prevalence is more than three times higher in individuals with type 1 diabetes and nearly twice as high in those with type 2 diabetes compared to those without [85]. The interaction between depression and diabetes is bidirectional; depression is significantly associated with poor adherence to diabetes treatment regimens, leading to poorer clinical outcomes [86]. Furthermore, in type 2 diabetes, acute hyperglycaemia can impair cognition and contribute to low mood, lethargy and increased anxiety [82].

From a pathophysiological perspective, there is a complex physical relationship between these conditions. Diabetes affects blood sugar, which can lead to inflammation and neurochemical changes impacting mood [83]. Evidence suggests a shared pathophysiology between diabetes and depression, necessitating an integrative approach to understanding depression in individuals with diabetes [85]. The impact of depression on motivation and the ability to perform activities of daily living, such as adhering to diabetic medication, likely involves changes in cortisol regulation, the stress response and the brain's reward system [87, 88], which can further affect blood glucose regulation.

A Biopsychosocial Approach to Complex Needs Case Study:

This is a fictitious case study, based on a composite of people seen in mental health services.

Jane – Depression and Type 2 Diabetes

Referral and Assessment

Jane, a 45-year-old divorced office manager and single mother of two teenagers, was referred by her general practitioner (GP), for suspected depression impacting poorly controlled type 2 diabetes.

Presenting complaints: Persistent low mood, fatigue, weight gain, difficulty concentrating, increased thirst and urination and social withdrawal.

Background

Medical: Type 2 diabetes (diagnosed 3 years ago), hypertension (diagnosed 1 month ago) and family history of type 2 diabetes (father).

Mental health: Persistent low mood, anhedonia, sleep disturbances, fatigue, feelings of worthlessness and difficulty concentrating. PHQ-9 score of 18 (moderately severe depression). Family history of depression (mother). No prior mental health diagnoses.

Social: Divorced 2 years ago, co-parenting challenges, high-stress job with increased responsibilities, reduced social interaction, financial concerns and first-generation immigrant from India experiencing cultural stigma around mental health.

Assessment (Biopsychosocial Perspective)

Biological:

BMI: 32 kg/m^2 (obese). Blood pressure (BP): 138/88 mmHg.
HbA1c: 69 mmol/mol (8.5%). Fasting glucose: 9.2 mmol/L. Lipid profile: Total cholesterol 5.7 mmol/L, LDL 3.6 mmol/L, HDL 1.0 mmol/L, triglycerides 2.4 mmol/L.
Slightly elevated ALT (45 U/L) and GGT (65 U/L). Moderately increased urine ACR (4.5 mg/mmol). Vitamin D insufficient (45 nmol/L). Other blood tests within normal limits.
Signs of insulin resistance (acanthosis nigricans), decreased sensation in feet (early neuropathy).

Psychological:

Depressed mood, flat affect, feelings of hopelessness and worthlessness. No suicidal ideation or psychosis. PHQ-9: 18.
Reports difficulty concentrating and forgetfulness.
Coping mechanisms: emotional eating and avoidance.
Low motivation and confidence in diabetes self-management, impacting daily functioning, work and parenting.

Social:

Limited support from ex-spouse.
Increased work stress and responsibilities.
Reduced social interactions and decreased participation in diabetes support group.
Financial concerns due to single income and debt.
Cultural stigma associated with mental health treatment.

Diagnosis:

ICD11 – 6A70.1 Single episode depressive disorder, moderate without psychotic symptoms
Type 2 diabetes mellitus (poorly controlled)
Hypertension
Obesity
Dyslipidaemia
Early diabetic nephropathy

Formulation/Plan (Integrated Biopsychosocial Approach)

Jane's depression is understood through a biopsychosocial lens. Predisposing vulnerabilities (family history, social stressors) have been worsened by precipitating factors such as increased work stress and poorly controlled diabetes. This cycle is maintained by negative self-talk, maladaptive behaviours, ongoing physical symptoms and limited social support. While Jane has engaged with some support services, further interventions addressing these interacting factors are crucial for her recovery and improved diabetes management.

   PLAN: Cognitive behavioural therapy (CBT) (12 weekly sessions) – focus on mood improvement, diabetes self-management, cognitive restructuring and coping strategies.

Biological:

Depression: If psychological interventions are insufficient, once physical health is optimised consider sertraline (starting 25–50 mg, titrating to 100 mg if tolerated). Emphasise discussion of risks and benefits including risk of dependence and withdrawal.
Diabetes: Continue metformin. Strong emphasis on lifestyle modifications (diet, exercise). Referral to dietitian for low glycaemic load diet advice. Re-engagement with diabetes support group. If no improvement, liaise with GP/specialist regarding SGLT2 inhibitors (e.g. empagliflozin) and potentially GLP-1 receptor agonists if needed after 3 months.
Hypertension: Jane to continue ramipril, monitor BP and liaise further in primary care if required.
Lipids: GP to consider statin (e.g. atorvastatin).
Vitamin D: GP to consider supplementation.

Social:

Explore family dynamics and offer signposting for parenting support.
Letter to employer regarding reasonable adjustments (Equality Act 2010).
Referral to social prescriber for social activity re-engagement.
Signposting to Citizens Advice for financial support.
Culturally sensitive mental health education and connection with relevant community organisations.

Integrated Care and Follow-Up

Coordinated care between GP, diabetes specialist, mental health team and third sector organisations.
Fortnightly follow-up for the first month, then monthly.
Regular monitoring of mood (PHQ-9), HbA1c, lipids, liver function, BP, medication efficacy/side effects, treatment adherence, social support and stressors.
Regular communication with psychological therapist.

Expected Outcomes

Improved mood and PHQ-9 scores within 10–12 weeks.
HbA1c <48 mmol/mol (6.5%) within 6 months.
5–10% weight loss within 6 months.
BP <130/80 mmHg.
Improved lipid profile.
Increased social engagement and work performance.
Enhanced family support.
Increased self-efficacy in managing depression and diabetes.

Consideration of Potential Challenges with Further Reviews and Outcomes

Medication side effects: Close monitoring and adjustment.
Treatment adherence: Motivational interviewing and medication reminders.
Poor engagement with therapy: Regular communication with therapist and consider alternatives.
Lifestyle changes: Gradual implementation and encouragement.
Cultural barriers: Cultural mediators and translated materials.
Work-life balance: Collaboration with employer and time management skills.

Long-Term Management

Consider maintenance therapy for depression in primary care (with careful review).
Ongoing diabetes education and specialist support.
Annual screening for diabetes complications.
Regular mental health check-ups.
Continued family and social support.
Career counselling.
Regular review and adjustment of treatment plan.

NICE guidelines recommend group exercise as a valuable intervention for depression, aligning with a biopsychosocial approach [89]. This recommendation is grounded in several key findings. First, exercise directly addresses the social component of well-being, which is particularly relevant given the established link between loneliness and depression [12, 90, 91]. Second, physical activity has been shown to significantly improve depressive symptoms and elevate mood, even in cases of major depressive disorder, while simultaneously providing benefits for individuals with type 2 diabetes. This evidence supports the effectiveness of exercise as an antidepressant treatment [3, 14, 92–94]. Recognising the importance of patient choice and minimising risks associated with medication, NICE emphasises discussing and offering all non-pharmacological options, including exercise, before considering antidepressants [54]. This holistic approach benefits the individual's overall well-being, encompassing both physical and mental health. Finally, it is important to note that psychological therapies have demonstrated comparable efficacy to pharmacological treatments and can be particularly effective when combined with other approaches, including exercise [25].

SYSTEMIC/ORGANISATIONAL IMPLICATIONS OF THE BIOPSYCHOSOCIAL MODEL

APMHs occupy a unique position within healthcare systems due to their holistic theoretical foundation, which spans all aspects of the biopsychosocial model. Their advanced training encompasses skills traditionally considered within both medical and psychological domains. This includes not only medical skills such as assessment, diagnosis and prescribing in some roles but also proficiency in psychological therapies like cognitive behavioural therapy (CBT) and dialectical behaviour therapy (DBT). This dual expertise distinguishes APMHs from other professionals and positions them as key figures in promoting integrative care delivery [78]. Furthermore, APMHs are distinguished by the fact that they have the ability to manage complete episodes of care, previously a level of autonomy that had been associated traditionally with medical roles [9, 26].

This autonomous and integrative capacity enables APMHs to provide crucial leadership at clinical, team and service levels, fostering collaboration across diverse disciplines and bridging the gap between primary and secondary care. By linking their leadership skills with a strong clinical focus, APMHs effectively function as 'clinical integration agents', ensuring seamless transitions and coordinated care for patients with complex needs. For example, an APMH might lead a multidisciplinary team meeting in their role with complete autonomy and oversight of the patient's episode of care. As part of this, they could develop a comprehensive care plan for a patient with comorbid depression and diabetes, ensuring effective communication and collaboration between GPs, diabetes specialists and social workers, psychiatrists, and junior mental health clinicians. This provides oversight of care, providing reassurance for the patient, improving efficiency, quality and safety. Furthermore, it provides support to junior colleagues, enabling confidence in decision-making, and education for others.

The Progression to Multi-professional Consultant Practice: Shaping Systemic Change

To further understand the systemic and organisational impact within mental healthcare, it is beneficial to consider multi-professional consultant practice as a distinct, further progression and developmental trajectory for APMHs. The urgent need for a whole-systems approach within health and social care, coupled with the demand for high-level, clinically driven system leadership, has been widely acknowledged [14]. This is where the roles of multi-professional advanced and consultant practitioners become crucial, enhancing the healthcare system at meso (service/organisational) and macro (system) levels.

While APMHs maximise their impact as 'clinical integration agents' at the micro (individual patient, team) and meso (service) levels, multi-professional consultant practitioners are specifically positioned to

40 Chapter 3 Holistic Care and the Biopsychosocial Framework

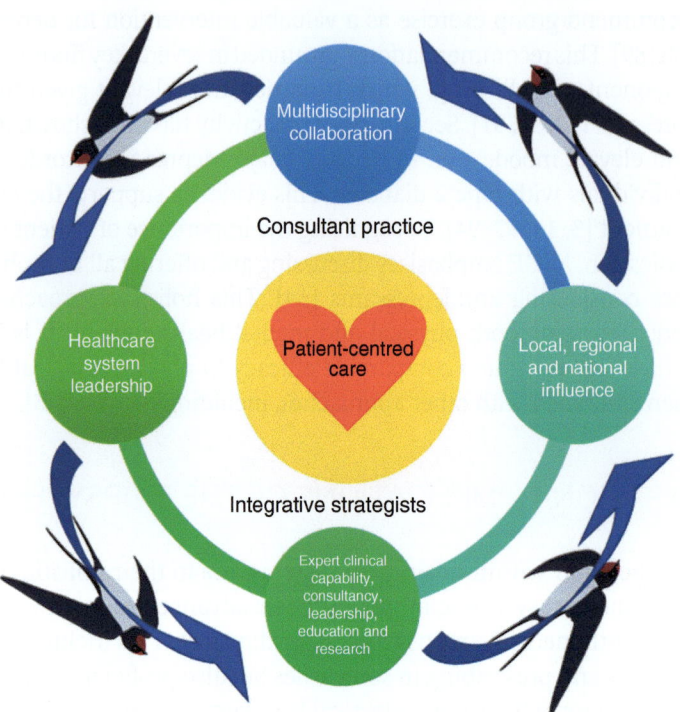

FIGURE 3.3 Model of multi-professional consultant practice to create an environment of integration as 'integrative strategists' within the healthcare system.

function as 'integrative strategists'. These roles are complementary, with consultant practitioners creating the environment for optimal healthcare delivery by explicitly linking the four pillars of advanced practice (clinical practice, leadership and management, education and research) to strategic system leadership.

Integrative strategists play a vital role in shaping policy and building system-wide connections. They bring their expert clinical practice and research expertise to policy discussions, bridging the gap between frontline practice and strategic decision-making. For instance, a multi-professional consultant practitioner involved in service redesign could use their clinical and research insights to advocate for integrated care pathways that prioritise patient-centred care and improve access to mental health services. Furthermore, they contribute to research that evaluates the effectiveness of integrated care models, providing evidence to support policy changes and service improvements. This ensures that services are developed and implemented in line with best practice guidelines and the needs of the local population, with advanced and consultant practice roles working together to drive positive change through healthcare transformation (see Figure 3.3).

Integrative Care

In order to define integrative care, the key output from an effective biopsychosocial model-based service, it is useful to first consider the definition of integrative care from the National Collaboration for Integrated Care and Support:

> 'I can plan my care with people who work together to understand me and my carer(s), allowing me control, and bringing together services to achieve the outcomes important to me' [14, 70].

A further definition of integrative care:

The process and approach to delivering the full range of treatment and therapeutic modalities coordinated in a person-centred way to promote healing of the whole individual and ensure health and well-being [95] (see Figure 3.4).

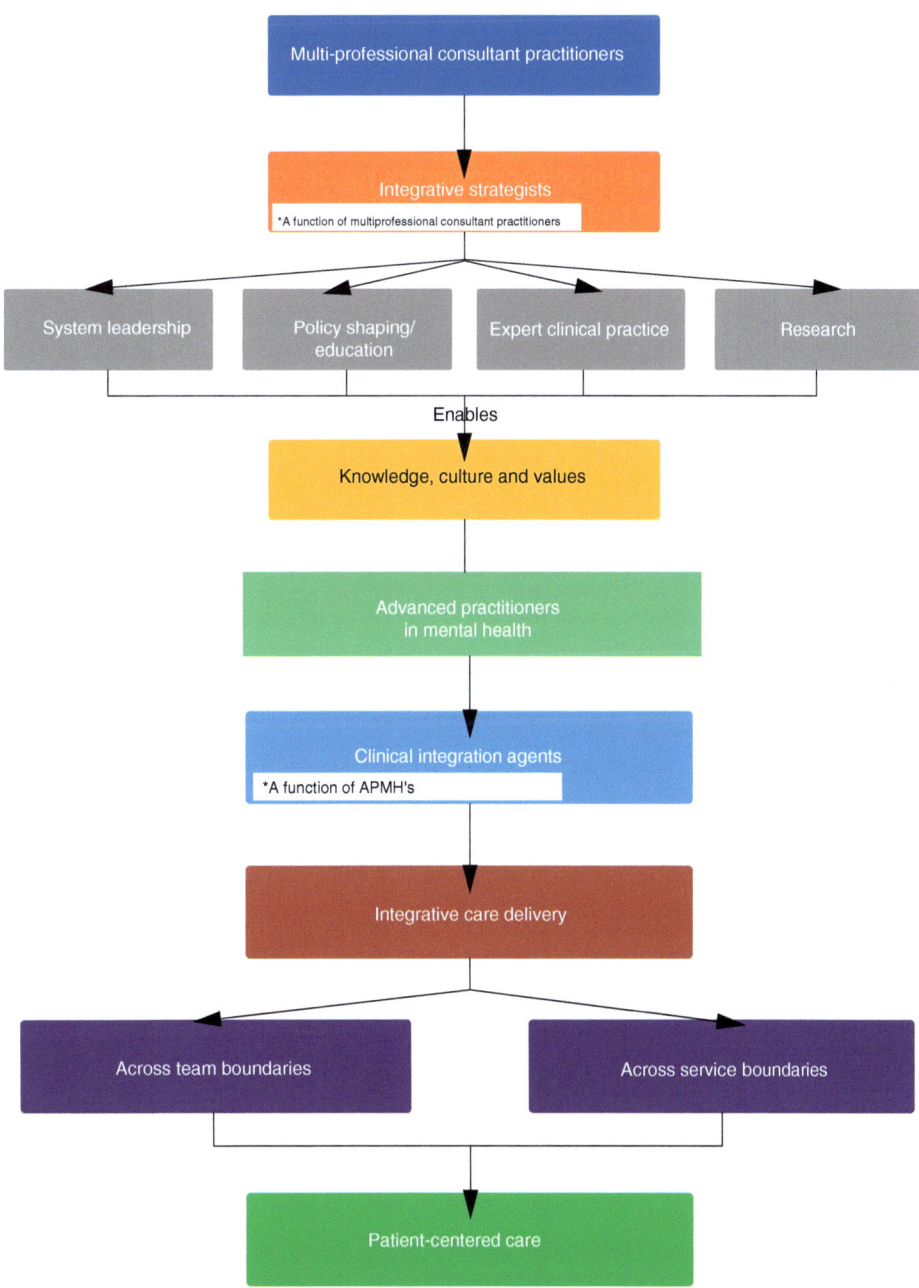

FIGURE 3.4 Integration of multi-professional consultant practice and advanced clinical practice to optimise integration across the system to maximise care delivery and patient outcomes.

CONCLUSION

The biopsychosocial approach has evolved significantly since Grinker first used the term in 1954 [20]. Initially, Grinker aimed to expand upon Freud's psychodynamic therapy by incorporating a biological basis, seeking to integrate medicine with the then-dominant psychological approach. Ironically, Engel's development of the biopsychosocial model in the 1970s [6] arose from a perceived overemphasis on the biomedical model. As a cardiologist with an interest in the influence of psychological factors on health, Engel sought to demonstrate the model's applicability to both physical and mental health settings [27]. This chapter has explored the historical interplay between these two perspectives – psychological and biological – and how this tension has shaped healthcare and service provision.

With the biopsychosocial model establishing holism as a core principle of modern healthcare delivery, this chapter has examined each of its three components – psychological, biological and social and considered their relevance, significance and application to advanced practice. This exploration highlighted the crucial role of advanced practitioners in mental healthcare in maintaining a balanced and holistic approach. These roles are essential for ensuring person-centred care and integrated service delivery. Finally, the chapter has examined the unique contributions of advanced practice in this context, demonstrating its importance in facilitating high-quality service delivery and promoting positive experiences for those accessing mental healthcare.

REFERENCES

1. Dossey, B.M. and Keegan, L. (2013). *Holistic Nursing: A Handbook for Practice*, 6th ed. Burlington, MA: Jones & Bartlett Learning.
2. Slater, V. (2005). Editorial: holistic nursing practice. *Journal of Holistic Nursing* 23 (3): 261–263. https://doi.org/10.1177/0898010105278885.
3. McColl, M.A. (1994). Holistic occupational therapy: historical meaning and contemporary implications. *Canadian Journal of Occupational Therapy* 61 (2): 72–77.
4. Asbjørnslett, M., Skarpaas, L.S., and Stigen, L. (2023). Being holistic is a lot to ask: a qualitative, cross-national exploration of occupational therapists' perceptions and experiences of holistic. *Practice* 2023: 2432879.
5. Royal Pharmaceutical Society England (2018). Utilising pharmacists to improve the care for people with mental health problems. https://www.rpharms.com/Portals/0/RPS%20document%20library/Open%20access/Policy/RPS%20England%20mental%20health%20policy%202018.pdf (accessed 13 April 2024).
6. Engel, G.L. (1977). The need for a new medical model: a challenge for biomedicine. *Science* 196 (4286): 129–136.
7. Shields, C. (2020). Aristotle's psychology. In: *The Stanford Encyclopedia of Philosophy* (ed. E.N. Zalta). Winter. https://plato.stanford.edu/archives/win2020/entries/aristotle-psychology/.
8. Nightingale, F. (1860). *Notes on Nursing: What It Is, and What It Is Not*. New York: D. Appleton and Company. https://digital.library.upenn.edu/women/nightingale/nursing/nursing.html.
9. NHS England (2021). Advanced practice mental health curriculum and capabilities framework. https://www.hee.nhs.uk/sites/default/files/documents/AP-MH%20Curriculum%20and%20Capabilities%20Framework%201.2.pdf (accessed 6 January 2023).
10. Health Education England and NHS England (2017). Multi-professional framework for advanced clinical practice in England. https://www.hee.nhs.uk/sites/default/files/documents/multi-professionalframeworkforadvancedclinicalpracticeinengland.pdf (accessed 11 July 2024).

11. The Code (2015). Read the code online. https://www.nmc.org.uk/standards/code/read-the-code-online/ (accessed 2 October 2024).
12. NHS England (2024). About AHPs. https://www.england.nhs.uk/ahp/about/ (accessed 13 April 2024).
13. The History of the Person-Centered Approach (2024). The association of the peron-centered approach. https://adpca.org/the-history-of-the-pca/ (accessed 2 October 2024).
14. WHO (2015). WHO global strategy on integrated people-centred health services 2016–2026. https://interprofessional.global/wp-content/uploads/2019/11/WHO-2015-Global-strategy-on-integrated-people-centred-health-services-2016-2026.pdf (accessed 20 April 2024).
15. Farre, A. and Rapley, T. (2017). The new old (and old new) medical model: four decades navigating the biomedical and psychosocial understandings of health and illness. 5 (4): 88.
16. Wade, D.T. and Halligan, P.W. (2017). The biopsychosocial model of illness: a model whose time has come. 31 (8): 995–1004.
17. Alexander, B.K. and Shelton, C.P. (2014). Empiricism: John Locke, David Hume, and experience as reality. In: *A History of Psychology in Western Civilization*, 257–332. Cambridge: Cambridge University Press.
18. Robinson, H. (2023). Dualism. In: *The Stanford Encyclopedia of Philosophy* (ed. E.N. Zalta and U. Nodelman). Spring Hutchinsons University Library London. https://plato.stanford.edu/archives/spr2023/entries/dualism/.
19. Ryle, G. (1949). *The Concept of Mind*. London: Hutchinson's University Library.
20. Grinker, R.R. (1964). A struggle for eclecticism. *American Journal of Psychiatry* 121 (5): 451–457.
21. Asokan, T. (2009). Towards an ideal paradigm. *Indian Journal of Psychological Medicine* 31 (2): 58–61.
22. Cambridge University Dictionary Eclecticism. https://dictionary.cambridge.org/dictionary/english/eclecticism (accessed 1 January 2024).
23. Blazer, D. (2010). Book review: the rise and fall of the biopsychosocial model: reconciling art and science in psychiatry. 40 (3): 361–362. https://ajp.psychiatryonline.org/doi/10.1176/appi.ajp.2010.10020268.
24. Lam, R.W., Levitt, A.J., Levitan, R.D. et al. (2006). The Can-SAD study: a randomized controlled trial of the effectiveness of light therapy and fluoxetine in patients with winter seasonal affective disorder. *American Journal of Psychiatry* 163 (5): 805–812.
25. Thornton, L. (2019). A brief history and overview of holistic nursing. *Integrative Medicine* 18 (4): 32–33.
26. Haddad, P., Reynolds, G., and Cooper, S. (2016). *BAP guidelines on the management of weight gain, metabolic disturbances and cardiovascular risk associated with psychosis and antipsychotic drug treatment*. British Association of Psychopharmacology. https://www.bap.org.uk/articles/bap-guidelines-metabolic/.
27. Ghaemi, S.N. (2009). The rise and fall of the biopsychosocial model. *The British Journal of Psychiatry* 195 (1): 3–4.
28. Engel, G.L. (1980). The clinical application of the biopsychosocial model. *American Journal of Psychiatry* 137 (5): 535–544.
29. Bolton, D. and Gillett, G. (2021). *The Biopsychosocial Model of Health and Disease: New Philosophical and Scientific Developments*, vol. 218. Royal College of Psychiatrists.
30. Psychiatric Times (2006). Introduction: an overview of psychotherapy integration. https://www.psychiatrictimes.com/view/introduction-psychotherapy-integration (accessed 1 January 2024).
31. Mehta, N. (2011). Mind-body dualism: a critique from a Health. *Perspective* 9 (1): 202.
32. Bates, V. (2017). Yesterday's doctors: the human aspects of medical education in Britain, 1957–93. *Medical History* 61 (1): 48–65.

33. Quinn, F., Chater, A.M., and Morrison, V. (2020). An oral history of health psychology in the UK. *Journal of Health Psychology* 25 (3). https://doi.org/10.1111/BJHP.12418.
34. Rakel, D. and Minichiello, V. (2023). *Integrative Medicine*, 5th ed. USA: Elsevier.
35. FPRCP (2023). Physician associate curriculum. https://www.fparcp.co.uk/file/image/media/653a42380d285_FPA_PA_curriculum_Sep_23_FINAL_WEB_VERSION.pdf (accessed 7 January 2024).
36. National Collaborating Centre for Mental Health (2022). The competence framework for physician associates in mental health supporting document. https://www.rcpsych.ac.uk/docs/default-source/improving-care/physician-associates/nccmh-the-competence-framework-for-physician-associates-in-mental-health-supporting-document.pdf?sfvrsn=53e8d0b4_4 (accessed 7 January 2024).
37. Faculty of Physician Associates Faculty of physician associates – quality health care across the NHS. https://www.fparcp.co.uk/about-fpa/news/the-faculty-of-physician-associates-launches-a-draft-physician-associate-curriculum (accessed 7 January 2024).
38. RCEM Emergency medicine – advanced clinical practitioners. https://rcem.ac.uk/emergency-care-advanced-clinical-practitioners/ (accessed 7 January 2024).
39. Scott, S. (2013). Development of advanced practice in the district nurse role: Sarah Scott's literature review illustrates the relationship between power and traditional hierarchies in the NHS. *Primary Health Care* 23 (8): 18–24.
40. Rust, J.E. (2004). Dr Hildegard Peplau. *Clinical Nurse Specialist* 18 (5): 262–263.
41. Hinchliff, S. and Rogers, R. (ed.) (2008). *Competencies for Advanced Nursing Practice*, 1st ed. Routledge https://doi.org/10.1201/b13538.
42. Kapur, S., Phillips, A.G., and Insel, T.R. (2012). Why has it taken so long for biological psychiatry to develop clinical tests and what to do about it. *Molecular Psychiatry* 17 (12): 1174–1179.
43. BMJ (2014). Neal Maskrey: treating the patient and not the disease. https://blogs.bmj.com/bmj/2014/11/17/neal-maskrey-treating-the-patient-and-not-the-disease/ (accessed 1 January 2024).
44. Ghaemi, S. (2007). *The Concepts of Psychiatry: A Pluralistic Approach to the Mind and Mental Illness*. Baltimore: Johns Hopkins University Press.
45. Hilton, C. (2016). Parity of esteem for mental and physical healthcare in England: a hundred years war? *Journal of the Royal Society of Medicine* 109 (4): 133–136.
46. Warrender, D., Connell, C., Jones, E. et al. (2024). Mental health deserves better: resisting the dilution of specialist pre-registration mental health nurse education in the United Kingdom. *Journal of Mental Health Nursing* 33 (1): 202–212.
47. Johnstone, L., Boyle, M., Cromby, J. et al. (2018). *The Power Threat Meaning Framework: Overview*. Leicester: British Psychological Society.
48. Jull, G. (2017). Biopsychosocial model of disease: 40 years on. Which way is the pendulum swinging? *British Journal of Sports Medicine* 51 (16): 1187–1188.
49. NHS (2019). The community mental health framework for adults and older adults. https://www.england.nhs.uk/wp-content/uploads/2019/09/community-mental-health-framework-for-adults-and-older-adults.pdf (accessed 1 June 2024).
50. Garratt K. (2023). Mental health policy and services in England. https://researchbriefings.files.parliament.uk/documents/CBP-7547/CBP-7547.pdf (accessed 1 June 2024).
51. NHS (2022). Myth-busting: advanced practice in mental health. https://advanced-practice.hee.nhs.uk/resources/mental-health-resources/myth-busting-advanced-practice-in-mental-health/ (accessed 21 April 2024).

52. Allabyrne, C., Chaplin, E., and Hardy, S. (2020). Advanced nursing practice in mental health: towards parity of esteem. *Nursing Times* 16 (12): 21–23.
53. Evans, C., Pearce, R., Greaves, S. et al. (2020). Advanced clinical practitioners in primary care in the UK: a qualitative study of workforce. *Transformation* 17 (12): 4500.
54. Scott, V.J. (2024). Assessing the benefits of advanced clinical practice for key stakeholders. *The British Journal of Nursing* 33 (6): 300–305.
55. The Guardian (2023). Most NHS staff say they don't have enough time to spend with patients. https://www.theguardian.com/society/2023/jul/24/most-nhs-staff-say-they-dont-have-enough-time-to-spend-with-patients (accessed 10 February 2024).
56. The nursing workforce. https://publications.parliament.uk/pa/cm201719/cmselect/cmhealth/353/35305.htm (accessed 24 February 2024).
57. Dixon-Woods, M., Summers, C., Morgan, M., and Patel, K. (2024). The future of the NHS depends on its workforce. *BMJ* 384 (384): https://www.bmj.com/content/384/bmj-2024-079474.
58. Hastings, P.D., Guyer, A.E., and Parra, L.A. (2022). Conceptualizing the influence of social and structural determinants of neurobiology and mental health: why and how biological psychiatry can do better at addressing the consequences of inequity. *Biological Psychiatry: Cognitive Neuroscience and Neuroimaging* 7 (12): 1215–1224.
59. Stein, D.J., Shoptaw, S., Vigo, D. et al. (2022). Psychiatric diagnosis and treatment in the 21st century: paradigm shifts versus incremental integration. *World Psychiatry* 21 (3): 393–414.
60. Remes, O., Mendes, J.F., and Templeton, P. (2021). Biological, psychological, and social determinants of depression: a review of recent literature. *Brain Sciences* 11 (12): 1633. https://doi.org/10.3390/brainsci11121633. PMID: 34942936; PMCID: PMC8699555.
61. RCPSYCH (2023). The role of genetic testing in mental health settings. https://www.rcpsych.ac.uk/improving-care/campaigning-for-better-mental-health-policy/college-reports/2023-college-reports/the-role-of-genetic-testing-in-mental-health-settings-(cr237) (accessed 11 July 2024).
62. Lake, J. (2012). *The Future of Mental Health Care Toward an Integrative Paradigm. Mental Illnesses – Evaluation, Treatments and Implications*. InTech. http://dx.doi.org/10.5772/30534.
63. RCPSYCH (2013). A competency based curriculum for specialist core training in Psychiatry. https://www.rcpsych.ac.uk/docs/default-source/training/curricula-and-guidance/core-psychiatry-curriculum-may-2019.pdf?sfvrsn=471d5223_6 (accessed 13 January 2024).
64. RCPSYCH (2022). Core psychiatry. Royal college of psychiatrists core training curriculum (CT1–CT3). https://www.rcpsych.ac.uk/docs/default-source/training/curricula-and-guidance/2022-curricula/core-psychiatry-curriculum-final-17-august-2022.pdf?sfvrsn=36b5ba25_10 (accessed 13 January 2024).
65. NHS (2019). NHS mental health implementation plan. https://www.longtermplan.nhs.uk/wp-content/uploads/2019/07/nhs-mental-health-implementation-plan-2019-20-2023-24.pdf (accessed January 2024).
66. Trimble, M.R. and George, M.S. (2009). *Biological Psychiatry*, 3rd ed. West Sussex: Wiley Blackwell.
67. Blows, W.T. (2021). *The Biological Basis of Mental Health*, 3rd ed. London: Routledge.
68. Malhi, G.S., Bell, E., Bassett, D. et al. (2021). The 2020 Royal Australian and New Zealand College of Psychiatrists clinical practice guidelines for mood disorders. *The Australian and New Zealand Journal of Psychiatry* 55 (1): 7–117. https://doi.org/10.1177/0004867420979353. PMID: 33353391.
69. Bolea-Alamanac, B., Nutt, D.J., Adamou, M. et al. (2014). Evidence-based guidelines for the pharmacological management of attention deficit hyperactivity disorder: update on recommendations from the British Association for. *Psychopharmacology* 28 (3): 179–203.

70. PWSA (2016). The mental health of people with Prader Willi Syndrome. https://irp.cdn-website.com/1b38aac2/files/uploaded/PWSA%20UK%20-%20The%20mental%20health%20of%20people%20with%20Prader-Willi%20Syndrome%202023.pdf (accessed 31 January 2024).
71. NICE (2014). Bipolar disorder. https://www.nice.org.uk/guidance/cg185/evidence/full-guideline-pdf-4840895629 (accessed 14 January 2024).
72. NIMH (2019). PANDAS – questions and answers. https://www.nimh.nih.gov/sites/default/files/documents/health/publications/pandas/pandas-qa.pdf (accessed January 2024).
73. Ghaemi, S.N. (2011). The biopsychosocial model in psychiatry: a critique. *Existenz* 6 (1).
74. BBC News (2024). Character.ai: Young people turning to AI therapist bots. https://www.bbc.com/news/technology-67872693 (accessed 14 January 2024).
75. NHS England (2018). The digital future of mental healthcare and its workforce: a report on a mental health stakeholder engagement to inform the Topol Review. https://topol.hee.nhs.uk/wp-content/uploads/HEE-Topol-Review-Mental-health-paper.pdf (accessed January 2024).
76. NHS England (2016). The five year forward view for mental health. https://www.england.nhs.uk/wp-content/uploads/2016/02/Mental-Health-Taskforce-FYFV-final.pdf (accessed January 2024).
77. Pryjmachuk, S. (2011). Theoretical perspectives in mental health nursing. In: *Mental Health Nursing: An Evidence Based Introduction* (ed. S. Pryjmachuk), 3–41. London: Sage Publications Ltd.
78. Mental Health Foundation (2024). Social determinants: statistics. Mental health statistics. https://www.mentalhealth.org.uk/explore-mental-health/mental-health-statistics/social-determinants-statistics (accessed 18 February 2024).
79. Compton, M.T. and Shim, R.S. (2015). The social determinants of mental. *Health* 13 (4): 419–425.
80. Marmot, M., Allen, J., Goldblatt, P. et al. (2024). Fair society, healthy lives: strategic review of health inequalities in England post 2010. https://www.instituteofhealthequity.org/resources-reports/fair-society-healthy-lives-the-marmot-review/fair-society-healthy-lives-full-report-pdf.pdf
81. Gureje, O. (2024). Deconstructing the social determinants of mental health. *World Psychiatry* 23 (1): 99–100.
82. NICE (2024). CKS is only available in the UK. https://www.nice.org.uk/cks-uk-only (accessed 20 February 2024).
83. Cleare, A.J., Pariante, C.M., Young, A.H. et al. (2015). Evidence-based guidelines for treating depressive disorders with antidepressants: a revision of the 2008 British Association for Psychopharmacology guidelines. *Journal of Psychopharmacology* 29 (5): 459–525.
84. Roy, T. and Lloyd, C.E. (2012). Epidemiology of depression and diabetes: a systematic review. *Journal of Affective Disorders* 142: S8–S21.
85. Gonzalez, J.S., Peyrot, M., Peyrot, M. et al. (2008). Depression and diabetes treatment nonadherence: a meta-analysis. *Diabetes Care* 31 (12): 2398–2403.
86. NICE (2022).Recommendations | Medicines associated with dependence or withdrawal symptoms: safe prescribing and withdrawal management for adults | Guidance | NICE. https://www.nice.org.uk/guidance/ng215/chapter/Recommendations#making-decisions-about-prescribing-and-taking-a-dependence-forming-medicine-or-antidepressant (accessed 20 February 2024).
87. Champaneri, S., Wand, G.S., Malhotra, S. et al. (2010). Biological basis of depression in adults with diabetes. *Current Diabetes Reports* 10 (6): 396–405.
88. Woo, Y.S., Lim, H.K., Wang, S.M., and Bahk, W.M. (2020). Clinical evidence of antidepressant effects of insulin and anti-hyperglycemic agents and implications for the pathophysiology of depression – a literature review. *International Journal of Molecular Sciences* 21 (18): 6969.

89. Sommerfield, A.J., Deary, I.J., and Frier, B.M. (2004). Acute hyperglycemia alters mood state and impairs cognitive performance in people with type 2 diabetes. *Diabetes Care* 27 (10): 2335–2340.
90. Pizzagalli, D.A. (2014). Depression, stress, and anhedonia: toward a synthesis and integrated model. *Annual Review of Clinical Psychology* 10 (1): 393–423.
91. Felger, J.C., Li, Z., Haroon, E. et al. (2016). Inflammation is associated with decreased functional connectivity within corticostriatal reward circuitry in depression. *Molecular Psychiatry* 21 (10): 1358–1365.
92. Royal Pharmaceutical Society England (2018). Utilising pharmacists to improve the care for people with mental health problems. https://www.rpharms.com/Portals/0/RPS%20document%20library/Open%20access/Policy/RPS%20England%20mental%20health%20policy%202018.pdf (accessed 13 April 2024).
93. Asbjørnslett, M., Skarpaas, L.S., and Stigen, L. (2023). Being holistic is a lot to ask: a qualitative, cross-national exploration of occupational therapists' perceptions and experiences of holistic practice. *Occupational Therapy International* 2023: 2432879.
94. NHS England (2022). Myth-busting: advanced practice in mental health. https://advanced-practice.hee.nhs.uk/resources/mental-health-resources/myth-busting-advanced-practice-in-mental-health/ (accessed 21 April 2024).
95. Cuijpers, P., Noma, H., Karyotaki, E. et al. (2020). A network meta-analysis of the effects of psychotherapies, pharmacotherapies and their combination in the treatment of adult depression. *World Psychiatry* 19 (1): 92–107.

CHAPTER 4

Physical Health and Integrated Care

Kirstie Tomlinson

Nottinghamshire Healthcare NHS Trust, Nottingham, UK

> **Aim**
>
> This chapter explores the role of the advanced practitioner in mental health (APMH) working directly at an advanced level with physical health issues that present in mental healthcare, viewed through the lens of integrated care and illustrated through the use of case examples. The chapter hopes to demonstrate how the APMH might structure and develop their knowledge base in this area of practice, emphasising how the skills of the APMH are ideally placed to contribute to high-quality physical healthcare.

LEARNING OUTCOMES

After reading this chapter, the reader will be able to:

- Understand the importance of promoting and supporting the physical health of people who use mental health services.
- Be aware of the wider integrated healthcare context of physical healthcare promotion in mental healthcare.
- Be aware of the importance of advanced assessment and management of long-term physical health conditions in people with a serious mental illness.
- Understand the importance of being able to recognise, respond and lead when a person's physical health is at risk of serious deterioration.
- Be able to reflect on the advanced practice role in the assessment and management of physical health issues in their own area of practice.

The Advanced Practitioner in Mental Health, First Edition. Edited by Clare Allabyrne.
© 2026 John Wiley & Sons Ltd. All rights reserved, including rights for text and data mining and training of artificial intelligence technologies or similar technologies. Published 2026 by John Wiley & Sons Ltd.

THE CONTEXT OF PHYSICAL HEALTHCARE IN MENTAL HEALTH SERVICES

The importance of healthcare professionals working in mental health services who can effectively assess, monitor and treat the physical health of the people who use their services has become an increasingly prominent agenda, reflected both in national policy frameworks [1] and in integrated care models, which focus on developing system-wide, integrated mental health and physical healthcare systems. National Health Service England (NHSE) acknowledges that, as people are living longer with more complex conditions, there must be increased consideration of the creation of joined up services that rethink how care is delivered [2]. The Darsi report [3] brought this into even sharper focus, warning that the NHS is in serious trouble, the health of the nation has deteriorated and that new multidisciplinary models of care are needed to bring together primary, community and mental health services if we are to remedy this.

In this social and political context, Integrated Care Systems are strongly encouraged to consider the physical health needs of all people severely affected by mental illness [4]. The Royal College of Psychiatrists [5] also emphasises the importance of an integrated approach to care for people with mental health problems, where care can be integrated more comprehensively into the wider health system to give better, more joined up care to people who use their services.

Evidence supporting the drive to develop better integrated mental and physical healthcare services points to the high rate of physical comorbidity in people with mental illness, physical health problems which often have poor clinical management and a subsequent reduced life expectancy for people with mental illness, increasing the personal, social and economic cost of mental illness across the lifespan [6].

However, critics suggest that despite this, integrated care remains challenged by current siloed practices and associated training [7], whilst others recognise that mental health practitioners may consider themselves unequipped to respond effectively in this area of practice [8]. The National Confidential Enquiry into Patient Outcomes and Death [9] highlights the importance of formalising clinical pathways between mental healthcare and physical healthcare, adding mental healthcare staff need support in providing physical healthcare and citing survey data where many mental healthcare professionals reported feeling less than fairly confident or competent in caring for patients with long-term conditions.

Attempting to address some of these concerns has led to the publication of important guidelines which aim to bridge the gap between psychiatric and physical health service provision [10]. A key objective of such guidelines and associated policy is to try to guide and enhance the knowledge and clinical decision-making skills of mental health professionals when assessing and treating physical healthcare-related presentations, thus improving integration of services more usually geographically and organisationally separate.

In this political and professional context, the training, competencies and role context of the advanced practitioner in mental health suggest they might be ideally trained and placed to address this agenda [11, 12]. The competencies they achieve include the development of clinical reasoning approaches to deal with differentiated and undifferentiated individual presentations and complex situations. Clinical reasoning is discussed in detail in Chapter 5. The APMH, therefore, could have a unique and exciting role to play in the promotion and management of the physical health of the people referred to their services, with an opportunity to lead on the development and embedding of a truly integrated approach to care.

This chapter focuses on two cases to attempt to illustrate how the APMH might apply their skills in integrated mental and physical healthcare. The first illustrates the ways in which an APMH can utilise their advanced knowledge and skills to work with people with serious mental illness (SMI) to support them to manage both their physical and mental health in the community, while the second case focuses on the role of an APMH in inpatient mental health services, where they might find themselves involved in assessing potentially complex comorbid presentations and may also have to respond to a patient who is physically deteriorating.

Clearly, it is not possible in a single chapter to describe all the facets of physical healthcare that an APMH may find themselves involved in whilst working with such a diverse group of patients, but by describing the events in each case, the chapter aims to illustrate the types of situation they might find themselves working within and how their particular skills might be ideally placed to respond to the integrated physical and mental healthcare agenda.

THE COMMUNITY MENTAL HEALTH ADVANCED PRACTITIONER – IMPROVING THE PHYSICAL HEALTHCARE OF THOSE WITH SERIOUS MENTAL ILLNESS

We know people living with SMI face one of the greatest health equality gaps in England. Their life expectancy is 15–20 years shorter than that for the general population [13], and this disparity is largely due to preventable physical illnesses [14]. In 2019, the Lancet Psychiatry Commission [6] identified the importance of protecting the physical health of people with mental illness, noting a 1.4-to 2-fold increased risk of obesity, diabetes and cardiovascular diseases compared to the general population. Although most evidence they evaluated related to SMI populations (particularly people experiencing psychotic disorders), the prevalence of cardiometabolic diseases was also similarly elevated across a broad range of other diagnoses, including substance use disorders and more common mental disorders.

From a UK policy framework perspective, Core20PLUS5 [15] attempts to address this, and other inequalities, setting an approach to inform action to reduce healthcare inequalities at both a national and a system level. It defines a target population: the most deprived 20% of the English population as identified by the National Index of Multiple Deprivation [16] and identifies '5' focus clinical areas requiring accelerated improvement, one of which is people with SMI. It sets out a target to ensure they have annual physical health checks to nationally set targets at the very least. Many people with SMI have difficulty accessing traditional health services, and it is incumbent on all of us in mental health services to take steps to address this barrier in the most person-centred way.

Why might the APMH role be well-placed to respond and lead on promoting this agenda? Following successful completion of training, an APMH will have developed skills in assessing differentiated and undifferentiated individual presentations and complex situations, to make appropriate, evidence-based judgements and/or diagnoses [12] and is ideally placed to provide a sensitive and timely physical assessment of people who access their services for support with their mental health. Paul's case (and Sally's later in the chapter) are adapted from examples drawn from clinical practice and illustrate how the APMH competency framework and associated skills might be weaved into everyday clinical practice. In line with Nursing and Midwifery Council (NMC) guidelines regarding confidentiality, these cases do not identify any individual person or their family [17].

Paul

Paul is a 49-year-old gentleman who has a diagnosis of paranoid schizophrenia. Paul has been involved with mental health services for many years, having had several inpatient admissions. His illness was successfully treated with clozapine, and maintaining his mental health is understandably extremely important to him. However, Paul does not like attending his GP services as he continues to hold a delusional belief that his GP wishes to control him, and he has never, therefore, felt able to return to these services for an annual review.

Paul has been referred to the advanced practitioner (AP) clinic for monitoring his mental health and treatment. He engages well with services, attending all of his appointments and annual checks and reporting that he finds support for his mental health problems very helpful.

One day, Paul attends clinic and reports to the APMH that he has been very troubled by what he calls his 'problem with checking'. He tells the APMH that this has been happening for some time (not long after he started taking clozapine) but that he has been too ashamed to talk about it before. He tells the APMH it can take up to one hour for him to get out of his flat as he has to keep repeatedly checking that the door is locked and the gas has not been left on. He does not want to check in this way and can't identify any trigger that would make him do it, but says he feels he has to, worrying something bad may happen if he doesn't.

This has led to Paul staying inside for much of the time in recent months, getting food delivered and not socialising in the way he used to. He is eating an unhealthy diet, is getting little exercise and he has gained weight.

Supporting Paul to Improve His Health Behaviours

The APMH is aware of the six elements of the annual health check for people with an SMI [4].

The 6 elements of the 'core' annual SMI physical health check:

- Alcohol consumption status
- Blood glucose or HbA1c test (as clinically appropriate)
- Blood pressure
- Body mass index (BMI)
- Lipid profile
- Smoking status

As a senior clinician in their mental health team, the APMH is able to involve the wider team to coordinate physical healthcare investigations for Paul in an environment and at a time most likely to engage him comfortably. The APMH can then review and synthesise the information gathered to support Paul in making decisions that support him to improve and maintain his physical health. Paul doesn't smoke or drink alcohol, but the APMH reviews his blood results and notes new concerns about hyperlipidaemia and an increase in BMI.

With physical inactivity and dietary risks elevated in research evidence across a broad range of mental health diagnoses [6], the APMH is aware that modifiable factors related to health behaviours are key. The APMH is also aware of the importance of adhering to the advice: don't just screen, intervene [4]. The APMH links in other healthcare professionals including a team dietician and a social prescriber to support Paul to improve his health behaviours in a way that he finds helpful. The APMH also contacts Paul's general practitioner (GP) with his permission to discuss the prescription of lipid-lowering therapy [18], and the GP is able to issue this prescription on repeat. Through comprehensive assessment, teamwork, effective delegation and coordination, the APMH has been able to apply their leadership skills to Paul's individual case in a way that has supported all involved to influence his engagement, empowerment and recovery [12].

Managing Medicines, Multimorbidity and Uncertainty

However, Paul remains understandably concerned about his 'problem with checking', and his social prescriber feels that this is continuing to act as a barrier to him improving his physical health. The APMH is concerned to hear about this ongoing impact and arranges an appointment to discuss this with Paul in more detail, showing professional curiosity in undertaking a comprehensive, person-centred history to critically assess complex information and identify those elements that may need to be pursued further [12]. A detailed history identifies that Paul has experienced these symptoms since he was initially prescribed clozapine, not before. They have worsened over time and now significantly impact on his life, making it hard for him to engage in social activities as he feels he can't leave his flat. He is ashamed of this problem but thankfully denies any suicidal ideation or thoughts of deliberate self-harm.

The APMH considers this problem and explores available evidence to try address Paul's concerns. Evidence identifies that people with a diagnosis of schizophrenia have a high lifetime risk for comorbid obsessive-compulsive symptoms [19], associated with pronounced positive and negative symptoms and lower levels of social functioning. Consequently, they have a less favourable prognosis. Hypotheses as to the aetiology of these symptoms suggest they might be a side effect of second-generation antipsychotics (SGAs), especially clozapine [19]. The APMH discusses this with Paul who says he would like to access some treatment for this and would prefer medication to treat it if possible. Kim et al. [20] note that selective serotonin reuptake inhibitors (SSRIs) can be effective in treating clozapine-induced obsessive-compulsive symptoms. The APMH discusses this suggestion with Paul, discussing the potential benefits and adverse effects of an additional prescription, and Paul agrees to trial a prescription of an SSRI, which the APMH then prescribes.

> **Paul**
>
> Paul attends a review in clinic with the APMH three months later. He reports that his 'problem with checking' has resolved completely. He no longer worries about going out of the house, his confidence has improved and he has joined a local photography group.
>
> When asked by the APMH, he denies any adverse effects from the medication prescribed. A review of his physical health notes his weight and his blood pressure have both reduced. An ECG reveals normal sinus rhythm with a QTc within normal range. Paul is pleased with his improvement.
>
> At the end of the appointment, Paul asks the APMH if he can ask a 'silly question'.
>
> He tells the APMH he has been wetting the bed at night and is very embarrassed about this.
>
> The APMH extends the clinic appointment to discuss Paul's incontinence and spends time encouraging him to talk about it in more detail. Paul becomes very upset when talking about it, worrying that he is 'behaving like a 2-year-old and that no-one will ever want to be his girlfriend'. In talking this through sensitively with Paul, the APMH is able to demonstrate expertise in establishing and maintaining a therapeutic relationship in the presence of sensitive information and distress [12].

The APMH is able to assess in more detail the unexpected physical health concern, in that Paul sleeps heavily throughout the night and wakes each morning having urinated in his sleep. He cannot remember anything else about this and has never been incontinent of urine before. Paul lives alone and does not have a family member who is able to provide collateral history. He does not drink excessive fluid before bed and does not drink caffeinated products. The APMH explores differentials for nocturia [21] and establishes there are no concerns about diabetes. The APMH then requests the team nursing associate to repeat Paul's bloods and finds bloods (and a subsequent urinalysis) are unremarkable.

There is no previous history of seizures, but the APMH is mindful of the onset of the problem with the change in medication. The APMH reflects on their own pharmacological understanding of both SSRIs and clozapine [22] but is also aware of the unusual nature of this presentation, noting the limits of their own competence and exercising professional judgement about when to seek help [12]. The APMH discusses this with the consultant psychiatrist and the team pharmacist. The pharmacist notes that, although not a common drug–drug interaction, both clozapine and SSRIs can lower the seizure threshold in an individual [22] and suggests that the combination of both clozapine and an SSRI might be leading to nocturnal seizures. The consultant psychiatrist advises, as the clozapine has been established for some years, to discontinue the SSRI as a precaution and keep Paul under close review.

Paul is disappointed that his SSRI has been discontinued. The APMH adjusts his clinic to spend some additional appointment time with Paul and explores other options to manage his obsessive-compulsive symptoms. Although Paul had not previously wanted to explore cognitive behavioural therapy (CBT), the APMH spends some time explaining therapeutic options and NICE guideline recommendations [23]; Paul agrees to trial it, and the APMH refers him for a course of therapy.

The nocturnal enuresis resolves when the SSRI is discontinued, and Paul has no previous history of seizures. However, the APMH notified Paul's GP about the events, so additional follow-up can be arranged if needed and links a team support worker with Paul to give him support to attend the GP surgery.

Paul's case illustrates how the physical and mental health of a person cannot and should not be viewed as separate aspects of healthcare. Physical health comorbidity and related poor outcomes are more prevalent in those with an SMI, and the treatment of a mental health problem can also, sometimes, result in physical healthcare complications that need to be recognised and addressed. In this case, the APMH was ideally placed to assess and engage Paul in improving and maintaining his physical health, engaging and coordinating teamwork across the fields of both mental and physical healthcare, critically assessing and appraising the evidence when clinical challenges arose and approaching interventions with a person-centred focus.

The APMH's flexible and responsive clinical role meant there were opportunities to monitor and intervene to maintain Paul's physical health, demonstrate their understanding of the impact of population health and take appropriate steps to address inequalities and vulnerabilities. The APMH was able to maintain a therapeutic relationship in the presence of sensitive information and distress, allowing Paul the space to talk about the issues that concerned him. The APMH was also able to demonstrate understanding of the interplay between the psychological, biological and social factors that affected Paul, recognising and addressing physical health issues within their scope of practice and referring, when required, for more specialist assessment and intervention. The APMH developed a co-produced management plan with Paul, taking into account the complexity of the risk related to treatment and Paul's preferences and wishes and was able to help him evaluate and modify a range of interventions when medication was no longer viable.

This case illustrates how the competencies of an APMH predispose them to being ideally placed to address the agenda of physical health comorbidities in people with SMI. It also offers an opportunity for the APMH to lead – not just in individual case management but also to apply their wider strategic knowledge in a senior clinical role. This presents an opportunity for them to impact on wider service delivery, building relationships that may help services develop more integrated strategies. APMHs might want to join and influence integrated care group meetings in their geographical area, and they might want to be involved in audits of physical health outcomes for people who use their services – just two examples that highlight how the APMH has a valuable role to play in the development of newer, better, multidisciplinary models of care.

THE ADVANCED PRACTITIONER IN INPATIENT MENTAL HEALTH – WORKING WITH COMPLEXITY AND RECOGNISING THE DETERIORATING PATIENT

APMHs working in inpatient mental health settings in the United Kingdom may be still relatively low in numbers, but this expanding area of advanced practice offers the APMH both challenge and opportunity. It asks them to work collaboratively at an advanced level with members of the multidisciplinary team (MDT) who have expertise in their own profession or area of practice, developing strategies to work with uncertainty in a fast-paced environment – both in mental health and wider healthcare. It also asks them to work with this uncertainty within themselves, whilst working in an area more traditionally in the realm of medicine.

The Care Quality Commission's (CQC) policy position on the provision of physical healthcare in inpatient mental health services proposes that a good service ensures that people with mental health needs receive the same standard of physical healthcare as any other member of society [24]. They acknowledge the complexity of delivering holistic healthcare and recognise services may deliver this through their own appropriately qualified and experienced staff or in partnership with other providers. Can the APMH then also contribute to this agenda in inpatient services?

The CQC suggests there are two main tasks for practitioners in mental health services when addressing physical healthcare needs:

→ Assessment to ensure physical illness is not causing the psychiatric presentation.
→ Monitoring for adverse physical effects of antipsychotic treatment or other causes of poor physical health.

The National Confidential Enquiry into Patient Outcomes and Death [9], reporting on physical healthcare in mental health inpatient settings, made more detailed recommendations that acknowledged patient complexity, the need for assessment and monitoring of patient deterioration, the monitoring of long-term physical health conditions and the need for development of integrated mental and physical healthcare pathways.

The remainder of this chapter attempts to illustrate these recommendations, and how they might translate into practice for the inpatient APMH, through the description of an inpatient case study, Sally.

Sally

Sally is a 69-year-old lady, who has a 30-year history of input from mental health services. She has a diagnosis of bipolar affective disorder which was successfully treated for many years with lithium. Unfortunately, 20 years ago, Sally developed kidney failure. Her lithium treatment was discontinued, and in the years that followed she received a kidney transplant.

Sally's mental health deteriorated following her kidney transplant, and she became depressed. An alternative mood stabiliser was prescribed, but she disliked the adverse effects. A lower dose was prescribed to try to reduce this, but unfortunately this led to Sally experiencing recurrent episodes of depression.

When Sally is depressed, she will take to her bed, have greatly restricted food and fluid intake and will need support with all aspects of care. The risk of acute kidney injury when her fluid intake is restricted means she has been prescribed electroconvulsive therapy (ECT) several times to treat her low mood. This treatment leads to a temporary improvement in mood, but she will relapse again quickly when she is discharged to her nursing care placement.

Sally is readmitted to the inpatient mental health ward, presenting with a recurrent depressive episode. She is bed bound, mute and has severely restricted food and fluid intake. Her daughter would like the inpatient team to consider maintenance (regular) ECT as she does not feel her psychiatric medication is helping.

Sally is a complex case, presenting with multiple physical healthcare comorbidities and a treatment-resistant psychiatric disorder. The APMH works in a multidisciplinary inpatient mental health team, with a Consultant Psychiatrist acting as Responsible Clinician. What role can the APMH fulfil in this complex presentation that will benefit both the patient and the team? Again, this case also illustrates the importance of not viewing a patient's physical healthcare as a separate entity from their mental health and illustrates how the APMH can play a vital and fluid role in jointly managing this complexity.

WHAT CAN AN APMH ROLE CONTRIBUTE IN A MENTAL HEALTH INPATIENT ENVIRONMENT?

The CQC [24] highlights the importance of assessment of patients for acute physical health conditions on arrival at a mental health inpatient setting, with a more detailed physical health assessment to be conducted once the patient is admitted. It emphasises that patients admitted for mental healthcare who are also physically unwell need complex care and may need a transfer to a physical health hospital for an acute condition. Equally, they may have at least one long-term physical health condition that needs monitoring.

Sally's Medical History
- 2023 Sepsis
- 2023 Fractured neck of femur
- 2022 Fragility fracture
- 2021 Chronic peripheral venous hypertension
- 2016 Renal transplant
- 2015 Lumbar spondylosis
- 2008 Osteoarthritis
- 2005 Chronic renal failure
- 2004 Hyperparathyroidism
- 1996 Bipolar affective disorder
- 1985 Hypothyroidism

At the point of admission, the APMH was asked to 'clerk in' or complete the admission processes for Sally. Experienced in psychiatric assessment, and having developed some experience and competency in physical examination [25] during training and the establishment of their APMH post, but having no prior experience of working with a patient with such a complex renal history, how is the APMH to ensure competence in assessing Sally?

> HAEMOGLOBIN 118 g/L [115–160]
> WBC 9.26 10 E9/L [4.00–11.00]
> PLATELETS 307 10 E9/L [150–450]
> RBC 3.98 10 E12/L [3.80–5.80]
> FERRITIN 74.0 micro g/L [5.0–204.0] TRANSFERRIN 2.1 g/L [2.0–3.6]
> NEUTROPHILS 6.41 10 E9/L [2.00–7.50]
> LYMPHOCYTES 2.04 10 E9/L [1.00–4.00]
> MONOCYTES 0.69 10 E9/L [0.20–1.00]
> EOSINOPHILS 0.10 10 E9/L [0.00–0.40]
> BASOPHILS 0.02 10 E9/L [0.01–0.15]
>
> *PTH 113 ng/L [15–68]
> *EGFR BY CKD-EPI/1.73M2 36 ml/min/1.73m[60–200]
> *UREA 16.7 mmol/L [2.5–7.8]
> *CREATININE 125 µmol/L [49–90]
>
> SODIUM 136 mmol/L [133–146]
> POTASSIUM 5.2 mmol/L [3.5–5.3]
>
> PHOSPHATE 1.38 mmol/L [0.80–1.50]
> *ALBUMIN 33 g/L [35–50]
> ADJUSTED CALCIUM 2.52 mmol/L [2.20–2.60]
> BICARBONATE 24 mmol/L [22–29]
>
> Impression:
> Raised eGFR, urea, creatinine consistent with known CKD, PTH consistent with secondary hyperparathyroidism in CKD
>
> *Awaiting tacrolimus level

In this complex context, the APMH is challenged to reflect on their broadened level of responsibility, the limits of their own competence and professional scope of practice in an undifferentiated medical environment [12]. They might want to address a knowledge gap by accessing learning around the complex medical history Sally presents with, including the ongoing management of her chronic kidney disease (CKD) and the implications of her taking immunosuppressant medication. The APMH needs to know where to access learning related to physical health, for example, they might revise the topic of CKD in a CPD resource such as BMJ Best Practice [26] or a learning module on the BMJ learning platform [27]. The APMH might want to explore the impact of taking antirejection drugs for Sally's physical health using a patient-centred online resource, such as the National Kidney Foundation [28]. Many resources are available that will equip the APMH to be informed when approaching Sally's admission, enabling them to work carefully within their own limitations, and it is crucial that the APMH in a developing role remains curious and open to challenge. In recognising their limitations, the APMH may want to assess Sally in conjunction with medical colleagues to ensure Sally's safety [12].

Following examination, the APMH completes a psychiatric and medical history and the nursing team takes Sally's bloods and physical observations. The resident doctor working with the APMH conducts a venous thromboembolism (VTE) assessment and commences Sally on prophylactic blood thinning medication to reduce the risk of VTE while she remains bed bound.

When available, the APMH interprets Sally's bloods and excludes any acute physical health presentation that may need transfer to acute hospital, utilising their knowledge of CKD, Sally's previous blood results and discussion with members of the medical team to establish that Sally's kidney function was presenting at its baseline (CKD stage 3b) [26]. The pharmacy team checks the drug card prescription and completes a medication reconciliation, and the nursing team compliments this integrated mental and physical health assessment with personal care and a skin integrity review.

Sally

Initial MDT discussion and collaborative care planning formulates that, as a consequence of her mental state and associated reduced fluid intake, Sally is at risk of severe physical health deterioration.

ECT is proposed by the consultant psychiatrist to treat her depressive episode.

Sally is assessed by the APMH as not having capacity to consent to this treatment, as she is unable to communicate her understanding and consent, and a course of ECT is planned under Section 62 of the Mental Health Act (MHA) [29].

Review of her hydration status, physical observations and repeat intervals for her bloods are care planned in conjunction to monitoring of her mental state.

The initial assessment and care planning during Sally's hospital admission illustrate the integrated and multidisciplinary nature of an inpatient psychiatric admission. As with all people who access help for their mental health, their physical health cannot and should not be separated from the psychiatric goals for admission, and the APMH is well-placed to understand the complex interplay between the psychological, biological and social factors that affect health [12]. In Sally's case, her mental health is placing her physical health at risk, and the complex nature of her medical history means that both must be managed simultaneously. While different healthcare professionals complete different aspects of the admission, formulation needs to be integrated and multidisciplinary. The APMH is ideally placed to work alongside the consultant, supporting the communication and synthesis of complex information and providing clinical leadership to ensure all members of the team are informed and understand the care plan.

Sally

Sally remains low in mood, bed bound and largely nonverbal, but her food and fluid intake improves with supported feeding from the nursing team. The APMH completes a psychiatric and medicines history by accessing Sally's historical medical records, and an alternative mood stabiliser is prescribed by the consultant psychiatrist to support treatment.

While completing personal care, the nursing team notes a large, raised lump on her left wrist and asked the APMH to review. A haematoma is identified, and on further examination of Sally's skin, multiple bruises are noted. A review of bloods identifies mild thrombocytopenia but nothing else of immediate concern.

The APMH reviews Sally's medical history, accessing her medical notes from an acute inpatient stay the previous year when she was treated for sepsis. During that admission, there is also a report of a large haematoma, and blood thinners are discontinued as they are suggested to be the causative agent. This adverse reaction was not documented in Sally's GP medical history or wider medical records.

> The APMH discusses this with the team resident doctor, discontinues the prophylactic blood thinners prescribed for Sally, informs Sally and her daughter of the adverse reaction, ensures a review and monitoring plan is initiated by the MDT and notifies the GP so that Sally's medical records can be updated.

One of the benefits of an APMH role in inpatient psychiatric services is the opportunity they provide in delivering consistency of care in a busy, dynamic, inpatient environment. Medical training means that resident doctors will frequently rotate between placements, and in the course of sometimes lengthy inpatient psychiatric admissions, several different medical professionals will be involved in treating a patient. An APMH based in an inpatient mental health service has the opportunity to provide oversight throughout the course of a lengthy psychiatric inpatient stay, exercising leadership to effectively promote patient safety, especially in the presence of multimorbidity, complexity and/or unpredictability [12]. In Sally's case, the APMH was able to access lengthy historical records from multiple sources, helping support the team formulation, identify the cause of her bruising and prioritise timely intervention in a situation where there was a changing priority in relation to Sally's physical health.

> **Sally**
>
> Sally's mental health continues to steadily improve, her dietary and fluid intake stabilises, she has regained capacity in relation to her medical treatment and is now accepting of her psychiatric medication. Discharge planning is in progress and, as Sally remains bed bound, a specialist nursing home placement is being explored in conjunction with Sally and her daughter's wishes.
>
> The CQC [24] recommends involving patients and their family in their physical healthcare, using inpatient admission as an opportunity to assess and involve patients in their general health. They identify that hospital admissions are an excellent opportunity to assess and help improve a patient's general physical health and including family can be a great form of support.
>
> Sally's daughter has supported her through different stages of Sally's life, while she lived independently at home and when she lived in a residential home. Her daughter reflects that Sally's mental state had deteriorated twice while she lived in a residential home, and her level of frailty has increased further during this admission. She tells the team that she feels Sally would now be best supported by a specialist nursing placement, and the MDT agreed that would be in Sally's best interests.
>
> As Sally awaits discharge, both her mental and physical health continue to be reviewed by the MDT. Routine physical observations, completed every 24 hours, indicate Sally is tachycardic, tachypnoeic and scoring 3 on the NEWS2 scoring system [30]. The APMH is asked to assess. On examination Sally has marked tenderness on palpation of the left lumbar region. It is thought she has not urinated in the last 6 hours.

Recognising the Deteriorating Patient

The CQC [24] recommends the ongoing physical healthcare of mental health inpatients should be monitored to prevent deterioration. NICE [30] recommends the National Early Warning Score 2 (NEWS2) scoring system is implemented in mental health inpatient settings to monitor for signs of patient deterioration, as it is a clear system for identifying those patients who are most physically unwell. Although Sally's NEWS2 score indicates only low to moderate risk, given Sally's history of right-sided kidney transplant, multiple acute hospital admissions over the past year and the geographical distance between the mental health hospital and an acute hospital should she deteriorate further and require transfer, the APMH contacts the local acute hospital admissions unit to discuss. The acute team agrees to an admission to the renal unit, and Sally is subsequently diagnosed with hydronephrosis, likely obstructive and caused by constipation.

In Sally's case, the CQC recommendations for good physical healthcare monitoring were actioned successfully. Her physiological observations were measured with appropriate frequency, deterioration recognised and care escalated promptly.

Although all members of the mental health MDT should be trained and be able to recognise and respond to a patient whose physical health is deteriorating, the APMH is well-placed to be able to exercise professional judgement and leadership to effectively promote patient safety [12]. Clear clinical leadership in the context of patient deterioration is crucial, and an APMH can demonstrate both clinical and leadership skills in this context, supporting the wider medical team, expanding physical healthcare provision and contributing to improved quality care in inpatient mental health services.

A NOTE ON THE LAW AND PHYSICAL HEALTHCARE FOR PATIENTS WITH MENTAL HEALTH PROBLEMS

Although these cases aim to illustrate the importance of mental health services recognising and addressing the physical healthcare needs of the people who are accessing support for their mental health, it is important for the APMH to be aware of the legal frameworks surrounding the assessment and treatment of physical health conditions in a mental health environment.

In the first instance, the APMH should use the same approach they would use to address any form of treatment with a patient and should aim to gain informed consent for any physical health interventions. But what if the patient refuses or lacks capacity to consent to a physical healthcare intervention?

While Section 63 of the MHA can be utilised to provide mental health treatment for a psychiatric inpatient who either refuses or lacks capacity to consent to treatment and is liable to be detained, physical healthcare can only be provided in this context if it is 'directly related to the mental disorder, or a manifestation or consequence of the mental disorder' [31].

If the physical healthcare treatment is unrelated to the mental disorder, and the patient does not have capacity to consent to this specific treatment, then the APMH should consider any such treatment under the framework of the Mental Capacity Act (2005) [32] considering carefully if the treatment is proportionate, necessary and in the patient's best interests. If a patient refuses a physical healthcare intervention, and has the capacity to do so, then their decision, even if it is an unwise decision, must be respected.

CONCLUSION

Both the Darsi report [3] and the CQC [24] emphasise the importance of formalised clinical pathways between mental healthcare and physical healthcare. The cases illustrated in this chapter demonstrate the multiple services and health professionals that may need to be involved to ensure a mental health patient receives the same standard of physical healthcare as any other member of society – either due to the complexity of supporting long-term conditions in conjunction with SMI or during an inpatient admission when physical healthcare complexity may be at its most acute.

An APMH may be ideally placed to advocate for their patient in this context – their training and experience mean they have the knowledge and skillset to be able to assess and formulate both mental and physical healthcare presentations, and patient care may benefit from a holistic APMH perspective and oversight. Both the patient and the MDT may also benefit from the APMH's ability to apply leadership and educational skills to promote a physical healthcare agenda, and the broad outlook of the APMH role may mean they are well-placed to lead on physical healthcare agendas in mental health services. However, given the increasing need to improve the health of the nation and the complexity that multi-morbid mental health and physical health presentations can bring, the APMH also needs to recognise when a presenting physical health problem sits outside the scope of their skills and experience, recognising when collaborative teamwork or specialist help is required.

The provision of good physical healthcare for people with SMI needs coordinated input from multiple specialities to be effective. Improvements in both physical and mental health service provision still need to be made before they can operate effectively through formalised pathways. The APMH role is an opportunity to influence and shape services to make sustained, positive change for the people who access our services, and we should lead on the development and embedding of a truly integrated approach to care.

> **Questions for Reflection**
> - What are the public health priorities of most importance or prevalence in your service?
> - What long-term physical health conditions commonly present in people who use your service?
> - How do you support your patients to manage any long-term physical healthcare conditions and what services are available to support this?
> - How might the APMH role help address any acute physical healthcare needs of the people who use your service?
> - How do you recognise and respond to a patient within your services whose physical health is deteriorating and what systems are in place to ensure safe and rapid response?
> - How can the APMH role add value to medication monitoring for people who use your service?
> - What services do you need to link in with to ensure the people who use your services access the same standard of physical healthcare as any other person?
> - What CPD do you need to access to ensure you remain competent in assessing and managing the physical healthcare needs of the people who use your services?
> - How might your research pillar promote and reflect the physical health agenda in mental healthcare?

REFERENCES

1. NHS (2019). NHS Long Term Plan. https://webarchive.nationalarchives.gov.uk/ukgwa/20230418145517/https://www.longtermplan.nhs.uk/ (accessed 16 February 2025)
2. NHS England (2024). NHS England 10 key actions: improving the physical health of people living with severe mental illness. https://www.england.nhs.uk/long-read/10-key-actions-improving-the-physical-health-of-people-living-with-severe-mental-illness/ (accessed 16 February 2025).
3. Department of Health and Social Care (2024). Summary letter from Lord Darzi to the Secretary of State for Health and Social Care. https://www.gov.uk/government/publications/independent-investigation-of-the-nhs-in-england/summary-letter-from-lord-darzi-to-the-secretary-of-state-for-health-and-social-care (accessed 16 February 2025).

4. NHS England (2024). Improving the physical health of people living with severe mental illness: guidance for integrated care systems. NHS England. https://www.england.nhs.uk/long-read/improving-the-physical-health-of-people-living-with-severe-mental-illness/ (accessed 16 February 2025).
5. Royal College of Psychiatrists (2019). Improving mental health services in systems of integrated and accountable care: emerging lessons and priorities. https://www.rcpsych.ac.uk/docs/default-source/improving-care/better-mh-policy/policy/rcpsych-improving-mental-health-services-in-icss-exec-summary-final.pdf (accessed 16 February 2025).
6. The Lancet Psychiatry Commission (2019). The *Lancet Psychiatry* Commission: a blueprint for protecting physical health in people with mental illness. The Lancet Psychiatry. https://www.thelancet.com/journals/lanpsy/article/PIIS2215-0366(19)30132-4/abstract (accessed 16 February 2025).
7. Sockalingam, S., Chaudhary, Z.K., Barnett, R. et al. (2020). Developing a framework of integrated competencies for adaptive expertise in integrated physical and mental health care. *Teaching and Learning in Medicine* 32 (2): 159–167. https://pubmed.ncbi.nlm.nih.gov/31482737/ (accessed 16 February 2025).
8. Attoe, C., Retter, S., Minster, R., and Parish, S. (2020). Developing the mental health workforce to meet the physical health needs of people with a serious mental illness. *BMJ Simulation and Technology Enhanced Learning* 6 (5): 297–299. https://pmc.ncbi.nlm.nih.gov/articles/PMC8936936/ (accessed 16 February 2024).
9. The National Confidential Enquiry into Patient Outcome and Death (2022). A picture of health? National Confidential Enquiry into Patient Outcome and Death: A Picture of Health? – HQIP. https://www.hqip.org.uk/resource/national-confidential-enquiry-into-patient-outcome-and-death-a-picture-of-health/ (accessed 16 February 2024).
10. Taylor, M., Gaughran, F., and Pillinger, T. (ed.) (2021). *The Maudsley Practice Guidelines for Physical Health Conditions in Psychiatry*. London: Wiley: Blackwell.
11. NHS England (2017). Multi-professional framework for advanced clinical practice in England. https://www.hee.nhs.uk/sites/default/files/documents/multi-professionalframeworkforadvancedclinicalpracticeinengland.pdf (accessed 16 February 2025).
12. Health Education England (2022). Advanced practice mental health curriculum and capabilities framework. https://www.hee.nhs.uk/sites/default/files/documents/AP-MH%20Curriculum%20and%20Capabilities%20Framework%201.2.pdf (accessed 16 February 2025).
13. Public Health England (2018). Severe mental illness (SMI) and physical health inequalities: briefing. GOV.UK. https://www.gov.uk/government/publications/severe-mental-illness-smi-physical-health-inequalities/severe-mental-illness-and-physical-health-inequalities-briefing (accessed 16 February 2025).
14. Office for Health Improvement & Disparities (2023). Premature mortality in adults with severe mental illness (SMI). GOV.UK. https://www.gov.uk/government/publications/premature-mortality-in-adults-with-severe-mental-illness (accessed 16 February 2025).
15. NHS England (2024). Core20PLUS5 (adults) – an approach to reducing healthcare inequalities. NHS England. https://www.england.nhs.uk/about/equality/equality-hub/national-healthcare-inequalities-improvement-programme/core20plus5/ (accessed 16 February 2025).
16. Ministries of Housing, Communities and Local Government (2019). English Indices of Deprivation. 2019. GOV.UK. https://www.gov.uk/government/statistics/english-indices-of-deprivation-2019 (accessed 16 February 2025).
17. Nursing and Midwifery Council (NMC) (2023). The Code: Professional standards of practice and behaviour for nurses, midwives and nursing associates. The Nursing and Midwifery Council. https://www.nmc.org.uk/standards/code/
18. NICE (2023). Cardiovascular disease: Risk assessment and reduction, including lipid modification. Overview | Guidance | NICE. https://www.nice.org.uk/guidance/ng238 (accessed 16 February 2025).

19. Schirmbeck, F. and Zink, M. (2012). Clozapine-induced obsessive-compulsive symptoms in schizophrenia: a critical review. *Current Neuropharmacology* 10 (1): 88–95.
20. Kim, D., Barr, A., White, R. et al. (2019). Clozapine-induced obsessive–compulsive symptoms: mechanisms and treatment. *Journal of Psychiatry and Neuroscience* 44 (1): 71–72.
21. BMJ Best Practice (2023). Enuresis – symptoms, diagnosis and treatment: BMJ best practice, Log in | BMJ Best Practice. https://bestpractice.bmj.com/log-in (accessed 16 February 2025).
22. Bhatti, M., Dorriz, P., and Mehndiratta, P. (2017). Impact of Psychotropic drugs on Seizure threshold. *Behavioral and Cognitive Neurology: Pharmacological Effects* P6: 311.
23. NICE (2005). Obsessive-compulsive disorder and body dysmorphic disorder: treatment. Clinical guideline [CG31]. Overview | Guidance | NICE. https://www.nice.org.uk/Guidance/CG31 (accessed 16 February 2025).
24. Care Quality Commission (2022). Brief Guide BG029: Physical healthcare in mental health settings v4. https://www.cqc.org.uk/sites/default/files/20191125_900852_briefguide-physical_healthcare_mental_health_settings_v4.pdf (accessed 16 February 2024).
25. HEE (2022). Advanced Clinical Practice in Older People Curriculum Framework. https://cpoc.org.uk/sites/cpoc/files/documents/2022-05/Advanced%20clinical%20practice%20older%20people%20curriculum%20framework%20%2027.04.pdf (accessed16 February 2024).
26. BMJ Best Practice (2024). Chronic Kidney Disease – Symptoms, diagnosis and treatment. BMJ Best Practice. https://bestpractice.bmj.com/topics/en-gb/84 (accessed 16 February 2025).
27. BMJ Learning (2024). Chronic Kidney Disease in Adults: diagnosis and management. bmj.cm. https://new-learning.bmj.com/course/5004312 (accessed 16 February 2025).
28. National Kidney Foundation (2024). Immunosuppressants. https://www.kidney.org.uk/kidney-topics/immunosuppressants-anti-rejection-medicines (accessed 16 February 2025).
29. Mental Health Act 1983, s.62. https://www.legislation.gov.uk/ukpga/1983/20/section/62.
30. NICE (2016) Suspected sepsis: recognition, diagnosis and early management. NICE guideline [NG51]. https://www.nice.org.uk/guidance/NG51 (accessed 16 February 2025).
31. Mental Health Act 1983, s.63. https://www.legislation.gov.uk/ukpga/1983/20/section/63.
32. Department of Health (2015). Mental Health Act 1983: Code of Practice, paragraph 13.37.

CHAPTER 5

Clinical Reasoning and Complexity: An Overview

James Tighe

Royal Marsden Hospital, London, UK

'As for the paradigms that guide our clinical thinking...they are necessary. They afford us, at a minimum, the comfort (and benefits) of being in error, rather than thrashing about in confusion...they provide us with the necessary consistency, coherence and vision'. [1, p. 27] *'... confrontation with one's existential situation reminds one that paradigms are self-created, wafer-thin barriers against the pain of uncertainty'* [2, p. 26].

Aim

To outline processes of clinical reasoning and complexity for advanced practitioners in mental health (APMH), enabling reflection on approaches to clinical assessment and planning care developed during core professional training and how this relates to clinical reasoning encountered in APMH practice. Thus, laying the foundation to thinking about complexity and more reflective clinical reasoning [3].

LEARNING OUTCOMES

After reading this chapter, the reader should be able to identify:

1. Where and how clinical reasoning sits within advanced practice and the influence of core professional and APMH training on the development of clinical reasoning.
2. The multifaceted nature of clinical reasoning including professional and patient contexts and the process of learning and applying clinical reasoning.

The Advanced Practitioner in Mental Health, First Edition. Edited by Clare Allabyrne.
© 2026 John Wiley & Sons Ltd. All rights reserved, including rights for text and data mining and training of artificial intelligence technologies or similar technologies. Published 2026 by John Wiley & Sons Ltd.

3. Basic and more sophisticated approaches to clinical reasoning and the cycle through the processes of learning and applying clinical reasoning.
4. Differences between complication and complexity and their applicability to clinical reasoning.
5. How to start integrating this learning into developing diagnostic formulations with patients.

MAPPING TO HEALTH EDUCATION ENGLAND ADVANCED PRACTICE MENTAL HEALTH CURRICULUM AND CAPABILITIES FRAMEWORK [4]

Aspects of clinical reasoning in mental health and their relationship to the HEE Advanced Practice Mental Health Curriculum and Capabilities Framework are mentioned in Table 5.1.

TABLE 5.1 Aspects of clinical reasoning in mental health and their relationship to the HEE Advanced Practice Mental Health Curriculum and Capabilities Framework.

Domain	
A1–A14	Effective clinical reasoning incorporates maximum information directly from the patient [5]
B 2,7 & 9	Recognising when capacity requires consideration [6]
B14 C1–4	Choosing appropriate assessments and investigations and making a shared formulation that recognises biopsychosocial [7] complexities [8]
D1–3, 7 & 8 D4–6 E1 & 7 F1	Formulation covers risk [9] and is a template for team intervention led by the APMH [10]
E 4–12	A critical part of clinical reasoning is identifying interventions, anticipating and evaluating their impact
F 2–8	APMH's clinical leadership role should promote development of colleagues' clinical reasoning and reflect on how service systems facilitate the process of clinical reasoning and the delivery of interventions

HOW THE CHAPTER ALIGNS TO THE FOUR PILLARS OF APMH [11]

Clinical Practice

Clinical reasoning is the heart of clinical practice and the rationale for all clinical interventions, where patient expertise is key but often unrecognised [5]. Becoming an advanced practitioner in mental health (APMH) is to step back and reflect on clinical reasoning, deepening it by analysing the process and broadening it by including assessments from other clinical approaches. This includes developing a more holistic approach, hearing the patient's voice, capturing risk and complexity, enabling better targeted more effective intervention.

Most advanced practice training in Europe and the United Kingdom [12] has focused on physical health and the extension of those skills rooted in core professional training. Their advanced practice training could be characterised as extending their knowledge upward like a well-rooted tree. However, APMH trainees are more heterogenous, while rooted in their core discipline, there is a grafting on of new shoots and extending laterally into other professional approaches. There are common processes in assessment across the core disciplines, but explicit teaching of clinical reasoning is not standard practice. An understanding of multidisciplinary assessment processes and where these and core professional assessment competencies sit within clinical reasoning is at the centre of the identity of the APMH.

Leadership and Management

Complexity and unpredictability are routine in clinical management [8]. Multidisciplinary team (MDT) approaches can both manage and exacerbate complexity [13]. Cross-speciality training for team leaders has been shown to reduce complexities generated from within MDTs [14]. The integrated clinical reasoning of APMH training creates a unique place in the mental health MDT, enabling insight into the assessment processes of colleagues from other professions and the creation of MDT-based formulations that reduce and address complexity, forming a clear vision of clinical leadership by APMHs.

Education

Professional role modelling is inherent in leadership enabling MDT's capacity to clinically reason together [10]. The APMH's core professional training includes distinct approaches to assessment, often with minimal conscious attention paid to the process of clinical reasoning. APMH training addresses this. Clinical education occurs both in lectures and in clinical practice where it utilises social learning [15]. This has demonstrated impact in developing both positive [16, 17] and negative [18] organisational traits. Importantly, this is where both leadership and education come together in the APMH role. The APMH's modelling of clinical reasoning includes not only the patient but also aspects of each part of the MDT contributing to an inclusive culture of well-coordinated intervention that respects and reflects the perspectives of each member of the MDT.

Research

The APMH is a discerning consumer of research, aware of how the evidence base not only can enhance clinical practice, identifying interventions that are effective, but can also restrict it through uncritical application [19]. Meta-analyses always reflect the exclusion criteria of the included trials. Exclusion criteria, while important in ensuring confounding and competing variables do not skew results, can also exclude groups encountered in clinical practice [20]. Additionally, randomised control trials (RCTs) cannot always detect differing outcomes between groups based on important demographics [21]. Hence, meta-analyses and RCTs can result in treatment algorithms that leave open the possibility of systemic discrimination [21]. An APMH does not simply follow a clinical algorithm. They bear in mind the risk group their patient comes from epidemiologically, possible exclusion criteria they may come under in trials and status of the evidence given their demographic group. The APMH needs the skills to navigate their way through this and apply adjustments to treatments in a thoughtful, transparent and auditable fashion [22].

As an APMH's practice develops, so does their knowledge of the gaps in the evidence base for different groups of patients. This knowledge and beginning to address it through small carefully targeted real-world research [23] was one of the Health Education England's (HEE) transition competencies from advanced to consultant practice [24].

CLINICAL REASONING

There are numerous definitions of clinical reasoning from discipline-specific concept analyses [25] to expert written definitions based on cross-discipline research such as:

> *'Clinical reasoning (or practice decision making) is a context dependent way of thinking and decision making in professional practice to guide practice actions. It involves the construction of narratives to make sense of the multiple factors and interests pertaining to the current reasoning task. It occurs within a set of problem spaces informed by the practitioner's unique frames of reference, workplace context and practice models, as well as by the patient's or client's contexts. It utilizes core dimensions of practice knowledge, reasoning and metacognition and draws on these capacities in others. Decision making within clinical reasoning occurs at micro, macro and meta levels and may be individually or collaboratively conducted. It involves meta skills of critical conversations, knowledge generation, practice model authenticity and reflexivity'* [26, p. 50].

This is a comprehensive definition based on a large body of research that can feel overwhelming. However, there are approaches to systematising areas of clinical reasoning from mnemonics to aid retention of factual information [27, 28]; through to guides to the process of learning clinical reasoning such as Krathwohl's [29] adaptation of Bloom's taxonomy [30] of knowledge when applied to clinical reasoning (Table 5.2). This demonstrates clinical reasoning's foundation on the factual and conceptual stages of clinical knowledge. Adding to and maintaining these is part of APMH training and continuing personal development. This develops into learning to apply these in practice in the procedural stage. Finally metacognition, that is thinking about thought processes in the moment or retrospectively considering what has been learnt and applied. The rest of this chapter focuses on making explicit how the factual, conceptual and procedural are used, with the aim of then enabling the APMH to engage in metacognition about their use of these processes, including identifying cognitive bias; both these cognitive processes are discussed in more detail in Chapter 6.

Dual Process Theory

In daily life and clinical practice, we encounter situations, make conclusions and reach decisions about actions to achieve outcomes. We wake up, conclude it is time to get up for work, decide coffee will help and fill and switch on the kettle to boil it. Such a string of inferences is a form of thinking, however fleeting. We go into this default mode in familiar situations. The default-mode network (DMN) in the brain, identified in the 1990s [31], is well-mapped. It is activated when we are not concentrating and deactivated when we need to analyse [31], and the salience network (SN) is triggered [32]. This is consistent with dual process theory (also known as System 1 and System 2 thinking) [31, 33] which is also discussed in Chapter 6 and with mindfulness [34].

TABLE 5.2 Bloom's cognitive taxonomy of learning as adapted to learning clinical reasoning adapted from Krathwohl [29].

Type of knowledge	Factual	Conceptual	Procedural	Metacognitive
Specifics to be known	• Terminology • Specific details • Elements	• Classifications • Categories • Principles • Generalisations • Theories • Models • Structures	• Subject-specific skills • Algorithms • Subject-specific techniques and methods • Criteria for determining when to use appropriate procedures	• Strategic knowledge • Cognitive tasks • Contextual and conditional knowledge • Self-knowledge
Example: working with depression	Core, cognitive, biological and psychotic symptoms of depression [31]	Differences between moderate and severe depression; biopsychosocial model of depression	NICE guidelines, use of PHQ-9, pharmacological and psychosocial interventions; integration of these and social approaches in one care plan Considering co-occurring diagnoses (PTSD, substance misuse) Considering issues of race, gender, sexuality and social class	Utilising personal experiences of low mood and personal adversity to enable empathy, while maintaining therapeutic boundaries Thinking about own internal representations of depression from experience of seeing multiple patients Considering what has worked and what has not worked with previous patients and similarities in presentation Reading source literature and research underlying guidelines and algorithms critically and applying this to clinical practice

Concrete Knowledge --
→ Abstract Knowledge

In System 1 thinking (DMN), a situation is recognised, identified as like the previous situations and acted on; this is pattern recognition [35]. In clinical reasoning, such patterns are often in the form of illness scripts [36] illustrated by typical presentations. These are consciously constructed mental representations of illnesses, developed with System 2 (SN) thinking, a conscious process in the mind of the clinician engaged in through the stages of learning acquired during academic and clinical experience [29].

Illness scripts consist of:

- Enabling conditions – risk factors for the condition.
- The actual pathology – the underlying cause of the condition.
- Signs/symptoms/investigation results – how is the condition identified.
- Treatment along with prognosis – treatments it will respond to and outcomes expected [37–39].

History-taking and examination hear the patient's script about symptoms (their experience) and fit this with the signs (clinician observations) into one of the clinician's illness scripts. This approach is used mostly in physical healthcare, but it has its place in APMH practice [40]. Core professional training develops scripts based on models that define the profession often about signs, symptoms and aspects such as social functioning and risk. APMH training provides the opportunity to develop further scripts based on the recognisable patterns of mental illness diagnoses (Table 5.3).

A diagnosis is an abstraction encapsulating the contents of the illness script. Terms like 'trauma', 'schizophrenia' or 'low mood' summarise collections of symptoms and signs [40, 41]. They are a shorthand to communicate what is believed to be happening to the patient and a guide to what should be done about it. In physical medicine most abstractions are uncontroversial – a fractured tibia can be obvious before an x-ray image; the presentation is mostly consistent.

In mental health this is more controversial. Two patients, one with auditory hallucinations and persistent persecutory delusions and the other with disorganised thinking and thought broadcasting, may both be diagnosed with schizophrenia. Two different presentations under the same diagnosis, fueling disputes about the causes of psychosis [42, 43].

In System 2 thinking, time is spent on analysing the interaction of the components of the situation, before choosing actions. While an APMH is building, editing and thinking about their illness scripts, they are engaging in System 2 (SN) thinking, and when they start applying illness scripts intuitively, they are applying System 1 thinking [35] (DNM).

In emergency situations where life is at risk, a well-trained and developed System 1 response is often preferable and a conscious choice [44]. Engaging in more System 2 thinking allows the refinement and development of illness scripts, while both System 1 and System 2 thinking are prone to error and cognitive bias, System 2 may maintain awareness of and reflection on this.

Cognitive load can impair System 2 thinking [45]. We store large amounts of information in our long-term memory in recognisable patterns like illness scripts. But working memory holds only 5–9 items and analyses only 2–4 at a time [45]. Information from working memory is temporary, either being renewed or stored in the long-term memory via linkage to information already stored [45] such as illness scripts. APMHs build a large reserve in their long-term memory, but each new assessment is a learning process, acquiring new patient-based information. The complexity of the new subject being learnt (the patient) is the *intrinsic* cognitive load, distractions from the environment are the *external* cognitive load and the complexity of processing or formulating is the *germane* cognitive load [45].

When the patient's presentation is complex (intrinsic), and circumstances do not allow space and time to fully assess (external) and formulate properly (germane), the best System 1 generated care and treatment is the default option.

TABLE 5.3 An example of an illness script for schizophrenia.

Enabling conditions:	Actual pathology:

Who (risk factors)?
 • Genetic vulnerability – first-degree relatives
 • Neurodevelopmental difficulties – motor skills, memory, attention and language. Neurocognitive decline leading up to the first episode
 • Birth complications (gestational diabetes, pre-eclampsia, emergency caesarean)
 • Early trauma (physical, sexual, emotional, neglect)
 • Gender/age – women in later life
 • Part of an immigrant community
 • Refugee
 • Raised in a city environment
 When (risk times)?
 • Stress vulnerability model
 • Substance misuse
 Symptoms and signs:
 What?
 Positive symptoms:
 • Hallucinations
 • Visual
 • Auditory
    ◦ Command
    ◦ Commentary
    ◦ Discussion
 • Somatic
 • Gustatory
 • Olfactory
 • Delusions
 • Beliefs
 • Thoughts
    ◦ Broadcast
    ◦ Insertion
    ◦ Withdrawal
 • Disorganised thoughts, neologisms, tangentiality, derailment
 Negative symptoms:
 • Flatness of affect
 • Incongruent emotion
 • Withdrawn
	Why?
	 Multiple biopsychosocial theories
	 Dopamine theory – very contested
	 Other possible pathologies:
	 • Endocrine – hypo/hyper thyroid, Cushing's, adrenal tumour
	 • Metabolic – porphyria, Niemann-Pick
	 • Autoimmune – lupus, thyroiditis, limbic encephalitis
	 • Infectious – cerebral malaria, toxoplasmosis, HIV, neurosyphilis, encephalitis
	 • Neuro – epilepsy, brain tumour, TIA, head injury, MS, Wilson's, Huntington's, Tay-Sachs
	 • Nutrition – Vit B1 and B12 deficient
	 • Cognitive – dementia or delirium
	 • Affective – bipolar, depression
	 Treatment:
	 • Early intervention psychosocial
	 • CBT for psychosis
	 • Family work on expressed emotion
	 • Antipsychotic medication
	 Investigations
	 Bloods – FBCs, U&Es, thyroid, CRP, LFTs
	 Tests and examinations – mental state examination, MoCA
	 Rule outs (see other pathologies above) PTSD, severe social anxiety, alcoholism, hallucinogen abuse
	 Red flags
	 Suicidal ideation
	     Passive
	     Active
	     Plan
	 Previous suicide attempts
	 Access to lethal means
	 Self-harm (frequency, duration, severity)
	 Command hallucinations – about who and to do what?

> **Reflection point:**
>
> Looking at Table 5.3:
> How useful is it?
> What else would you need in terms of knowledge if you were working with someone with schizophrenia?
> What illness scripts or pattern recognition were you taught in your core professional training?
> Using the headings:
>
> 1. Enabling conditions
> 2. Actual pathology
> 3. Signs/symptoms/investigation results
> 4. Final treatment along with prognosis
>
> Can you write an illness script for any of the following conditions: PTSD, anorexia or depression. How useful is this? What does it leave out?

Basic Moves in Clinical Reasoning

The space to formulate properly allows System 2 thinking. Applying factual and conceptual knowledge [29] in clinical reasoning can be seen as a procedure with three types of inference: deductive, inductive and abductive. How these interact becomes clear as clinical reasoning is explored more deeply with associated metacognition about personal practice.

The examples used in this section and summarised in Table 5.4a and 5.4b are intentionally simplistic and intended, to some extent, to mimic the reasoning of a student clinician who is just beginning to develop into the procedural stage of Krathwohl's [29] clinical adaptation of Bloom's taxonomy. They are intended as illustrations rather than actual examples of clinical reasoning.

In Table 5.4a the example is of a patient who presents as hypervigilant and easily startled following a car accident, and a family member is concerned they might have post-traumatic stress disorder (PTSD).

In Table 5.4b there is an example of a patient who presents in clinic with a body mass index (BMI) <18.5 with a family member concerned that this may be due to anorexia. This example demonstrates how deductive reasoning can lose its way. However, the deductive reasoning though faulty reaches a conclusion that is supported by inductive and abductive reasoning.

Deductive Reasoning

Deductive arguments have two basic forms either *affirming the antecedent* or *denying the consequent* [46]. These are simpler than they sound.

Affirming the antecedent structure:

1. If A, then B
2. A
3. Therefore, B

TABLE 5.4a Comparison between the different types of approaches in clinical reasoning.

Deductive: Affirming the antecedent	Deductive: Denying the consequent	Inductive	Abductive
Major premise: If patient had a traumatic event *and* is re-experiencing this, *then* they have post-traumatic stress disorder (according to ICD-11).	**Major premise:** If the trauma only happened a week ago, *then* it is too early to say if this is PTSD and could be an acute stress reaction.	**Major premise:** Many people who have had a traumatic experience and have a history of anxiety disorder will develop PTSD.	**Observation:** This person had a traumatic experience and is re-experiencing it.
Minor premise/observation: This patient had a traumatic experience *and* is re-experiencing this.	**Minor premise/observation:** The trauma happened 28 days ago.	**Minor premise/observation:** This patient had a traumatic experience and has a history of anxiety disorder.	**Conclusion:** This patient probably has PTSD.
Conclusion: Therefore, this patient has post-traumatic stress disorder (according to ICD-11).	**Conclusion:** Therefore, the re-experiencing is not due to acute stress reaction.	**Conclusion:** Therefore, this patient probably has PTSD.	**Explanation:** Because PTSD is the best explanation for re-experiencing after trauma. Especially, given the deductive rule outs and the inductively known risk factors.

TABLE 5.4b How a logical fallacy can appear valid in clinical reasoning when other approaches support the conclusion.

Deductive: Affirming the antecedent	Deductive: Denying the consequent	Inductive	Abductive
Major (False) premise: If the person has a BMI less than 18.5 and a fear of weight gain, *then* they have anorexia (according to ICD-11).	**Major premise:** If there is a thyroid-stimulating hormone (TSH) level higher than 4.0 mU/L, *then* the BMI less than 18.5 is due to hyperthyroidism.	**Major premise:** Most people with a BMI <18.5 and a fear of weight gain have anorexia.	**Observation:** This person has a BMI under 18.5 and has a fear of weight gain.
Minor premise/observation: This patient has a BMI less than 18.5 and a fear of weight gain.	**Minor premise/observation:** The TSH is not higher than 4.0 mU/L.	**Minor premise/observation:** This patient has a BMI <18.5 and a fear of weight gain.	**Conclusion:** This patient probably has anorexia.
Conclusion: Therefore, this patient has anorexia.	**Conclusion:** Therefore, the BMI <18.5 is not due to hyperthyroidism.	**Conclusion:** Therefore, this patient probably has anorexia.	**Explanation:** Because anorexia is the best explanation for the conjunction of a BMI below 18.5 and a fear of putting on weight. Especially, given the deductive rule outs and the inductively known risk factors.

For our patient in Table 5.4a who may have PTSD, the deductive reasoning may look like this:

1. *If* they had a traumatic event *and* are re-experiencing this, *then* they have PTSD.
2. This patient had a traumatic event *and* is re-experiencing this.
3. Therefore, this patient has PTSD.

It is occasionally this simple in physical healthcare but rarely in mental health. While the diagnosis of PTSD may be correct, it is never this straightforward. It is arguable that the term *PTSD* is just shorthand for re-experiencing after a traumatic event, making the two features so close in meaning that they add no new or usable knowledge to the situation.

Advocates of deductive reasoning argue it provides a testable theory that can be shown to be wrong. One way of doing this is use of *denying the consequent*, a move useful in sorting differential diagnoses.

Denying the consequent is structured as follows:

1. If A, then B
2. Not B
3. Therefore, not A

This is used to exclude differential diagnoses. Using the PTSD example, the possibility of acute stress reaction would be ruled out as follows:

1. *If* the trauma happened only a week ago, *then* it is too early to say if this is PTSD. It could be an acute stress reaction.
2. The trauma happened 28 days ago.
3. Therefore, the re-experiencing is not due to acute stress reaction.

This is simplified, and there are several possible differentials to rule out before a diagnosis of PTSD can be made.

Caution with Deductive Reasoning

A warning comes with deductive reasoning, as it can be used to make false arguments sound perfectly logical. These are known as fallacies. The examples in Table 5.4 are syllogisms, a form of reasoning in which a conclusion is drawn from two given or assumed propositions:

1. Major premise (rule, if. . .then)
2. Minor premise (observation)
3. Conclusion/consequent

If the major and minor premises are true, then the conclusion is the only one that can be drawn. There are syllogisms that can look logical and have plausible major and minor premises as well as a true conclusion; but though the conclusion looks as if it follows, it does not. For example, in a patient presenting with possible anorexia 'affirming the antecedent' *could look like this*:

1. *If* the person has a BMI <18.5 and a fear of weight gain, *then* they have anorexia (according to ICD-11).

2. This patient has a BMI <18.5 and a fear of weight gain.
3. Therefore, this patient has anorexia.

However, they could be malnourished and concerned about re-feeding syndrome [47]. This is the fallacy of 'false premise', one of many used in convincing arguments about clinical problems to know and be wary of [46]. For the APMH recognising these moves in their own clinical reasoning, that of colleagues and an awareness of their uses and limitations is foundational to clinical reasoning.

Inductive Reasoning

While deductive reasoning starts from a general theory and ends in an observation; inductive reasoning runs in the opposite direction [46], starting from a series of observations and ending in a specific hypothesis about one case. The moves in inductive reasoning are:

1. Most A's are B.
2. This is an A.
3. Therefore, this is probably a B.

The conclusion does not logically follow from the premises, but there is support for the conclusion, crucially based on a series of previous observations.

So, staying with our anorexia example while the deductive syllogism may be based on a false premise, the inductive syllogism as follows may be correct:

1. Most people with a BMI <18.5 and a fear of weight gain have anorexia.
2. This patient has a BMI <18.5 and a fear of weight gain.
3. Therefore, this patient probably has anorexia.

However, if the APMH knows extra information about the patient and their circumstances, they may reasonably use this in their assessment. For instance, if the patient has hyperthyroidism, this may rule out anorexia unless the patient values it for its weight-limiting effects.

The validity of inductive inferences relies on the quality of the previous observations. Personal experience of previous cases can also generate cognitive bias and is not the same as a series of carefully designed cohort studies establishing risk factors.

Risk Factors for Depression: An Example for Inductive Reasoning

A recent umbrella review of depression [48] synthesised the findings of 134 meta-analyses finding 108 associations between biopsychosocial factors and depression. When the papers were whittled down to high-quality prospective studies, the number of risk factors dropped to six variables:

- Widowhood
- Childhood physical abuse
- Four to five metabolic factors
- Sexual dysfunction
- Job strain

An example of how easy it is to find associations and the rigour needed to identify real risk factors.

Relying solely on the risk factors in illness scripts is a part of pattern recognition, APMHs working with a specific under researched population may lead to them being aware of risk factors yet to be identified within the research base. Only well carried out epidemiological research will establish whether this is an insight or a cognitive bias. Carefully judging the results of research that identify risk factors and applying them is the beginning of critical thinking about the evidence base and its gaps.

In earlier parts Kohler et al's [48] data exclusion process meant other risk factors for depression were relegated as the studies they came from were less stringent. These were being:

- A Gulf War veteran
- The victim of intimate partner violence if female
- The victim of childhood emotional and sexual abuse
- Diagnosed with psoriasis
- Being diagnosed with Sjogren's syndrome (an autoimmune condition affecting the body's production of fluid such as saliva and tears)

When faced with a patient with low mood considering the presence of these risk factors in history taking is relevant.

Abductive Reasoning

Deductive and inductive reasoning give clear pathways from major premises to observations and conclusions; clinical reasoning is rarely this straightforward. Abductive reasoning starts from an unexplained observation and tries to find a major premise that best explains as much as possible of what is observed [41]. Returning to the anorexia patient an abductive approach might be as follows:

1. **Observation:** This person has a BMI <18.5 and has a fear of weight gain.
2. **Conclusion:** This patient probably has anorexia.
3. **Explanation:** Because anorexia is the best explanation for the conjunction of a BMI below 18.5 and a fear of putting on weight. Especially given the deductive rule outs and the inductively known risk factors.

Hence, abductive reasoning is often known as inference to best explanation [49]. It can be argued that deductive and inductive reasoning are moves in an overall abductive argument, or that abductive reasoning is all that is left when deductive and inductive approaches have run their course without a clear conclusion.

This can feel vague in comparison to deductive and inductive reasoning, but much in life and clinical mental health practice can only be explained this way. When we see a patient responding to hallucinations, there are theories about causes we use to make deductions from [42, 43, 50] and many observational studies we use to identify risk factors, making inductive inferences [51, 52]; but only through abductive reasoning can we conclude whether the behaviour of the patient (signs) and their own report (symptoms) are indicative of hallucinations.

There are times when abductively arrived at conclusions are presented as deductive, to make the conclusion appear more certain than it is. This is not clinical reasoning but persuasion and is often when fallacy syllogisms such as 'false premise' are used. Spotting and challenging this may lead to honesty about how the conclusion was reached, which is positive. But it might not change the conclusion unless a better alternative abductive argument can be made. How to choose between alternative abductive arguments is challenging, and alternative views may depend on differing theoretical viewpoints or paradigms [53] that are not easily resolved. Cognitive bias may also influence choices between explanations.

Deduction, Induction and Abduction: The Cycle of Clinical Reasoning

Whether arrived at deductively, inductively or abductively (or by all these), eventually a conclusion is drawn that guides intervention. So far deductive, inductive and abductive reasoning have been discussed only in relation to diagnosis. But for all clinicians in both mental and physical health, the definition of clinical reasoning at the beginning of this section is a reminder that it includes decision-making in professional practice to guide practice actions [26]. Diagnosis is useful to illustrate the thinking processes, but as in clinical practice, it is also only a beginning point. In addition from inference to best explanation, the APMH has to make an inference to the safest and most effective intervention.

This is in effect a testable theory which predicts a desired outcome from an intervention. A deductive inference is being proposed, but instead of looking backwards to explain a presentation, it is being made forwards to predict the effect of an intervention. If this works, then the conclusion is supported, and if not or not as well as anticipated, then there will be a return to the process of clinical reasoning and other differential diagnoses or alternative formulations that could be considered. This makes every treatment intervention a pragmatic trial of treatment. It is often the only way to choose between abductively reached conclusions.

This assumes only one intervention when pharmacological, psychological and social interventions are often blended. Designing interventions with clarity about the outcomes, how and why each intervention contributes and what constitutes success are essential parts of the rigour of clinical reasoning. This is founded on the rigour and clarity of the diagnostic/formulation process.

Learning Clinical Reasoning: From System 2 Thinking to System 1 Thinking

The process of learning to clinically reason starts with taking the knowledge learned in non-clinical environments and applying it under the guidance of clinical mentors [41]. The learner then actively engages in System 2 thinking to make sense of what they observe and reflects on this with their clinical mentor. From this use of deductive, inductive and abductive reasoning, the clinician develops their illness scripts. These include 'Other Possible Pathologies' to be ruled out by 'denying the consequent' and inductively established 'Risk Factors' (see Table 5.3) indicating a raised probability of the condition.

While there are times when illness scripts can be used to plan based on symptoms and signs and pattern recognition, there are other times when risk factors and rule outs are sorted and searched through to find and establish a diagnosis. When this happens, they are being used to find the best explanation for the clinical observations and so are reasoning abductively. This could be argued to represent a transitional moment between System 1 and System 2 thinking.

The Role and Place of Formulation

Diagnoses are abstractions encapsulating the contents of illness scripts. Terms like, trauma, schizophrenia or low mood, summarise collections of symptoms and signs [40, 41]. This approach is subject to criticism, arguing that psychiatric diagnoses suggest a spurious level of scientific accuracy [42, 43], fail to take account of the context of the patient's life, cause stigma and denude the patient of the meaning they make of their experiences. Johnstone [54] and Vertue and Haig [55] propose formulation as the alternative. This is an agreement about causes and more pertinently 'maintainers' [56, p. 174] of mental health problems, constructed by patient and therapist effectively joining together in System 2 thinking. Vertue and Haig [55] convincingly argue case formulation is a process of making a chain of abductive inferences with the patient about their problems; they also claim abductive inference and case formulation as exclusive methods of psychological therapy. However, abductive inference is used in physical healthcare [26, 57–59], and both deductive and inductive reasoning also have their place in psychological therapy [40].

Formulation is not just confined to psychology; psychiatrists [60], nurses [61] and occupational therapists [62] have long used formulation models to explain presentations and collaboratively plan and deliver interventions. Every formulation is based on a theory [42, 43, 54, 61] which is part of a network of theories that have a number of fundamental principles about the world in common otherwise known as a paradigm [53]. Inevitably these generate their own abstractions as shorthand for the complex ideas being communicated. Johnstone's [54] approach is trauma based; trauma is an abstraction, used in differing but overlapping ways by both psychiatrists and psychologists [63]. The APMH when using abstractions as either diagnostic or formulatory terms should reflect on how they would explain such a term to a patient.

Nonetheless, abductive reasoning leaves more space for patient participation in making meaning and finding explanation. Hence, it is well suited to case formulation approaches, upon which inferences to best and safest treatment can be made.

Cause and Explanation: Post-traumatic Stress Disorder (PTSD)

The APMH engaging in System 2 Thinking about the patient in Table 5.4a who might have PTSD may go through a series of deductive 'denying the consequent' moves to rule out other differentials [64]. Given the diagnostic criteria, uncomplex trauma can be a more straightforward diagnosis to make, despite debates about what is classified as a traumatic event [65]. The APMH may also look for risk factors that provide inductive support for a diagnosis [66, 67].

They will then engage in a series of decisions, each abductively reached by inferring to best explanation [49]. In doing so, they will often base their decisions on a number of theories or paradigms [53], each one of which they believe provides the best explanation for each aspect of the patient's presentation and for why they think a given intervention will work. The reality is that there are usually a number of competing paradigms, hence a biopsychosocial [7] approach, which is described in detail in Chapter 3. Since Engel [7] first developed this approach, it has attracted supporters [68], critics and counter critics [68–70]. I would argue that this debate has obscured the more fundamental challenge of defining 'explanation' or the unavoidable deeper debate about the definition of 'cause' in clinical reasoning. This fundamental debate will not be resolved here, but having some understanding of these debates enables the APMH to deepen their reflection and metacognition on clinical reasoning.

Cause, described as the cement of the universe [71], is woven into life's daily patterns and regularities guiding our actions. Yet it is elusive, usually referring to an observed regularity, that can be described, even quantified but without ultimate explanation. Snooker balls colliding regularly and reliably lead to the first ball stopping and the second ball moving [72] as described by Newton's third law [73], a fundamental principle in engineering and science. Though described as a law, the support for it is through inductive reasoning; albeit about the strongest inductive support possible, despite exceptions [74]. This strongly supported regularity and predictability of Newton's third law means it is relied on as an explanation with the cause of the movement of the second snooker ball attributed to the first snooker ball.

However, as with many fundamental principles, how it explains or attributes cause is debated. Whether as down to a divine being, a construct that accounts (abductive) for numerous observations (inductive) or just a principle so fundamental that it has no further explanation [75]. A challenge to such a fundamental principle can lead to a major change in how we explain the world, known as a paradigm shift [53].

The point of this for the APMH is that there is more than one paradigm in mental health assessment that can guide assessment and hence the biopsychosocial approach [7]. An understanding of the issues around cause and explanation can enable a better understanding of how each paradigm sees the clinical problem and the contribution it makes to guiding treatment and recovery.

Continuing with the example of PTSD, the relationship between bio-psycho-social factors can be seen and their relationship with cause, explanation and inference to best explanation and intervention illustrated. It must be pointed out that as with all examples in this chapter, much has been simplified and explained only in the most basic of terms to enable illustration. Experts in PTSD will no doubt have views on details missed in this most basic of outlines.

In the biological part of a biopsychosocial approach, PTSD has identified neurological pathways in the amygdala [76] and hippocampus [77] down to the level of neurons and their electro-chemical mechanisms [76], moving in waves move down neurons due to changes in the charges of atoms, determined by imbalances between electrons and protons in the atoms [78]. These predictable regularities are described using terms like 'strong attraction' and 'action potential', yet the root causes are debated by physicists [79] in terms of the arrangement of sub-atomic particles called 'quarks' [80]. This approach to cause, known as reductionism, proposes that all ultimate causes are physical, and as understanding descends to lower levels of cause, it is both simpler and more potent [8]. This is reflected in the structure of introductory medical textbooks organised from atoms to cells to organs to systems [78]. However, this paradigm has not led to consistently effective pharmacotherapy for PTSD [81] yet. The key to addressing PTSD has come from approaches that bridge the biological to the psychological.

Early psychological interventions in PTSD by pioneers of cognitive behavioural therapy (CBT) [82] were based on a number of potential theories about how traumatic memories were stored and processed [83]. Brewin [84] focused initially on how memories are experienced by a traumatised person, identifying verbally accessible memories (VAMs) of trauma as the aspects of the experience the person can access in a controlled way and situationally accessible memories (SAMs) which are experienced as flashbacks. This initially informed cognitive behavioural intervention in PTSD [83]. Later the VAMs were reconceptualised as contextualised representations or C-Reps and SAMs as sensation near representations or S-Reps. The key to this was linking C-Reps and S-Reps to neural pathways in the brain; C-Reps via the ventral visual pathway to the temporal lobe and S-Reps via the dorsal visual pathway via the amygdala, potentially accounting for the role of S-Reps in flashbacks [84]. The empirical evidence to support this is developing [77].

It is notable that VAMs and SAMs were developed through clinical observation with theories about the neurological correlates and proved useful in cognitive behavioural approaches [84, 85]. It was later that the neurological connection began to emerge via C-Reps and S-Reps. What is already a complicated subject can be made more complicated when the discovery of new knowledge is not linear but more of a mosaic with the true picture still only emerging.

> **Reflection point:**
>
> If the dorsal visual pathway via the amygdala 'accounts' for S-Reps and flashbacks in PTSD – how does it explain them?
>
> Can this be a cause of PTSD?
>
> If the empirical evidence to support S-Reps and flashbacks is developing – does this make it an inductively or deductively reached conclusion.
>
> Is the following syllogism a deductively valid argument or a fallacy?
>
> 1. If there is ventral visual activation through the amygdala, then the person has PTSD.
> 2. There is ventral visual activation through the amygdala.
> 3. Therefore, this person has PTSD.

This leaves the social part of the biopsychosocial approach to PTSD. Primarily of course an awareness of the impact of PTSD on personal and social function and the impact of this on the patient's quality of life, and their risk to themselves or from or to others. But there is also the need for an interpersonal connection to be able to address and ameliorate the experience of PTSD.

During the process of developing theories about the processes involved in PTSD, researchers in CBT were also making an early impact on the symptoms of PTSD through face-to-face therapy [82]. Over time the approach moved from exposure therapy [86] through cognitive re-processing [87] to integration of these approaches to cognitive behavioural approaches that encourage emotional re-processing [88, 89] and on to third-wave approaches [90].

Figure 5.1, for all its omissions, shows the outline of a hierarchy of the biopsychosocial model in PTSD. The cause is external to this hierarchy; the traumatic event could be biological (cancer or a natural disaster) or psychosocial (interpersonal violence or humiliation). The reality is that most traumas will be a mixture.

The problem is that Figure 5.1 is itself a simplistic abstraction of an infinitely complex process, that is as likely to start from the formulation.

One approach to pinning down cause is the idea of necessity. The traumatic event is to PTSD what the first snooker ball is to the second snooker ball in the illustration near the beginning of this section. The relationship though is not like that between a BMI <18.5 and anorexia in the earlier examples. Having a BMI <18.5 is not a cause of anorexia.

One explanation is in knowing the regularities in the process from cause to effect, often called 'understanding'. The point for the APMH is that knowing the regularities between cause and effect hopefully allows for more effective System 2 Thinking and fuller more informed formulation, specifically knowing where in the chain of regularities between cause and effect to intervene.

Identifying where the most effective intervention point in the chain is a major reason for the success of CBT. In CBT formulation, the cause is relevant, but the maintainer of the problem is at the heart of the formulation [56] and the starting point for intervention. This is in contrast to insight-based approaches where the formulation can be the end point of therapy [91] cited in [92].

Even when simplified the PTSD example is complicated, but it lends itself to being used as an illustration as many other common presentations in mental health have highly disputed theories about causal pathways such as depression [93, 94] and psychosis [43, 95], making the kinds of reasoning outlined here even more challenging.

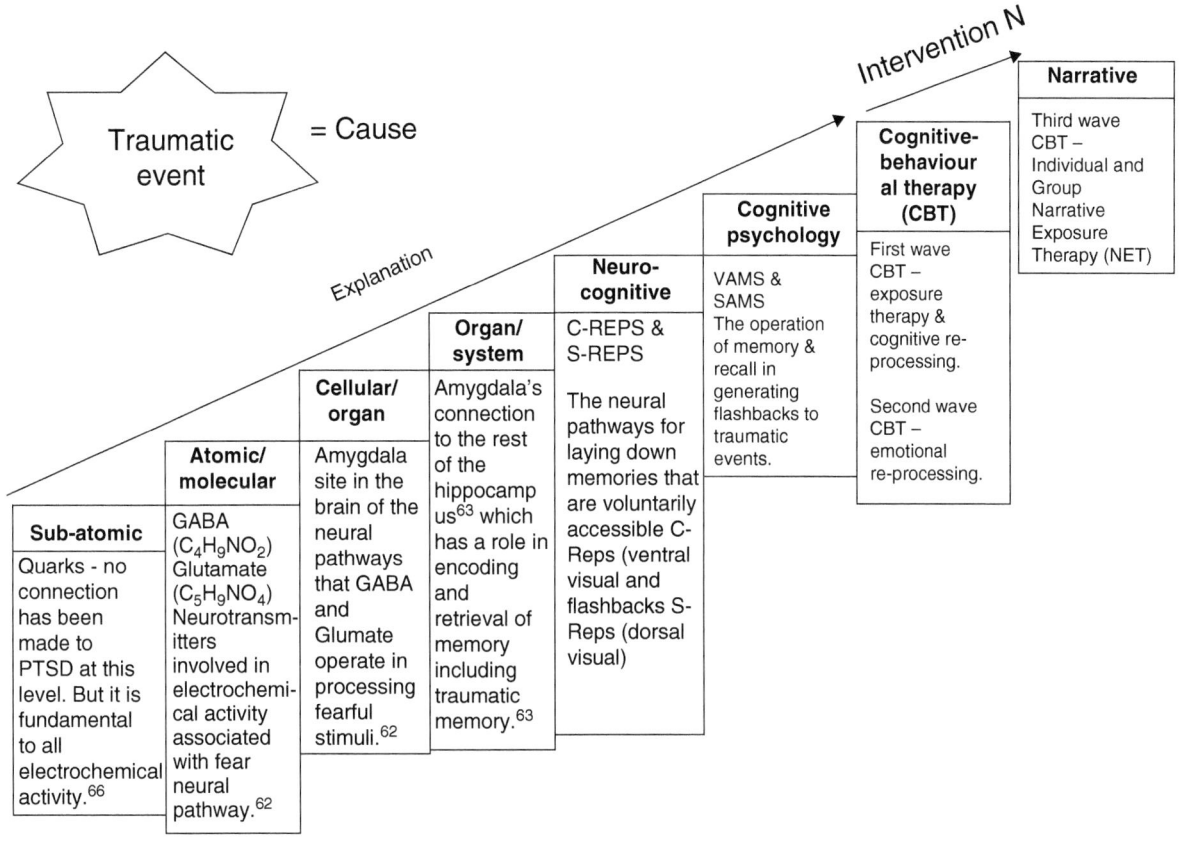

FIGURE 5.1 A biopsychosocial illustration of cause, explanation and intervention in PTSD.

A Note on Metacognition: From System 1 Thinking Back to System 2 Thinking

Many clinical situations, especially in mental health settings, present with such levels of complexity that the usefulness of illness scripts is limited. This is when the APMH stands back, thinking about their thinking in the given situation, consciously dropping illness scripts, reverting to System 2 thinking and trying to make sense of the situation. This can feel vulnerable, and there is evidence at least in physical healthcare that some experienced clinicians continue to search their illness scripts just with more vigour, while less-experienced clinicians find it easier to revert to System 2 thinking [41]. While a large reserve of comprehensive and sophisticated illness scripts is part of the equipment of the effective clinical reasoner, being too reliant on or committed to them can make an inflexible clinical reasoner. Regular practice at stepping outside of illness scripts is preparation for situations when the usefulness of the illness script runs out.

As all illness, mental or physical occurs within the context of the patient's life, they are the person best placed to understand their complex situation, even if the knowledge to achieve this is only implicit at first. Case formulation developed empathically is the most effective abductive approach to arriving at a mutual understanding between patient and clinician. In a cognitive behavioural formulation, for instance, it is the patient's rules that are discerned (if...then) through Socratic questioning, once made explicit and shared between therapist and patient a series of deductions can be made that make sense of the patient's presentation [56].

Using this kind of abductive reasoning with patients to form chains of inferences to explain complexity should be informed by some basic understanding of the nature of complexity.

Complication and Complexity

Complication

A system is one part of the world with a boundary around it that has some form of internal mechanism, for instance a wind-up wristwatch. These can be increasingly complicated dependent on how many parts there are; a jet engine is more complicated still. Both are determinate, when there is a problem, there is also an equation underlying the system that guides tracking the problem down.

Complication in terms of the number of parts there are to a potential problem is an important part of an APMH's daily practice. Where to limit scope or boundary of an assessment, detail and amount of information within that boundary is a daily challenge for an APMH. A recent causal mapping exercise of risk pathways to suicide by Giabbenelli et al. [96] found 361 points of information to consider.

Complexity

The complexity of a system determines how its parts interact. The interaction of cogs is predictable, whereas the interaction of the parts of complex systems less so. Molecules, cells, organs, people, communities, IT systems and power grids, all respond to both internal (self-organising) and external changes (perturbations) interacting with and responding to each other (interdependence). This leads to unpredictable outcomes (emergence) which are more than the sum of their parts (irreducible). Two complex interdependent systems can 'co-evolve' in response to a perturbation, effectively becoming sub-systems of a larger system. Hence, complex systems are further differentiated from complicated ones by looser boundaries. These responses and outcomes are often the result of long causal chains. So, change in a complex system can be a response to both the system's history and its environment [97, 98].

While it is difficult to identify clear goals for complex systems, they all respond to maintain internal balance and stability known as stasis [98] or homeostasis when referring to a functioning body [78]. Hence, 'self-organising' is the first noted aspect of a complex system. There are times when it is unable to achieve this (dissipative) due to an internal response or a perturbation that destabilises it. This can settle after a reorganisation of the system emerges (adaptation). Sometimes the change needed in response to the instability is too rapid, and the existence of the system is threatened (self-organised criticality) [98]. For example, people are complex systems with consciousness and intentional behaviours (self-organised). They form many kinds of relationships (interdependence and the basis of a wider system of community). If a person suffers PTSD (perturbation), they may self-medicate with alcohol and become addicted (emergence); if the trauma is across their community ('perturbation' of a wider complex system), interpersonal aggression may arise due to raised levels of arousal and a wider substance misuse problem (both emergent and irreducible). A local healthcare system may need to develop a new skill set to deal with this issue; this co-evolvement enables a further system to bring the dissipative community system and the people in it back into stasis.

It is worth reflecting that the 361 points in the Giabbenelli et al. [96] study mentioned previously noted 946 significant interactions between points that led to increased risk of suicide. In the example of PTSD illustrated in Figure 5.1 moving from PTSD to complex PTSD would double the number of factors involved to consider from 3 to 6 [99], changing the number of combinations of factors from 7 to 720. A clear illustration of the difference between the complicated and the complex.

For APMH's exploring clinical reasoning, complicated systems can be represented by some external model that allows some level of prediction, such as an illness that can be summarised by an abstraction diagnosis. However, moving from complication to complexity, because either:

- the systems within the patient are interacting in an unpredictable way – for instance the patient with stable schizophrenia on insulin who is now on steroids to reduce inflammation secondary to meningitis or;
- their psychosocial context – for instance the depressed patient, experiencing domestic abuse, resorting to illicit drugs and alcohol to cope and in turn committing crime to fund this, while looking after their children or;
- both above – for instance the teenage patient with complex PTSD who self-harms and lives a chaotic lifestyle and is diagnosed with breast cancer requiring surgery, radiotherapy and chemotherapy and then long-term maintenance on tamoxifen which has mood swings and depression as a side effect.

In these circumstances, while illness scripts have their place it is very limited, and the levels of System 2 thinking and the sophistication of the abductive approach needed go beyond psychological case formulation requiring very active patient engagement placing them, if possible, at the centre of multidisciplinary decision-making.

This starts with the patient's presentation, clinicians may instinctively make System 1 inferences to an abstraction/diagnosis via an illness script on history taking and examination. Part of metacognition is to recognise this and if necessary, put it to one side to engage in System 2 approaches. This is also a key strategy in avoiding cognitive bias. However, before going straight to an abductive approach, the process of creating and ruling out differentials (deductive reasoning using 'denying the consequent') and considering what risk factors the patient has (applying inductive reasoning) brings a focus to the assessment and allows what can be known with some objective proof to be identified.

Part of going beyond the illness script is to note that the risk factors being considered are not those connected to one diagnosis. Part of the metacognitive process is retaining the list of risk factors but detaching them from the illness scripts; one way of approaching this is for the APMH to consider themselves as working on a new, as yet unnamed illness script.

Reflection point:

Think about the simplest and least challenging patient you have ever worked with.

- What complications were there?
- Why was it easy for you to deal with this?
- What complications could have arisen but didn't?

Now think about the most complex and challenging case you have ever worked with:

- Try to list the complexities?
- Try to draw a diagram with each complexity on it and lines between them showing the relationships?
- How does it look?

> Rating your easiest case as = 0 and your most complex as = 10:
>
> - Think of a case that = 5 on this scale.
> - What would change with this case to decrease or increase its score?

Diagnostic Formulation; The Application of Abductive Reasoning to Complexity

Diagnostic Formulation

Starting from the left in Figure 5.2, many clinicians intuitively identify potential abstractions from illness scripts that fit the initial information about the patient yielding some initial diagnoses, hopefully more than one to avoid cognitive bias and allow a process of sorting diagnoses. These go through the sieve of deductively reached rule outs (denying the consequent) and inductively identified risk factors. A single diagnosis is rarely identified; choices may need to be made abductively; contextual information developing a formulation informs this process. It allows the patient's voice to be heard and for them to make sense of their experience. The formulation in Figure 5.2 is cognitive behavioural, but any other theoretical approach could be placed here.

Once abstraction has been acknowledged, a proper set of differentials has been established using signs, symptoms and risk factors, there will be a final (hopefully short) list of differentials. The abductive approach in physical medicine might be to then chose whichever diagnosis appears to explain most of the signs and symptoms and treat it. If this does not work, then treatment of the diagnosis with the next best explanation may be tried; alternatively, the co-existence of differential diagnoses may be considered. A move also open to APMHs, for instance depression with psychotic features, may also be post-psychotic depression. But the other option open to the APMH is to explore further how the signs and symptoms

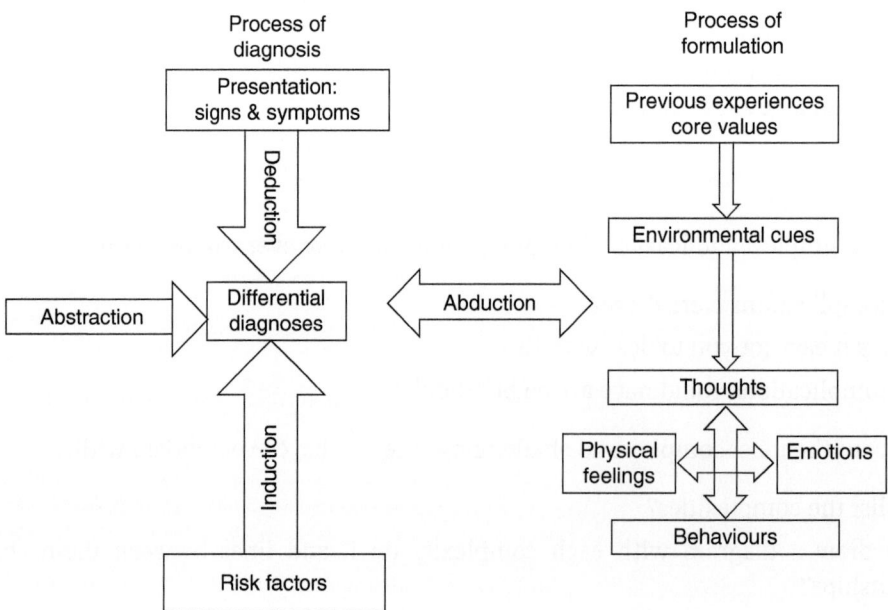

FIGURE 5.2 The relationships between the processes in this chapter.

relate to each other in the daily life of the patient and how they relate to historical risk factors. This is the beginning of a formulation which also adds the value of bringing into awareness the impact of the problem on the patient.

CONCLUSION

Clinical reasoning is the heart of clinical practice, from which the four pillars of APMH grow. The APMH training fosters reflection by being explicit about the process and by introducing multidisciplinary approaches. Learning clinical reasoning is a Type 2 (conscious) thinking activity initially teaching illness scripts. These reflect the theoretical foundation of core disciplines, generating their own abstractions. When the same term is used for two abstractions from different theories, confusion ensues. As experience develops, more patterns are recognised and Type 1 thinking (intuitive) develops. The presentation of a complex patient triggers reflection. One approach is to keep searching the illness scripts for a solution; another is to re-engage System 2 thinking, potentially leading to a new illness script.

Understanding clinical reasoning by moving from deductive reasoning, through inductive reasoning to abductive reasoning is the map, but the map is not the territory. This orderly progression is not reflected in clinical practice. Dealing with clinical complexity requires flexibility in moving between reasoning approaches. As every patient brings their own unique complexity, the learning process of clinical reasoning never stops. The three approaches could be argued to represent three points on a scale (deductive, inductive, abductive) moving from more to less certainty but also from less to more meaning.

REFERENCES

1. Dumont, F. (1993). Inferential heuristics in clinical problem formulation: selective review of their strengths and weaknesses. *Professional Psychology: Research and Practice* 24 (2): 196–205.
2. Yalom, I.D. (1980). *Existential Psychotherapy*. Basic Books.
3. Parkinson, S., Shenfield, M., Reece, K., and Fisher, J. (2011). Enhancing professional reasoning through the use of evidence-based assessments, robust case formulations and measurable goals. *British Journal of Occupational Therapy* 74 (3): 148–152.
4. Health Education England (2020). Advanced practice mental health curriculum and capabilities. https://www.hee.nhs.uk/sites/default/files/documents/AP-MH%20Curriculum%20and%20Capabilities%20Framework%201.2.pdf
5. Sturgiss, E.A., Peart, A., Richard, L. et al. (2022). Who is at the centre of what? A scoping review of the conceptualisation of 'centredness' in healthcare. *BMJ Open* 12 (5): e059400.
6. Keene, A.R., Terrell, M., Marin, M., and Ashton, G.R. (2018). *Mental Capacity: Law and Practice*. United Kingdom: LexisNexis.
7. Engel, G.L. (1977). The need for a new medical model: a challenge for biomedicine. *Science* 196: 129–136.
8. Anjum, R.L., Copeland, S., and Rocca, E. (ed.) (2020). *Rethinking Causality, Complexity and Evidence for the Unique Patient: A CauseHealth Resource for Healthcare Professionals and the Clinical Encounter*. Cham: Springer International Publishing. https://link.springer.com/10.1007/978-3-030-41239-5 (accessed 18 December 2023).
9. Hawton, K., Lascelles, K., Pitman, A. et al. (2022). Assessment of suicide risk in mental health practice: shifting from prediction to therapeutic assessment, formulation, and risk management. *Lancet Psychiatry* 9 (11): 922–928.

10. McTiernan, K., Jackman, L., Robinson, L., and Thomas, M.A. (2021). Thematic analysis of the multidisciplinary team understanding of the 5P team formulation model and its evaluation on a psychosis rehabilitation Unit. *Community Mental Health Journal* 57 (3): 579–588.
11. NHS (2017). Multi-professional framework for advanced clinical practice in England.
12. Higgins, A., Kilkku, N., Kristofersson, G.K., and editors. (2022). *Advanced Practice in Mental Health Nursing: A European Perspective*. Springer Nature.
13. Mitchell, R. and Boyle, B. (2021). Too many cooks in the kitchen? The contingent curvilinear effect of shared leadership on multidisciplinary healthcare team innovation. *Human Resource Management Journal* 31 (1): 358–374.
14. Bäker, A., Maisano, F., and Mestres, C.A. (2023). Enabling leaders of multispecialty teams via cross-training. *BMJ Lead* 7 (1): 45–51.
15. Rumjaun, A. and Narod, F. (2020). Social learning theory—albert bandura. In: *Science Education in Theory and Practice: An Introductory Guide to Learning Theory* (ed. B. Akpan and T.J. Kennedy), 85–99. Springer International Publishing.
16. Stanley, M.J., Banks, S., Matthew, W., and Brown, S. (2020). Operationalization of bandura's social learning theory to guide interprofessional simulation. *Journal of Nursing Education and Practice* 10 (10): 61.
17. Wenger-Trayner, E., Wenger, E., and Wenger-Trayner, B. (2020). *Learning to Make a Difference: Value Creation in Social Learning Spaces*. Cambridge University Press.
18. Lian, H., Huai, M., Farh, J.L. et al. (2022). Leader unethical pro-organizational behavior and employee unethical conduct: social learning of moral disengagement as a behavioral principle. *Journal of Management* 48 (2): 350–379.
19. Copeland, S. (2020). The guidelines challenge. Rethinking causality, complexity and evidence for the unique patient. In: *A CauseHealth Resource for Healthcare Professionals and the Clinical Encounter* (ed. R.L. Anjum, S. Copeland, and E. Rocca), 95–110.
20. Kennedy-Martin, T. (2015). A literature review on the representativeness of randomized controlled trial samples and implications for the external validity of trial results. *Trials* 16: 495.
21. Vyas, D.A. (2020). Hidden in plain sight – reconsidering the use of race correction in clinical algorithms. *The New England Journal of Medicine* 383: 874–882.
22. Wiltsey Stirman, S., Baumann, A.A., and Miller, C.J. (2019). The FRAME: an expanded framework for reporting adaptations and modifications to evidence-based interventions. *Implementation Science* 14 (1): 58.
23. Blonde, L., Khunti, K., Harris, S.B. et al. (2018). Interpretation and impact of real-world clinical data for the practicing clinician. *Advances in Therapy* 35 (11): 1763–1774.
24. HEE (2020). Consultant practice capability and impact framework. Consultant Practice Capability and Impact Framework (6).pdf.
25. Simmons, B. (2010). Clinical reasoning: concept analysis. *Journal of Advanced Nursing* 66 (5): 1151–1158.
26. Higgs, J., Jensen, G.M., Loftus, S., and Christensen, N. (2018). *Clinical Reasoning in the Health Professions*. Elsevier.
27. Bostwick, J.M. and Rackley, S. (2012). Recognizing mimics of depression: the '8 Ds': this mnemonic helps recall conditions that may make medically ill patients appear depressed. *Current Psychiatry* 11: 30–35.
28. Kadiyala, P.K. (2020). Mnemonics for diagnostic criteria of DSM V mental disorders: a scoping review. *Gen Psychiatry*. 33 (3): e100109.
29. Krathwohl, D.R. (2002). A revision of bloom's taxonomy: an overview. *Theory into Practice* 41 (4): 212–218.

30. Hoy, A.W. (2019). *Educational Psychology*, 4the, 1. New York: Pearson.
31. Smallwood, J., Bernhardt, B.C., Leech, R. et al. (2021). The default mode network in cognition: a topographical perspective. *Nature Reviews. Neuroscience* 22 (8): 503–513.
32. Stein, J., Korb, F.M., Goschke, T., and Zwosta, K. (2025). Salience network resting-state functional connectivity predicts self-controlled decision-making. *Scientific Reports* 15 (1): 16332.
33. Kahneman, D. (2011). *Thinking Fast and Slow*. London: Penguin.
34. Guertin, R., Malo, M., and Gilbert, M.H. (2023). Switching off automatic pilot to promote wellbeing and performance in the workplace: the role of mindfulness and basic psychological needs satisfaction. *Frontiers in Psychology* 6 (14): 1277416.
35. Tay, S.W., Ryan, P., and Ryan, C.A. (2016). Systems 1 and 2 thinking processes and cognitive reflection testing in medical students. *Canadian Medical Education Journal* 7: e97–e103.
36. Custers, E.J.F.M. (2015). Thirty years of illness scripts: Theoretical origins and practical applications. *Medical Teacher* 37 (5): 457–462.
37. Nordick, C.L. (2021). Integrating strategies for improving diagnostic reasoning and error reduction. *Journal of the American Association of Nurse Practitioners* 33 (5): 366–372.
38. Higgins, K. and Nesbitt, C. (2022). Learning illness scripts through drawing. *The Journal of Nursing Education* 61 (10): 603–603.
39. Si, J. (2024). Fostering clinical reasoning ability in preclinical students through an illness script worksheet approach in flipped learning: a quasi-experimental study. *BMC Medical Education* 24 (1): 658.
40. Fernando, I., Cohen, M., and Henskens, F. (2013). A systematic approach to clinical reasoning in psychiatry. *Australasian Psychiatry* 21 (3): 224–230.
41. Ten Cate, O., EJFM, C., and Durning, S.J. (ed.) (2018. Innovation and Change in Professional Education). *Principles and Practice of Case-based Clinical Reasoning Education*, vol. 15. Cham: Springer International Publishing. http://link.springer.com/10.1007/978-3-319-64828-6 (accessed 26 Auguest 2023).
42. Howes, O.D. and Kapur, S. (2009). The dopamine hypothesis of schizophrenia: version III – the final common pathway. *Schizophrenia Bulletin* 35 (3): 549–562.
43. Hengartner, M.P. and Moncrieff, J. (2018). Inconclusive evidence in support of the dopamine hypothesis of psychosis: why neurobiological research must consider medication use, adjust for important confounders, choose stringent comparators, and use larger samples. *Frontiers in Psychiatry* 1 (9): 174.
44. Mishra, J.L., Allen, D.K., and Pearman, A.D. (2015). Understanding decision making during emergencies: a key contributor to resilience. *EURO Journal on Decision Processes* 3 (3–4): 397–424.
45. Mancinetti, M., Guttormsen, S., and Berendonk, C. (2019). Cognitive load in internal medicine: What every clinical teacher should know about cognitive load theory. *European Journal of Internal Medicine* 60: 4–8.
46. Copi, I.M., Cohen, C., and MacMahon, K. (2014). *Introduction to Logic: Pearson New International Edition*, 14e, 640. Harlow: Pearson Education Limited (Pearson custom library).
47. Mehanna, H.M., Moledina, J., and Travis, J. (2008). Refeeding syndrome: what it is, and how to prevent and treat it. *BMJ* 336 (7659): 1495–1498.
48. Köhler, C.A., Evangelou, E., Stubbs, B. et al. (2018). Mapping risk factors for depression across the lifespan: an umbrella review of evidence from meta-analyses and Mendelian randomization studies. *Journal of Psychiatric Research* 103: 189–207.
49. Lipton, P. (2017). Inference to best explanation. In: *A Companion to the Philosophy of Science*, 2nde (ed. W.H. Newton-Smith), 184–193. Wiley-Blackwell.
50. Cardinal, R.N. and Bullmore, E.T. (2011). *The Diagnosis of Psychosis*. Cambridge University Press.

51. Kupper, Z. and Tschacher, W. (2002). Symptom trajectories in psychotic episodes. *Comprehensive Psychiatry* 43 (4): 311–318.
52. So, S.H.W., Peters, E.R., Swendsen, J. et al. (2013). Detecting improvements in acute psychotic symptoms using experience sampling methodology. *Psychiatry Research* 210 (1): 82–88.
53. Kuhn and Thomas, S. *The Structure of Scientific Revolutions: 50th Anniversary Edition*. United Kingdom: University of Chicago Press.
54. Johnstone, L. (2018). Psychological formulation as an alternative to psychiatric diagnosis. *Journal of Humanistic Psychology* 58 (1): 30–46.
55. Vertue, F.M. and Haig, B.D. (2008). An abductive perspective on clinical reasoning and case formulation. *Journal of Clinical Psychology* 64 (9): 1046–1068.
56. Kennerley, H., Kirk, J., and Westbrook, D. (2017). *An Introduction to Cognitive Behaviour Therapy: Skills and Applications*. United Kingdom: SAGE Publications.
57. Chiffi, D. and Andreoletti, M. (2022). Abduction in prognostic reasoning. In: *Handbook of Abductive Cognition* (ed. L. Magnani), 1–23. Cham: Springer International Publishing. https://link.springer.com/10.1007/978-3-030-68436-5_11-1 (accessed 3 July 2024).
58. Stanley, D.E. and Nyrup, R. (2020). Strategies in abduction: generating and selecting diagnostic hypotheses. *The Journal of Medicine and Philosophy* 45: 159–178.
59. Montgomery, K. (2013). *How Doctors Think: Clinical Judgement and the Practice of Medicine*. Oxford Universtiy Press.
60. Baird, J., Hyslop, A., Macfie, M. et al. (2017). Clinical formulation: Where it came from, what it is and why it matters. *BJPsych Advances* 23 (2): 95–103.
61. Fawcett, J. (2016). *Applying Conceptual Models of Nursing Quality Improvement, Research, and Practice*. Springer Publishing Company.
62. Taylor, R., Bowyer, P., and Fisher, G. (2023). *Kielhofner's Model of Human Occupation*. Wolters Kluwer Health.
63. Busch, B. and McNamara, T. (2020). Language and trauma: an introduction. *Applied Linguistics* 41 (3): 323–333.
64. NICE (2018). Post-traumatic stress disorder. Diagnosis _ Diagnosis _ Post-traumatic stress disorder _ CKS _ NICE.pdf.
65. Marx, B.P., Hall-Clark, B., Friedman, M.J. et al. (2024). The PTSD criterion a debate: a brief history, current status, and recommendations for moving forward. *Journal of Traumatic Stress* 37 (1): 5–15.
66. Wild, J., Smith, K.V., Thompson, E. et al. (2016). A prospective study of pre-trauma risk factors for post-traumatic stress disorder and depression. *Psychological Medicine* 46 (12): 2571–2582.
67. Trickey, D., Siddaway, A.P., Meiser-Stedman, R. et al. (2012). A meta-analysis of risk factors for post-traumatic stress disorder in children and adolescents. *Clinical Psychology Review* 32 (2): 122–138.
68. Lugg, W. (2022). The biopsychosocial model – history, controversy and Engel. *Australasian Psychiatry* 30 (1): 55–59.
69. Roberts, A. (2023). The biopsychosocial model: its use and abuse. *Medicine, Health Care, and Philosophy* 26 (3): 367–384.
70. Smith, R.C. (2021). Making the biopsychosocial model more scientific – its general and specific models. *Social Science & Medicine* 272: 113568.
71. Mackie, J.L. (1980). *The Cement of the Universe: A Study of Causation*. Clarendon Press.

72. Hume, D. and Millican, P.J.R. (2007). *An enquiry concerning human understanding.* Oxford New York: Oxford University Press (Oxford world's classics).
73. Newton, I. (1687) Translated by Taylor, M (2023) Principles of Natural Philosophy. Flame Tree. 451.
74. Sochi, T. (2024). The epistemology of contemporary physics: classical mechanics II. *arXiv.* http://arxiv.org/abs/2411.10022 (accessed 4 June 2025).
75. Stan, M. (Forthcoming). Laws and natural philosophy. In: *The History and Philosophy of Science* (ed. S. M), 1450–1750. Bloomsbury Press Accessed at: Stan Laws and natural philosophy final.
76. Šimić, G., Tkalčić, M., Vukić, V. et al. (2021). Understanding emotions: origins and roles of the amygdala. *Biomolecules* 11 (6): 823.
77. Clancy, K.J., Devignes, Q., Ren, B. et al. (2024). Spatiotemporal dynamics of hippocampal-cortical networks underlying the unique phenomenological properties of trauma-related intrusive memories. *Molecular Psychiatry* 29 (7): 2161–2169.
78. Widmaier, E.P., Raff, H., Strang, K.T., and Shoepe, T.C. (2022). *Vander's Human Physiology: The Mechanisms of Body Function.* McGraw Hill Education.
79. Drukarch, B., Wilhelmus, M.M.M., and Shrivastava, S. (2022). The thermodynamic theory of action potential propagation: a sound basis for unification of the physics of nerve impulses. *Reviews in the Neurosciences* 33 (3): 285–302.
80. The NNPDF Collaboration, Ball, R.D., Candido, A. et al. (2022). Evidence for intrinsic charm quarks in the proton. *Nature* 608 (7923): 483–487.
81. Burback, L., Brémault-Phillips, S., Nijdam, M.J. et al. (2024). Treatment of posttraumatic stress disorder: a state-of-the-art review. *Current Neuropharmacology* 22 (4): 557–635.
82. Monson, C.M., Friedman, M.J., and La Bash, H.A.J. (2007). A psychological history of PTSD. In: *Handbook of PTSD; Science & Practice* (ed. J. Friedman, P.A. Resick, and T.M. Keane), 37–52. Guilford.
83. Cahill, S.P. and Foa, E.B. (2010). Psychological theories of PTSD. In: *Handbook of PTSD: Science and practice*, 55–77. The Guilford Press.
84. Brewin, C.R. (2014). Episodic memory, perceptual memory, and their interaction: foundations for a theory of posttraumatic stress disorder. *Psychological Bulletin* 140: 69.
85. Vasterling, J.J. and Brewin, C. (ed.) (2005). *Neuropsychology of PTSD: Biological, cognitive, and clinical perspectives.* Guilford Press.
86. Foa, E.B., Hembree, E.A., and Rothbaum, B.O. (2007). *Prolonged exposure therapy for PTSD: emotional processing of traumatic experiences: therapist guide*, 146. Oxford; New York: Oxford University Press (Treatments that work).
87. Resick, P.A., Monson, C.M., and Chard, K.M. (2017). *Cognitive Processing Therapy for PTSD: A Comprehensive Manual.* New York, NY: Guilford Press.
88. Ehlers, A., Clark, D.M., Hackmann, A. et al. (2005). Cognitive therapy for post-traumatic stress disorder: development and evaluation. *Behaviour Research and Therapy* 43 (4): 413–431.
89. Ehlers, A. and Clark, D.M. (2000). A cognitive model of posttraumatic stress disorder. *Behaviour Research and Therapy* 38 (4): 319–345.
90. Lely, J.C.G., Ter Heide, F.J.J., Moerbeek, M. et al. (2022). Psychopathology and resilience in older adults with posttraumatic stress disorder: a randomized controlled trial comparing narrative exposure therapy and present-centered therapy. *European Journal of Psychotraumatology* 13 (1). https://www.tandfonline.com/doi/full/10.1080/20008198.2021.2022277 (accessed 8 July 2025).

91. Ruggiero, G.M., Caselli, G., and Sassaroli, S. (ed.) (2021). Case formulation as an outcome and not an opening move in relational and psychodynamic models. In: *CBT Case Formulation as Therapeutic Process*, 217–232. Springer Nature.
92. Ruggiero, G.M., Caselli, G., and Sassaroli, S. (ed.) (2021). *CBT Case Formulation as Therapeutic Process*. Cham: Springer International Publishing. https://link.springer.com/10.1007/978-3-030-63587-9 (accessed 10 July 2025).
93. Moncrieff, J., Cooper, R.E., Stockmann, T. et al. (2023). The serotonin theory of depression: a systematic umbrella review of the evidence. *Molecular Psychiatry* 28 (8): 3243–3256.
94. Jauhar, S., Arnone, D., Baldwin, D.S. et al. (2023). A leaky umbrella has little value: evidence clearly indicates the serotonin system is implicated in depression. *Molecular Psychiatry* 28 (8): 3149–3152.
95. Moncrieff, J. (2006). Does antipsychotic withdrawal provoke psychosis? Review of the literature on rapid onset psychosis (supersensitivity psychosis) and withdrawal-related relapse. *Acta Psychiatrica Scandinavica* 114 (1): 3–13.
96. Giabbanelli, P.J., Rice, K.L., Galgoczy, M.C. et al. (2022). Pathways to suicide or collections of vicious cycles? Understanding the complexity of suicide through causal mapping. *Social Network Analysis and Mining* 12 (1): 60.
97. Heino, M.T.J., Knittle, K., Noone, C. et al. (2021). Studying behaviour change mechanisms under complexity. *Behavioral Science* 11 (5): 77.
98. Manson, S.M. (2001). Simplifying complexity: a review of complexity theory. *Geoforum* 32 (3): 405–414.
99. Brewin, C.R., Cloitre, M., Hyland, P. et al. (2017). A review of current evidence regarding the ICD-11 proposals for diagnosing PTSD and complex PTSD. *Clinical Psychology Review* 58: 1–15.

CHAPTER 6

Cognitive Bias and Heuristics

Steve Bown
Sheffield Hallam University, Sheffield, UK

Aim

The aim of this chapter is to explore the effect of heuristics and cognitive biases on advanced practitioners working with complex mental health scenarios. We should at the outset recognise that heuristics and the intuitions we derive from them have real value in complex health and social care settings decision-making [1]. However, the potential for heuristics and intuition to develop into cognitive biases if left unchecked suggests the adoption of an active process of critical thinking is imperative in advanced practice. The recognition of this need leads us to an exploration of metacognition as an active and conscious process aimed at understanding heuristics and mitigating the negative effects of cognitive biases.

LEARNING OUTCOMES

After reading this chapter, the reader will be able to:

1. Understand the origin of heuristics and their role in effective advanced assessment and decision-making in health and social care settings.
2. Understand cognitive biases as distinct from heuristics and their potential negative effect on advanced practice decision-making.
3. Understand the role of metacognition in mitigating the effects of cognitive biases and supporting critically considered decision-making in health and social care settings.
4. Explore models of metacognition that can be employed in practice scenarios.

The Advanced Practitioner in Mental Health, First Edition. Edited by Clare Allabyrne.
© 2026 John Wiley & Sons Ltd. All rights reserved, including rights for text and data mining and training of artificial intelligence technologies or similar technologies. Published 2026 by John Wiley & Sons Ltd.

INTRODUCTION

As we delve into biases, heuristics and metacognition, we must clarify that our scope allows us only to provide an introduction. The concepts we will introduce have been extensively covered in academic and popular literature, spanning disciplines from statistics to civic planning. Here, we aim to pragmatically introduce these concepts in relation to advanced practice in mental healthcare.

To accept heuristics, we must acknowledge that many of our thoughts and emotions operate beyond our immediate control and awareness. At times, we may act against our better judgement without realising it.

Cognitive psychology, influenced by Kahneman and Tversky's work [2], has firmly established the scientific basis for identifying thinking errors and biases. Pinker summarises their central message, laying the groundwork for the discussion in this chapter.

'... human reason left to its own devices is apt to engage in a number of fallacies and systematic errors, so if we want to make better decisions in our personal lives and as a society, we ought to be aware of these biases and seek work arounds'. (2 para 1.)

We can begin by broadly defining heuristics as mental shortcuts for interpreting complex information [3]. In this we can start to see both their value if used insightfully and potential risks if used uncritically. Before moving towards a clinical perspective, let's consider an everyday example:

When driving you might feel more caution on the motorway than in your local area. It's possible that you will have had the visceral and upsetting experience of seeing the aftermath of a crash on the motorway. If not directly, you will have seen this in films or television. It's possible on reading the words 'crash on a motorway' that you automatically experienced an image or a mild dread placing the thought into an immediate emotional context. The immediacy and availability of these sensations might lead you quite sensibly to approach motorway driving with caution and focus. This can be understood as a useful heuristic or shortcut [3]. We need not engage in each experience afresh to know the dangers. Active consideration is not required. We feel the need to employ caution at the outset. The mental shortcut or heuristic does its job of keeping us safe.

Such experiences might lead you to assume a higher likelihood of crashing on a motorway due to driving at high speed, than in comparison to your local area. Statistically speaking, this is not the case. A survey [4] in 2004 found that 77% of crashes occurred close to home on familiar roads. Here we can observe a cognitive bias developing from misapplying the heuristic 'speed equals danger' to a situation with additional variables. Pedestrians, two-way traffic, roundabouts, driveways, etc., are not accounted for in the model we used to assess motorway risks. By applying this heuristic uncritically to other driving scenarios, we prioritise speed as the main concern, overlooking other factors and potentially forming a bias. Our attention is focused on emotionally loaded factors that do not reflect new situations we find ourselves in. Upon exiting the motorway and reducing speed, our perception of risk and the need for concentration may decrease due to reduced anxiety. To counteract this bias, we might acknowledge the change in key variables and adapt our response accordingly. This effort demonstrates a basic form of metacognition, acknowledging that a previously, potentially valid assessment doesn't fit a new situation.

The aforementioned example illustrates 'The Availability Heuristic' [5] Here, we base the likelihood of an event on its ease of recall. This doesn't require actual personal experience; emotional impact can outweigh factual accuracy. Culture and media significantly influence this process, evident in biases like stereotypes [6]. In stereotyping, we see the use of emotionally loaded, highly context specific information being generalised to reduce complex socio-cultural information into a simple, emotionally coherent narrative [6].

What causes flawed decisions regarding bias and heuristics? Drawing from evolutionary psychology principles, we know that our thinking evolved to meet ancient priorities, which may not reflect our current complex needs [7].

Kahneman [8] describes two forms of reasoning, Systems 1 and 2 or Dual Process thinking. System 1 is fast, automatic and emotionally loaded, it is through this that we form heuristics. System 2 is slower due to a process of conscious judgement. It is suggested that System 1 predates us as humans, whereas system 2 is present only in humans. It is System 2 that allows us to engage in abstract reasoning and constructing hypotheses [9].

A useful example of our tendency to think non rationally is found in research, indicating that we base judgements of positive social traits such as trustworthiness on peoples' facial features [10]. The suggestion here is that complex social decisions and judgements may more be borne from immediate and emotionally satisfying judgements rather than rational painstaking consideration. The fact that attractive individuals tend to earn more than their less attractive counterparts [11] evinces the persistence of biased and irrational decisions in complex, rational, interconnected systems.

To embrace and confront this susceptibility to bias and irrationality, it's crucial to cultivate awareness of our own thought processes. Metacognition involves the deliberate reflection on how we think. This comprises two key components, understanding cognition and regulating cognition [12]. This requires us to be critically aware of the thinking patterns we employ and to employ tools to enhance or counteract them. This, however, is not an automatic process.

Working in a field where self-awareness is paramount [13], we might assume we are already proficient in this. However, research into self-assessment bias in mental health practice [14] noted 25% of mental health professionals rated themselves in the top 10% in relation to their skill base. None viewed themselves as below average.

Similarly, research into the Dunning-Kruger effect [15] identifies a tendency for individuals lacking competence in a particular area to overestimate these abilities in self-assessment. From this we should acknowledge that a simple self-assessment will be coloured by the very biases it purports to uncover.

'The first principle is that you must not fool yourself, and you are the easiest person to fool' [16, p. 313].

HEURISTICS AND BIASES AND METACOGNITION AND THE APMH ROLE

Table 6.1 identifies role descriptors from The Advanced Practice Mental Health Curriculum and Capabilities Framework [17] in relation to the advanced practitioners in mental health's (APMH) responsibility to recognise biases and heuristics. This relates not only to one's own practice but to the practice of colleagues whom we supervise or have managerial responsibility. You may wish to reflect on the suggested considerations in relation to your APMH practice.

As given earlier, we propose that identifying and managing heuristics and biases is an essential aspect of the APMH role. As such, we emphasise the necessity of cultivating effective metacognitive skills as a vital component to fulfil both clinical and leadership responsibilities.

TABLE 6.1 The APMH Framework with considerations for APMH practice.

Descriptor	Considerations
1.14 Act on professional judgement about when to seek help, demonstrating *critical reflection on their own practice, self-awareness, emotional intelligence and openness to change*.	Are we aware of the parts of ourselves we bring into the process of clinical decision-making? Are we able to change and challenge our practice or are we emotionally attached to certain ways of thinking and doing because they make us feel secure?

(Continued)

TABLE 6.1 (Continued)

Descriptor	Considerations
3.2 Develop differential judgements, recognising key biases and common errors, including diagnostic overshadowing and the issues relating to diagnosis in the face of ambiguity and incomplete data.	Are we critically aware of the diagnostic models we use with a view to their potential bias? Are we able to tolerate clinical uncertainty?
6.3 Critically explore and analyse systems and practices in identifying, influencing and challenging unconscious bias, stigma and discrimination.	Are we able to identify biases within the teams we work in and in doing so provide constructive challenge?
6.6 Receive, lead and exemplify a culture of critically reflective clinical practice supervision.	Are we using our influence to develop higher thinking or metacognition in teams via effective dialogue and supervision?

Source: Adapted from Health Education England [17].

COMMON HEALTH-SPECIFIC BIASES AND HEURISTICS

We'll now examine particular heuristics and biases, exploring their potential impact on the delivery of effective mental healthcare by the APMH. It's crucial to emphasise that our approach here intends pragmatic application and academic understanding. This distinction is important, as significant advancements in comprehending biases and heuristics stemmed from decision-making processes grounded in statistical utilisation within research contexts [18]. Clinical situations in which the APMH operates are likely to be more dynamic than research settings. In developing a research question or hypothesis, the steps towards its resolution often become evident. However, this clarity does not extend to situations involving mental health comorbidity, where a complex interplay of fluid and interdependent biopsychosocial factors is at play [19].

The clinical sphere is dynamic and constantly evolving, resistant to being encapsulated by a single framework of knowledge [20]. As we move forward, it is crucial to heed Korzybski's maxim that 'The map is not the territory' ([21], p. 58). This reminds us to resist the temptation to perceive biases and heuristics as rigid, unified realities, but rather as flexible frameworks for comprehending the intricacies of our own and others' thinking. With this in mind, the heuristics and biases discussed here are included for their relevance to complex mental health, conceptual clarity and ease of understanding.

Anchoring Bias

This is a cognitive bias where individuals rely heavily on the first piece of information encountered (the 'anchor') when making subsequent judgements or decisions, even if this information is irrelevant to the larger situation [8].

Consider a scenario where a client comes to our attention having displayed anger in a local pharmacy. Our initial insight into the situation reveals that the client has directed verbal abuse towards the staff. The nature of this verbal aggression could significantly influence our perception of the client. If the abuse appears to be indiscriminate, it may facilitate our identification of mitigating circumstances, such as an ongoing experience of chronic pain and the accompanying frustration caused by delays or alterations in their pain medication. Understanding these underlying factors can foster empathy towards the client's situation. Yet, if instead we learn that the abuse was racist, we may find ourselves unwilling to consider other factors and struggle to see the client holistically. Rightfully, we condemn such behaviour, but our natural aversion to it might inadvertently shape our perception of the client in a broader sense. This information might anchor our understanding of the client in a specific context. Critical factors such as occupation, mental state and support networks may be viewed through this lens, influencing our subsequent interventions and decisions.

This is not to downplay the repugnance of racism; the example is deliberately provocative to highlight a crucial point. The management of our biases and heuristics, intertwined with our values, can lead to cognitive dissonance as we strive for internal psychological coherence [22]. Cognitive dissonance will be a factor we return to repeatedly as we recognise the emotional security of biases in comparison to the inherent uncertainty in deliberate system 2 thinking.

Confirmation Bias

Continuing with the importance of beliefs, confirmation bias is a tendency for individuals to favour information that confirms existing beliefs while downplaying contradictory evidence [23]. This leads people to seek out, interpret or remember information that aligns with their preconceptions, reinforcing their initial views. It is important to note that evidence suggests much of our values and beliefs are formed unconsciously. Such factors may lie outside of our awareness, whilst significantly influencing the decisions we make [24]. Thus, the confirmation bias hampers objective evaluation, influences decision-making and perpetuates misconceptions.

This tendency may be evident in situations where we encounter ethical dilemmas and need to believe that our actions are morally good. In instances where we struggle to collaborate effectively with the client, this perceived inability could stem from various factors, such as concerns about risks to the client, others or our reputation as an effective practitioner.

When justifying the use of restrictive practices for example, we might emphasise factors that align with our decision such as appreciation of risk and potential harm to the client, whilst downplaying contradictory information [25]. We might concentrate on historical or diagnostic factors, which, although relevant, should be critically evaluated in the context of the client's current presentation. Alternatively, we might adopt the opposite approach, prioritising the client's current behaviour as indicative, while dismissing historical factors as irrelevant. In essence we might unconsciously eschew the full complexity of the situation and focus on factors that fit our assumptions and provide us a sense of emotional coherence and security.

Representativeness Heuristic

When acting under the representativeness heuristic, we make judgements based on how closely a situation resembles an existing mental categorisation leading to perceived similarities being favoured over other information [8]. Regarding clients with a diagnosis of Emotionally Unstable Personality Disorder, we may take core diagnostic descriptors (such as impulsivity, unpredictability and quarrelsomeness) [26] as more representative or valid than the individual's own expressions. Here a small contextually significant set of factors may colour our interactions, assessment and planning. In effect we might view the client's biopsychosocial complexity through the prism of diagnostic descriptors that can if we are not careful be reduced to negative personality traits. Instead of asking ourselves, 'Have I seen this before?' (system 2), we might assert, 'I have seen this before', (system 1) thereby simplifying the complexity of the situation to fit neatly into a model we perceive as a valid representation. In our efforts to uphold our representative model, we may downplay opposing information, such as legitimate forms of social support and networks that don't easily align with, for example, a biomedical or risk management model. Consequently, approaches centred on collaboration and co-production, which could hold significant value, might be perceived as irrelevant when compared to sources and factors that seem more concrete.

These sources, such as diagnostic criteria and descriptors, are often seen as more representative of crucial situational factors. It's essential to acknowledge that these approaches don't directly characterise the client; instead, they represent a dataset to which we are linking this specific client [27]. This dataset or criteria doesn't encapsulate the client's intricate biopsychosocial profile or the practical, tangible factors pertinent to the client and the situation. Instead, they represent abstractions of past clinical encounters.

Our own experience will be key here as noted regarding the availability heuristic. Our most easily accessible clinical experience may well be our most troubling and traumatic. In having engaged with clients with Emotionally Unstable Personality Disorder in the midst of a crisis, we may struggle to consider the client in a noncrisis oriented manner. The potential to devise controlling interventions to manage risk or laissez faire interventions to absolve ourselves of responsibility may be sought over engagement with the client which will require us to engage with uncertainty.

The six category intervention analysis model as devised by Heron [28] provides a useful tool to understanding how this heuristic might affect our clinical working (see Table 6.2).

It suggests interventions tend to be authoritative or facilitative in style. In seeking a solution that fits with our pre-existing representation of the situation we may limit the extent to which we seek further, confounding information. In such situations we may authoritatively provide the client with the information we believe is key; prescribe interventions that we feel will resolve the represented problem and challenge the client when the plan is not followed or resisted. The converse of this is the use of facilitative interventions which recognise the client's role in decision-making and seek collaborative and co-produced action. We might find such an approach provokes anxiety as it requires the handing over of control and security for collaboration and uncertainty.

While the representativeness heuristic can assist in making decisions during crises, in more nuanced and complex situations, it can result in errors by disregarding crucial information that doesn't align with our mental framework. Recognising the influence of this heuristic promotes a more rational approach to decision-making processes.

The representativeness heuristic may also become a factor in clinical situations where we are dealing with socio-clinical contexts with which we have limited experience such as different cultures and different points in the life course. In such situations the ability to seek and apply expertise other than our own may be the key effective intervention.

TABLE 6.2 Six category intervention analysis.

Authoritarian	Facilitative
Prescriptive 'I make the decision'	Cathartic 'How does this feel?'
Informative 'I hold the information'	Catalytic 'What might you be able to do?'
Confronting 'This must happen, if not ...'	Supportive 'How can we help you?'

Source: Adapted from Heron [28].

Cognitive Biases and Mitigation

We've delved into various heuristics and biases, considering their potential influence both in clinical settings and in everyday life. While it's not feasible to cover all biases comprehensively, Table 6.3 aims to summarise the biases we've discussed so far and others that warrant further examination beyond this chapter. It includes indicators suggesting caution, outlines the clinical risks associated with each bias and proposes basic steps grounded in sound clinical practice to mitigate their impact.

TABLE 6.3 Common biases and issues.

Availability Bias:	Overestimating the importance of information that is easily recalled. Overemphasis on recent or vivid examples [29]. 'This is just like that time…' The risk – overestimation of the likelihood of certain clinical factors or outcomes based on vivid or recent cases either directly encountered or encountered through media and culture rather than considering a broader range of factors. **Mitigating Strategies** The use of evidence-based practice. Willingness to seek diverse perspectives. Critically evaluating information may serve to mitigate the effect of information that is easily available and emotionally loaded.
Anchoring Bias:	Relying too heavily on the early information encountered. Biasing subsequent judgements towards information (anchor), even if no longer relevant [30]. 'I spotted this straight away'. The risk – if the client is understood in reference to a specific symptom early in the assessment process, the clinician may anchor their subsequent evaluations and interventions around this initial information. More complex nuanced factors around the client's recovery could be overlooked. **Mitigating Strategies** Gathering comprehensive information from multiple sources. Regularly reassessing hypotheses and treatment plans to ensure they remain flexible and responsive to evolving clinical needs. Critically considering one's understanding of the client.
Confirmation Bias:	Interpreting and favouring information that confirms preexisting beliefs. Downplaying contradictory evidence [31]. 'This just proves I was right all along'. The risk – this bias can skew assessment of a patient's condition, potentially resulting in poorly planned or inappropriate interventions. Additionally, it may influence how we interpret client behaviours and interactions, leading to the reinforcement of stereotypes or the misinterpretation of clinical indicators. **Mitigating Strategies** Remaining aware of our biases. Actively seek out diverse perspectives and information sources. Critically evaluate evidence to ensure a comprehensive and balanced approach to patient care.

(Continued)

TABLE 6.3 (Continued)

Overconfidence Bias:	Excessive confidence in one's knowledge or judgements. Overestimating likelihood of success [32]. 'I don't see what all the fuss is about. Luckily for you I'm here to sort this out'. The risk – practitioners may feel overly confident in their understanding of a clinical situation, leading them to overlook or downplay important clinical factors. The ineffective assessment of risk is an easily understood example. This can result in delayed or inaccurate diagnoses, potentially compromising patient outcomes. Additionally, the bias may influence treatment decisions, as practitioners may be more inclined to pursue certain interventions or approaches without fully considering alternative options or seeking additional input from the client, colleagues or specialists. **Mitigating Strategies** Cultivating self-awareness. Acknowledging the limitations of our knowledge and expertise. (This may be an uncomfortable process due to the resulting dissonance and uncertainty the process may raise).
Loss Aversion Bias:	Strongly focusing on avoiding losses over the potential for gains [33]. Whilst this bias tends to be understood best in terms of resources, its application in mental health can be informative in considering the need to maintain the stability of a client, over making and promoting efforts for increased self-efficacy and recovery. 'I know better than him and this has to happen'. The risk – the practitioner may be hesitant to change a treatment plan as it provides stability for the client. Whilst this is sometimes appropriate, potential gains for the client may be downplayed. This might in turn lead to the practitioner resisting the need to work collaboratively with the client leading ultimately to a breakdown in therapeutic engagement. **Mitigating Strategies** Critical awareness of how one manages clinical boundaries. Identify potential over-involvement and recognising the risks caused by this [34].
Recency Bias	Similar to the availability bias. Weighing recent events or information more heavily than older ones. Overlooking long-term trends or patterns [35]. 'This is the situation now'. The risk – we may see this in tandem with the availability bias in regard to significant recent clinical incidents. Such events may alter or prevent the use of normally effective clinical skills and interventions. We may see it independently in relation to recently acquired clinical knowledge becoming key to decision-making, not due to its validity and applicability but the recency with which it was learned. **Mitigating Strategies** Effective clinical supervision and post-incident debrief. Practice of critical reflection in relation to decision-making [36].

TABLE 6.3 (Continued)

Bandwagon Effect Bias:	Adopting certain beliefs or understandings because many others are doing so rather than considering them rationally [37]. 'They can't all be wrong'; 'I don't want to be the odd one out'. The risk – in responding to the bandwagon effect bias, practitioners are subject to social pressure and the need to conform. Considered from a team perspective, we can imagine how more forceful individuals are able to reductively interpret complex clinical scenarios in order to provide the team a sense of certainty or clarity. **Mitigating Strategies** Identifying and maintaining core clinical and ethical values.
Hindsight Bias:	The tendency to perceive past events as having been more predictable than they actually were. This can lead to an overestimation of one's own foresight or knowledge. This can be understood as an overlap between the availability bias and the representativeness bias that we have previously discussed [38]. 'I knew it all along'. The risk – the hindsight bias can lead to an undue overly simplistic negative appraisal of the self or others in regard to clinical decision-making. Multivariate and dynamic clinical situations can be erroneously reduced in hindsight to the key factors observed in the outcome. In simpler terms, once the situation is concluded and static, it is possible to define and understand the key factors and their effect. Whilst the situation is in play, such factors are difficult to prioritise and disentangle. **How to mitigate** Effective debriefing strategies providing a safe space whilst looking at how services can improve [39]. This is important both as individual practitioners taking stock of a situation and as clinical leads guiding a team through a difficult or aversive outcome.

Source: Adapted from Kahneman [18].

Learning Event 1

Let's consider how biases might affect how we manage our clinical boundaries. In intense interactions, we may either become too controlling, draining our energy and fostering a fear of loss, or too laissez faire, potentially overlooking others' needs when they challenge or do not tally with ours [34].

Let's consider this in relation to the boundary seesaw model. This model uses a seesaw as a metaphor for the dynamic and shifting nature of boundary management in therapeutic settings identifying the need for the practitioner to shift in relation to the client to maintain a sense of balance [34]. Whilst this model was developed in relation to personality disorder, it usefully illustrates the value of effective boundary management in complex clinical decision-making.

Consider this adapted boundary seesaw model in Figure 6.1 in regard to a clinical situation you have found difficult.

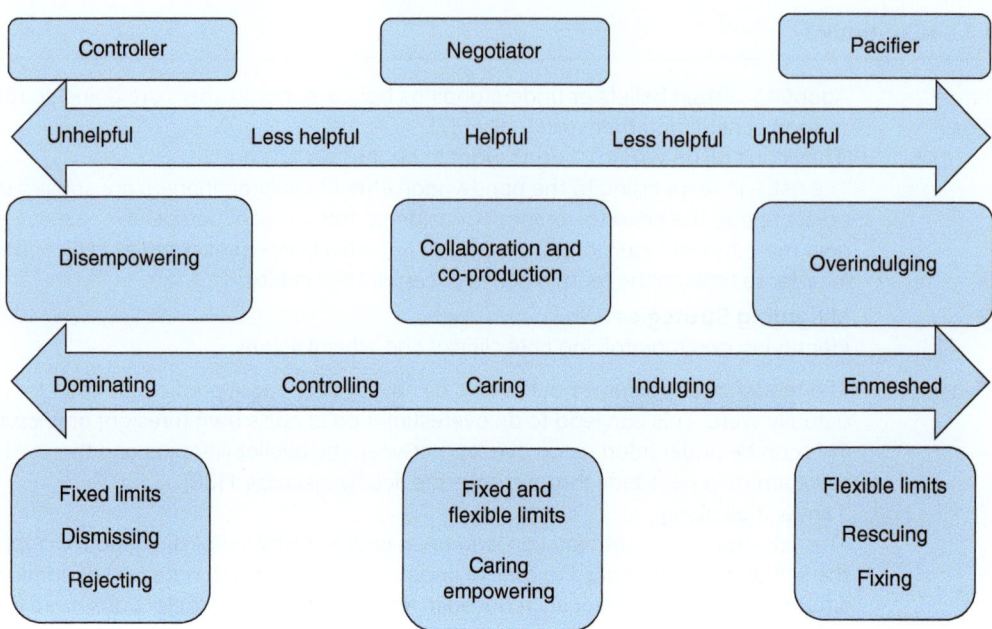

FIGURE 6.1 The boundary seesaw model. Source: Adapted from Hamilton [34].

Did you feel the need to control or pacify the client?

Did you feel the need to dominate the decision-making or did you feel enmeshed within and dominated by the decision?

Were you able offer both fixed and flexible limits? Here, consider whether there were aspects of the decision you could accept change and uncertainty in and others where you were clear about what needed to happen.

Were you able to negotiate?

Did you tend towards controlling the situation or stepping back?

In considering the aforementioned, reflect on what heuristics/biases may have influenced your thinking?

METACOGNITION

Metacognitive Knowledge

As previously mentioned [12], there exists a distinction between metacognitive knowledge and metacognitive regulation. When discussing metacognition in a clinical context, it is challenging to separate one from the other. Awareness of metacognition within a practice setting naturally prompts a process of regulation and exploration of strategies to manage its effects and outcomes. Consequently, some overlap is inevitable as we apply these concepts clinically. In the following section, we will explore methods for fostering metacognitive knowledge.

Metacognitive knowledge can be understood as consisting of three types of awareness [40].

1. Declarative knowledge – knowledge of things that can be explicitly stated.
2. Procedural knowledge – knowing how to do things. Strategies.
3. Conditional knowledge – choosing when to use different types of knowledge.

TABLE 6.4 The Johari Window.

	Known to self	Not known to self
Known to others	Arena What we present and take	Blind Spot What others see
Not known to others	Facade What we conceal	Unknown What no one sees

Source: Adapted from Luft and Ingham [41].

In delving deeper into metacognition, it's crucial to understand it as a higher-order cognitive process. The prefix 'meta' denotes something beyond or above. Hence, metacognition involves a form of thinking that transcends our typical cognitive processes, aiming to examine the thoughts and cognitions underlying them. The key question is 'what are you thinking about what you're thinking?' A central aspect of metacognition lies in understanding oneself and the factors that impact one's performance [12].

Acknowledging that our thinking can be influenced by internal and external factors and being open to scrutinising these factors is crucial to this process. Once more, biases like self-assessment bias and the Dunning-Kruger effect might impede our progress if we're not prepared to engage in an honest assessment of our thinking and comprehension of the situation [14, 15].

A method of commencing this process is to accept that we only partly know ourselves. Utilising a tool like the Johari Window in Table 6.4 may help illustrate parts that we do not readily see [41].

The four quadrants depicted earlier represent different aspects of oneself: arena (known to both self and others), blind spot (known to others but not to self), facade (known to self but not to others) and unknown (neither known to self nor others). The overarching goal is to extend awareness from the arena into the blind spot and unknown, fostering deeper self-understanding into the facade to nurture genuine interpersonal connections. For our purposes here we will focus on the blind spot as it is unknown to us but accessible through our interactions with others [42]. It is of course of note that maintaining the blind spot might be motivated in order to maintain a positive self-image and enhance self-worth [43]. We may have experience of this due to peer appraisals where we might be upset to find that an attribute we pride ourselves in having is not perceived by others. The extent that we are actively willing to accept feedback may be key to this [44].

The process of developing self-awareness, both personally and professionally is fraught with challenges and blocks. It is certainly easier to turn from one's faults to those of another. As La Rochefoucauld noted, 'If we had no faults, we should not take so much pleasure in noting those of others'. ([45], p. 24.) The ability to actively engage in such a process requires us to accept that it may make us feel vulnerable. In considering the necessary constituents of wisdom and self-awareness, we should include the ability to accept uncertainty as being key [46]. It is perhaps the ability to tolerate and accept this that enables us to follow through when we make the decision to examine our thinking and decision-making.

Metacognitive Self-awareness in Clinical Practice

As previously mentioned, Heron's 6 category intervention [28] provides a tool for us to examine how we interact with clients and supervisees in the clinical sphere. It is considered here as a framework to investigate interpersonal competence in the caring professions [47].

It may be useful to consider whether our interactions with clients are facilitative or authoritarian. We may find ourselves being prescriptive, telling clients what they need to do, taking the view that our knowledge and understanding is key and making challenges to ensure our guidance is followed.

Authoritarian and controlling interventions have a place in emergency situations. In such situations, a facilitative approach where we explore the emotional meaning of the situation for the client, supporting them to develop their own solutions whilst foregoing our own, might place the client at undue risk or allow the situation to deteriorate further. We can understand how we act in such a situation as reflecting the value of expert intuition, this is when the system one thinking described previously is effective. In such situations, say for example, effective interaction with an agitated and distressed client we may find it difficult to explain how we knew what we knew, how we knew the right moment to speak or when to hold back. Kahneman [17] suggests that in such situations where we have developed expertise, we effectively recognise patterns and alter our approach accordingly without the need for slow, laborious system two thinking. Such patterns may be based around the client's tone of voice, physical gestures or a wealth of other data that we struggle to identify in hindsight. Similarly, Dreyfus and Dreyfus [48] in their model of skill acquisition, note intuition as

'…the product of deep situational involvement and recognition of similarity [48 p. 29]'.

However, this in itself is not enough, as they note that such an approach works effectively when things are proceeding as normal but potentially not when unknown variables are waiting to come into play. Regarding this they note

'When time permits and much is at stake, detached deliberative rationality….can enhance the performance of even the intuitive expert' [48, p. 40].

Through reflection we might consider whether the situations we are engaged in need an immediate resolution. Will they be resolved by a technical or linear process or is there a need for further exploration of the problem. Have we defined the situation collaboratively to move away from our biases? In such situations a consideration of complex or "wicked problems" would note the act of framing the problem, in effect attempting to understand it from the different perspectives of those involved will be the first necessary step for leaders [49]. Whilst "wicked problems" have previously been the province of complex system management, there is evidence to suggest their value in considering complex problems in mental health settings [20].

A facilitative approach, used in response to a more complex and open problem, may mitigate the effect of biases by removing from us the role of solution provider. Rather than hearing ourselves say at all costs this must happen and subscribing to the loss aversion bias or thinking we've gone too far to turn back now and acting under the sunk cost fallacy, we might be able to work to mitigate the effect that our biases are placing on the clinical encounter [20, 49, 50].

We can further consider the value of such an approach in supervising colleagues. In such situations, as the supervisee outlines a clinical situation the availability heuristic may take effect. In supervising our colleague, we might assume we know what's going on here and rather than listening further to details that do not marry with our understanding, await the opportunity to provide our solution. It may be that we fall victim to the anchoring bias and in hearing the immediate clinical details say to ourselves "I spotted this straight away." It may be that we engage in overconfidence and hear ourselves "thinking lucky for you I was here." It's important here to recognise the emotional meaning of such certainty and confidence as it enables us to feel secure in situations that question our control.

Common with all of these is the belief that we must have a solution. This need to provide a solution may be independent of our scope or responsibility to provide a solution. In taking a facilitative approach we can find space to accept the uncertainty and dissonance previously noted and allow space for a conversation that prevents us from misusing shortcuts and rendering them as biases [46].

Learning Event 2

Building on the previous learning event, consider another client or staff interaction (Table 6.5) in light of the six category intervention analysis.

TABLE 6.5 Questions to support meta cognition.

Were you able to be facilitative or authoritarian?

Were you able to allow the individual to express emotion and how comfortable did you feel with this?

Were you confident in generating solutions with and from the client?

Were you able to support the individual in plans they developed?

Was the situation one that needed an emergency response due to potential risks and losses, or was their scope to allow exploration and time?

We've examined the significance of metacognitive knowledge and initiated our exploration into applying metacognitive regulation. Moving forward, our focus will be on delving deeper into the mechanics of metacognitive regulation in order to provide a practical understanding.

Metacognitive Regulation

Schraw [12] suggests the advancement of metacognitive regulation through the implementation of a regulatory checklist. This checklist emphasises the crucial steps of planning the intended action, monitoring its progress and evaluating its outcomes. He underscores the significance of factors such as comprehending the nature of the task, defining one's goals, assessing available resources and gauging personal understanding.

While this framework offers a solid foundation for grasping metacognitive regulation, it's important to note that the checklist is primarily designed for learners in educational settings. This focus does not fully capture the intricacies of the clinical context we've previously explored.

The Berlin Wisdom Paradigm [46, 51] offers a conceptual framework of wisdom that could guide us in determining what aspects to plan, monitor and evaluate within the clinical domain. It suggests that wisdom might be understood as expertise in the practical matter of living [46]. Such expertise is not limited to one field but requires the integration of cognitive, reflective and affective components, as well as the ability to balance what is taking place within with the broader context outside of ourselves [46, 51].

This model encapsulates wisdom and wise decision-making within five dimensions, outlined as follows:

Factual knowledge: Are we equipped with pertinent factual information? In the clinical sphere this encompasses clinical evidence and relevant theories. It involves grasping the client's presentation, devising a treatment plan and offering referrals or recommendations based on evidence indicating potential benefits.

Procedural knowledge: Do we comprehend how the aforementioned strategies will function in real-world scenarios? Specific policies and guidelines might cause delays in initiating treatment or hinder the client's acceptance of it. In instances where the client faces barriers in accessing services, solely relying on factual knowledge may prove inadequate in addressing the situation effectively [51].

Lifespan context: Do we grasp the broader context of the client's life journey? Are they at a stage where significant changes, as proposed, are feasible? Factors such as lifestyle choices valued by a couple wishing to start a family are likely to be different to those of a couple approaching retirement. We can suggest that each life stage carries its own existential challenges and resolutions and that the assessing and planning of care needs to not merely acknowledge but engage these [52].

Value relativism: Do we grasp the socio-cultural values and beliefs of the client? Are we mindful of our own socio-cultural beliefs and how they shape our clinical outlook, potentially diverging from those of the client? While our interventions may emphasise stability and support, the client's values may lean towards self-determination and self-reliance. Conversely, we might advocate growth and positive risk-taking, whereas the client's expectations of care may revolve around security and safety [53].

Recognition and management of uncertainty: Can we embrace and acknowledge ambiguity in client-centred clinical engagement? Are we capable of tolerating uncertain outcomes and making informed decisions despite having incomplete or conflicting information? Can we maintain appropriate boundaries in the midst of uncertainty, avoiding becoming overly involved and controlling or conversely, disengaged and laissez-faire? [34].

Case Scenario

This case scenario has been written in adherence to the Nursing and Midwifery Guidelines [54] to ensure the privacy and confidentiality of all involved parties. Personal information and identifying details have been anonymised to protect the identities of patients and healthcare providers.

Background: Mark H. is a 35-year-old man diagnosed with schizophrenia. He has a long history of mental health issues, including suicidal ideation and substance misuse. Mark lives with his parents, Dan (70 years old) and Margaret (68 years old), but expresses a wish to move out of the family home and live independently as he notes the home environment as stressful. His parents have been his primary caregivers, providing emotional and financial support. Mark reports a history of domestic violence from his father towards his mother when Mark was a teenager. Dan and Margaret have discussed this with previous care coordinators and both parties deny this took place. These discussions have been a significant source of conflict. When unwell, Mark has previously threatened his father.

Medical history: Mark was first diagnosed with paranoid schizophrenia during his first year of university aged 18. He has since that time been hospitalised on 5 occasions. The most recent of these approximately 1 year ago was under the Mental Health Act (2007) [55] and required a 2-week stay in a psychiatric intensive care unit due to threatening behaviour.

Mark has been prescribed Risperidone 25 mg IM fortnightly to manage his symptoms of schizophrenia.

Substance misuse history: Mark has a history of substance misuse, including crack cocaine and cannabis. He has been in contact with substance misuse services in the past for support and treatment. Despite efforts to address his substance use, Mark has struggled to maintain sobriety. Drug tests carried out by substance misuse services have occasionally come back positive for both substances.

Notably, Mark has refused to allow his parents to be informed of these results under the grounds of confidentiality.

Legal history: Mark has a history of offending behaviour, including a recent incident of common assault prior to his last admission. His behaviour has led to legal involvement, and he was admitted under Section 3 of the Mental Health Act (2007) [55] for treatment and assessment. Mark has also threatened his father with a knife in the past leading to police involvement; however, his father declined to press charges.

Current challenges: Mark's desire to move out of his family home presents challenges for his treatment and support. While he expresses a desire for independence, there are concerns about his ability to manage daily living tasks and adhere to his treatment plan outside of a structured environment.

His history of substance misuse and offending behaviour further complicates his transition to independent living.

First Thoughts – Cognitive Awareness

What are your immediate concerns regarding this situation?
Does it call to mind a similar situation you have been involved with?
What is are your first thoughts as to next steps? To be clear, you may well revise and revisit these, but what parts of the situation really felt key or important?
Have you seen this before?

Next Steps – Cognitive Regulation

How might you explore the situation with Mark?
How might you do this in an authoritarian manner?
How might you do this in a facilitative manner?
What might be different in this situation to similar ones you have managed before?
How will you take these differences into consideration?
What might make it easier or more difficult to maintain the role of negotiator?
What are your fixed limits?
What are your flexible limits?

Wisdom

What is the factual knowledge you require? What will you need to know?
What is the procedural knowledge you require? How will things happen?
Where does the situation sit in relation to the life course of the individuals involved? How might you find this out?
Where does the situation sit in relation to the values of the individuals involved including yours? How might you explore this?
What uncertainty might you be left with? Are there things you can accept being uncertain about? Are there things you cannot?

The aforementioned model, naturally, is not a cure-all; indeed, we might have to concede at this juncture that no such universal remedy exists. As Kant drily observed, 'Out of the crooked timber of humanity, no straight thing was ever made'. ([56], p. 47).

CONCLUSION

While this might initially sound pessimistic, such an interpretation is not the intention here. Instead, we must acknowledge, both as clinicians and as human beings, that we are not flawless rational agents nor should we aspire to be. We possess intuitions in the form of heuristics that assist us in comprehending complex situations and making intricate decisions. However, with humility, we should recognise that these heuristics and resultant unconscious cognitive biases, without the application of a guiding framework like metacognition, may inherently lead us astray. Our clinical decision-making process must integrate both elements for us to truly achieve advanced practice.

REFERENCES

1. Dale, J.C., Drews, B., Dimmitt, P. et al. (2013). Novice to expert: the evolution of an advanced practice evaluation tool. *Journal of Pediatric Health Care* 27 (3): 195–201.
2. Observer, T. D. (2014). Kahneman changed the way we think about thinking. But what do other thinkers think of him? The Observer. https://www.theguardian.com/science/2014/feb/16/daniel-kahneman-thinking-fast-and-slow-tributes#:~:text=I%27ve%20called%20Daniel%20Kahneman (accessed 29 February 2024).
3. Tversky, A. and Kahneman, D. (1974). Judgment under Uncertainty: Heuristics and Biases: Biases in judgments reveal some heuristics of thinking under uncertainty. *Science* 185 (4157): 1124–1131.
4. Autoweek (2002). Survey finds vehicle crashes most likely to occur close to home. Autoweek. https://www.autoweek.com/news/a2108966/survey-finds-vehicle-crashes-most-likely-occur-close-home/
5. Tversky, A. and Kahneman, D. (1973). Availability: a heuristic for judging frequency and probability. *Cognitive Psychology* 5 (2): 207–232.
6. Rothbart, M., Fulero, S., Jensen, C. et al. (1978). From individual to group impressions: availability heuristics in stereotype formation. *Journal of Experimental Social Psychology* 14 (3): 237–255.
7. Pinker, S. (2012). *The Better Angels of Our Nature: Why Violence Has Declined*. Penguin Books.
8. Kahneman, D. (2003). A perspective on judgment and choice: mapping bounded rationality. *American Psychologist* 58 (9): 697.
9. Evans, J.S. (2003). In two minds: dual-process accounts of reasoning. *Trends in Cognitive Sciences* 7 (10): 454–459.
10. Todorov, A. (2008). Evaluating faces on trustworthiness: an extension of systems for recognition of emotions signaling approach/avoidance behaviors. *Annals of the New York Academy of Sciences* 1124: 208–224.
11. Gehrsitz, M. (2014). Looks and labor: do attractive people work more? *Labour* 28 (3): 269–287.
12. Schraw, G. (1998). Promoting general metacognitive awareness. *Instructional Science* 26: 113–125.
13. Eckroth-Bucher, M. (2001). Philosophical basis and practice of self-awareness in psychiatric nursing. *Journal of Psychosocial Nursing and Mental Health Services* 39 (2): 32–39.
14. Walfish, S., McAlister, B., O'Donnell, P., and Lambert, M.J. (2012). An investigation of self-assessment bias in mental health providers. *Psychological Reports* 110 (2): 639–644.
15. Dunning, D. (2011). The Dunning–Kruger effect: on being ignorant of one's own ignorance. In: *Advances in Experimental Social Psychology*, vol. 44 (ed. J.M. Olson and M.P. Zanna), 247–296. Academic Press.
16. Feynman, R.P. (2010). *"Surely You're Joking, Mr. Feynman!": Adventures of a Curious Character: Adventures of a Curious Character*. WW Norton & Company.
17. HEE (2022). Advanced Clinical Practitioner Mental Health Curriculum and Capabilities Framework.
18. Kahneman, D. (2011). *Thinking, Fast and Slow*. Macmillan.
19. Williams, J., Cain, R., Arnone, D., and Kyratsous, M. (2020). The one and the many: a case highlighting comorbidity and complexity in psychiatry. *BJPsych Bulletin* 44 (4): 169–173.
20. Hannigan, B. and Coffey, M. (2011). Where the wicked problems are: the case of mental health. *Health Policy* 101 (3): 220–227.
21. Korzybski, A. (1933). *Science and Sanity: An Introduction to Non-Aristotelian Systems and General Semantics*. International Non-Aristotelian Library Publishing Company.
22. Festinger, L. (1962). Cognitive dissonance. *Scientific American* 207 (4): 93–106.

23. Klayman, J. (1995). Varieties of confirmation bias. *Psychology of Learning and Motivation* 1 (32): 385–418.
24. Bargh, J.A. and Morsella, E. (2008). The unconscious mind. *Perspectives on Psychological Science* 3 (1): 73–79.
25. Muir-Cochrane, E., O'Kane, D., and Oster, C. (2018). Fear and blame in mental health nurses' accounts of restrictive practices: implications for the elimination of seclusion and restraint. *International Journal of Mental Health Nursing* 27 (5): 1511–1521.
26. World Health Organization (2021). *International Statistical Classification of Diseases and Related Health Problems*, 11th ed. ICD-11; World Health Organization.
27. Kapadia, M., Desai, M., and Parikh, R. (2020). Fractures in the framework: limitations of classification systems in psychiatry. *Dialogues in Clinical Neuroscience* 22 (1): 17–26.
28. Heron, J. (1976). A six-category intervention analysis. *British Journal of Guidance and Counselling* 4 (2): 143–155.
29. Tversky, A. and Kahneman, D. (1973). Availability: a heuristic for judging frequency and probability. *Cognitive Psychology* 5 (2): 207–232. https://doi.org/10.1016/0010-0285(73)90033-9.
30. Furnham, A. and Boo, H.C. (2011). A literature review of anchoring bias. *The Journal of Socio-Economics* 40 (1): 35–42. https://doi.org/10.1016/j.socec.2010.10.008.
31. Nickerson, R.S. (1998). Confirmation bias: a ubiquitous phenomenon in many guises. *Review of General Psychology* 2 (2): 175–220.
32. Pallier, G., Wilkinson, R., Danthiir, V. et al. (2002). The role of individual differences in the accuracy of confidence judgments. *The Journal of General Psychology* 129 (3): 257–299. https://doi.org/10.1080/00221300209602099. PMID 12224810. S2CID 6652634.
33. Kahneman, D. and Tversky, A. (1977). Prospect Theory. An Analysis of Decision Making Under Risk. https://doi.org/10.21236/ada045771.
34. Hamilton, L. (2010). The boundary seesaw model: Good fences make for good neighbours. In: *Using Time, Not Doing Time: Practitioner Perspectives on Personality Disorder and Risk*. (ed. A. Tennant and K. Howells), 181–194. Wiley.
35. Turvey, B.E. and Freeman, J.L. (2012). Jury psychology. In: *Encyclopedia of Human Behavior (Second Edition)* (ed. V.S. Ramachandran), 495–502. Academic Press.
36. Rolfe, G. and Freshwater, D. (2020). *Critical Reflection in Practice: Generating Knowledge for Care*. Bloomsbury Publishing.
37. Lammers, J., Bukowski, M., Potoczek, A. et al. (2022). Disentangling the factors behind shifting voting intentions: the bandwagon effect reflects heuristic processing, while the underdog effect reflects fairness concerns. *Journal of Social and Political Psychology* 10: 676–692.
38. Blank, H., Musch, J., and Pohl, R.F. (2007). Hindsight bias: on being wise after the event. *Social Cognition* 25 (1): 1–9.
39. Kolbe, M., Eppich, W., Rudolph, J. et al. (2020). Managing psychological safety in debriefings: a dynamic balancing act. *BMJ Simulation & Technology Enhanced Learning* 6 (3): 164.
40. Jacobs, J.E. and Paris, S.G. (1987). Children's metacognition about reading: issues in definition, measurement, and instruction. *Educational Psychologist* 22 (3–4): 255–278.
41. Luft, J. (1963). The Johari Window: a graphic model of awareness in interpersonal relations. In: *Group Processes: An Introduction to Group Dynamics*, 10–16. Palo Alto (CA): National Press.

42. Neubauer, A.C., Pribil, A., Wallner, A., and Hofer, G. (2018). The self-other knowledge asymmetry in cognitive intelligence, emotional intelligence, and creativity. *Heliyon* 4 (12): e01061. https://doi.org/10.1016/j.heliyon.2018.e010.1. PMID: 30603696; PMCID: PMC6307038.
43. Vazire, S. and Carlson, E.N. (2011). Others sometimes know us better than we know ourselves. *Current Directions in Psychological Science* 20 (2): 104–108. https://doi.org/10.1177/0963721411402478.
44. Facteau, C.L., Facteau, J.D., Schoel, L.C. et al. (1998). Reactions of leaders to 360-degree feedback from subordinates and peers. *The Leadership Quarterly* 9 (4): 427–448.
45. La Rochefoucauld, F., De, D., and Stevens, F.G. (1943). *The maxims of François duc de La Rochefoucauld*. London: H. Milford.
46. Baltes, P.B., Glück, J., and Kunzmann, U. (2003). Wisdom: its structure and function in regulating successful lifespan development. In: *Handbook of Positive Psychology* (ed. C.R. Snyder and S.J. Lopez), 327–347. New York: Oxford University Press.
47. Sloan, G. and Watson, H. (2001). John Heron's six-category intervention analysis: towards understanding interpersonal relations and progressing the delivery of clinical supervision for mental health nursing in the United Kingdom. *Journal of Advanced Nursing* 36 (2): 206–214. https://doi.org/10.1046/j.1365-2648.2001.01961.x. PMID: 11580795.
48. Dreyfus, H.L. and Dreyfus, S.E. (1986). *Mind Over Machine: The Power of Human Intuition and Expertise in the Era of the Computer*. New York: The Free Press.
49. Grint, K. (2010). Wicked problems and clumsy solutions: the role of leadership. In: *The New Public Leadership Challenge*, 169–186. London: Palgrave Macmillan UK.
50. Samuriwo, R. and Hannigan, B. (2020). Wounds in mental health care: the archetype of a 'wicked problem of many hands' that needs to be addressed? *International Journal of Mental Health* 49 (1): 81–96.
51. Kunzmann, U. and Baltes, P.B. (2005). The psychology of wisdom: theoretical and empirical challenges. In: *A Handbook of Wisdom: Psychological Perspectives* (ed. R.J. Sternberg and J. Jordan), 110–135. Cambridge University Press.
52. Erikson, E.H. and Erikson, J.M. (1997). *The Life Cycle Completed*. New York: W.W. Norton.
53. Snowden, L.R. and Yamada, A.M. (2005). Cultural differences in access to care. *Annual Review of Clinical Psychology* 27 (1): 143–166.
54. Nursing and Midwifery Council (2018). *Code of Professional Conduct*. London: Nursing & Midwifery Council.
55. Mental Health Act (2007). https://www.legislation.gov.uk/ukpga/2007/12/contents.
56. Kant, I. (1991). Idea for a universal history with a cosmopolitan purpose. In: *Kant: Political Writings* (ed. H.S. Reiss), 41–53. Cambridge: Cambridge University Press (Cambridge Texts in the History of Political Thought).

CHAPTER 7

Advanced Practice in Mental Health and Trauma-Informed Care

Rachael Smith[1], Alicia Bailey[2] and Elizabeth Hearn[3]
[1] Essex Partnership Foundation Trust, Essex, UK
[2] Alder Hey Children's Hospital Trust, Liverpool, Merseyside, UK
[3] St George's, Epsom, and St Helier University Hospitals and Health Group, London, UK

Aim

This chapter provides an overview of how trauma develops across one's lifespan, including the impact of early relationships and the developing brain. It will introduce the concept of trauma-informed care (TIC) and how advanced practitioners in mental health (APMHs) can identify trauma through assessment and use of appropriate screening tools.

In accordance with TIC, further thought and consideration will be given to the notion of vicarious trauma and the impact this can have on healthcare professionals and those caring for people suffering from trauma.

The integration of TIC within advanced practice is a crucial evolution in healthcare that enhances patient care by acknowledging and addressing the profound impact of trauma on health. APMHs are particularly well-positioned to implement TIC due to their advanced knowledge, skills, clinical expertise and leadership roles.

LEARNING OUTCOMES

After reading this chapter, the reader will be able to:

1. Have a critical understanding of trauma across the lifespan.
2. Understand a wide range of validated assessment and interventional theories related to trauma.
3. Have developed awareness of the impact of trauma on health and consideration of associated health inequalities and vulnerabilities.

The Advanced Practitioner in Mental Health, First Edition. Edited by Clare Allabyrne.
© 2026 John Wiley & Sons Ltd. All rights reserved, including rights for text and data mining and training of artificial intelligence technologies or similar technologies. Published 2026 by John Wiley & Sons Ltd.

4. Consider diagnostic overlaps between trauma and other health complaints.
5. Have knowledge of vicarious trauma and the impact that can have on self and others.

This chapter embodies the following competences within the curriculum and capabilities framework of advanced practice in mental health [1] (see Table 7.1).

TABLE 7.1 How this chapter meets the APMH curriculum and capabilities framework.

Clinical practice

1. Work autonomously within professional, ethical codes and legal frameworks, being responsible and accountable for their decisions, actions and omissions at this level of practice.
2. Demonstrate the underpinning psychological, biological and social knowledge required for advanced practice in mental health.
3. Demonstrate comprehensive knowledge of and skills in systematic history taking and clinical examination of patients who are culturally diverse and/or have complex needs in challenging circumstances to develop a co-produced management plan.
4. Utilise clinical reasoning and decision-making skills to make a differential diagnosis and provide rationales for person-management plans, through critically reflecting on and evaluation of their own role in relation to challenging traditional practices, new ways of working and the impact on the multidisciplinary team.
5. Initiate, evaluate and modify a range of interventions, which may include therapies, medicines, lifestyle advice and care.

Leadership and management

1. Exercise professional judgement and leadership to effectively promote safety in the presence of complexity and unpredictability.
2. Demonstrate team working, leadership, resilience and determination, managing situations that are unfamiliar, complex or unpredictable.

Education

1. Effectively utilise a range or evidence-based educational strategies/interventions to support person centred with individuals, their families and carers and other healthcare colleagues.

Research

1. Critically appraise and apply the evidence base in influencing engagement, recovery, shared decision-making, transference and safeguarding.

Source: Adapted from [1].

INTRODUCTION

Understanding and defining trauma is essential for advanced practitioners in mental health (APMHs) for several reasons; it directly impacts patient care, treatment outcomes and overall healthcare quality. APMHs need to understand and define trauma to provide high-quality, effective and empathetic care; thus, enhancing diagnostic accuracy, enabling improved treatment outcomes, improved patient trust and a supportive healthcare environment. By integrating trauma-informed (TI) principles into their practice, APMHs can significantly improve the overall health and well-being of their patients, particularly those with trauma histories.

According to The Diagnostic and Statistical Manual of Mental Disorders (DSM-5) [2] trauma and related mental health conditions can be triggered by external traumatic events, including exposure to actual or threatened death, serious injury or sexual violence, through direct or indirect experiencing or witnessing of the event(s).

The Substance Abuse and Mental Health Services Administration (SAMHSA) [3, p. 1] defines trauma as an 'event, series of events, or set of circumstances experienced by an individual as physically or emotionally harmful or life-threatening, with lasting adverse effects on the individual's functioning and mental, physical, social, emotional, or spiritual well-being'.

Therefore, trauma can be defined as any event that lies outside the range of typical human experience overwhelming an individual's ability to cope [4]. The broader definition emphasises the subjectivity of trauma. Individuals respond differently to trauma and what may be traumatic for one person may not be traumatic for another. The effects of trauma can vary in intensity and duration, further impacting a person's mental, emotional and physical well-being.

However, concerns persist among some survivors that adopting a broad conceptualisation of trauma may dilute its meaning. It is argued that the gravity of experiences and effects should be considered, allowing individuals to develop their own narratives [5].

Global research [6, 7] shows approximately 70% of adults have experienced at least one form of trauma in their lifetime, with 30% experiencing 4–5 incidents. This is much higher in certain vulnerable populations such as women, LGBTQ+, ethnic minorities and those with mental health issues [8]. Further evidence suggests that being exposed to any form of abuse in childhood increases the risk of interpersonal partner violence and sexual assault later in life due to the psychological effects of early victimisation, increasing vulnerability to further abuse.

Consequently, adults encountering mental health services have an increased likelihood of having been through traumatic experiences, that may or may not be included within their clinical formulation and they might not associate their symptoms/challenges with their trauma history. For example, adults with bipolar personality disorder (BPD) are more likely to have experienced abuse when compared to others in both the mental health setting and the general population. People with BPD are thirteen times more likely to have experienced childhood maltreatment, thirty times more likely to be recipients of emotional abuse and seven times more likely to have been the victim of physical or sexual abuse [9].

Evidence [4] suggests that people with a diagnosis of psychosis or schizophrenia can have neurodevelopmental changes in the brain following exposure to trauma, further emphasising the need to identify and treat trauma early.

THE DEVELOPMENT OF TRAUMA

Early Life Experiences and Predisposing Factors

It is essential to distinguish between isolated traumatic events and the effects of cumulative trauma. Unlike specific incidents, which occur as singular, identifiable traumatic events, cumulative trauma arises from repeated or prolonged exposure to stressful situations. This type of trauma can have a profound impact on an individual's mental and physical health, as the stress accumulates over time and overwhelms their ability to cope [10].

Trauma can occur at any stage of life; literature particularly focuses on the profound impact of early life experiences and its direct correlations to identified traumas [11]. Early life experiences wield a profound influence on mental health, with childhood and adolescence shaping cognitive, social and emotional development. As an advanced practitioner, understanding a patient's adverse childhood experiences (ACEs) and the quality of relationships with caregivers and significant others (attachments) is imperative to treating them holistically. Furthermore, understanding how secure attachments can mitigate ACEs is crucial as this may play a protective role, helping to buffer individuals against the impact of traumatic event(s).

Attachment and Relationships

Early attachments to caregivers significantly impact one's ability to form healthy adult relationships. Secure attachments foster trust and emotional security, while insecure attachments may lead to challenges in forming and maintaining relationships, potentially resulting in mental health difficulties. Attachment style can also influence the formation and efficacy of therapeutic relationships [12, 13].

Adversity

Traumatic events during childhood, including neglect, exposure to parental violence or abuse, can leave enduring imprints on mental health. Individuals who undergo adversity face an elevated risk of developing post-traumatic stress disorder (PTSD), anxiety and depression [2].

The impact of early experiences can be mitigated or modified through supportive relationships, therapy and positive life experiences later in life [14]. Early intervention and support for those who have faced adversity play a pivotal role in promoting mental well-being and resilience.

Adverse Childhood Experiences

ACEs encompass stressful or traumatic events in childhood [15] and can significantly impact a child's well-being with potential long-term consequences for physical and mental health. ACEs are typically categorised into three groups:

Abuse

- Being the victim of physical, sexual and/or emotional abuse.

Neglect

- Being the victim of physical and emotional neglect.

Household dysfunction

- Parental mental health issues
- A household member being in prison
- Parental alcohol and drug use
- Domestic violence
- Parental abandonment

Research demonstrates that individuals experiencing four or more ACEs are at an increased risk of mental health disorders, substance abuse, chronic physical conditions and early mortality [15]. Efforts to prevent and address ACEs involve interventions promoting supportive and nurturing environments for children and young people, as well as providing resources and support for families and caregivers [16].

The development of trauma is a complex process influenced by biological, psychological, social and environmental factors including natural disasters, violence, abuse and other life-threatening events [17].

Having an awareness of trauma development equips APMHs with the knowledge and skills to provide compassionate, effective and comprehensive care, ultimately leading to better outcomes for patients. APMHs should be mindful of the following events:

Experience of a Traumatic Event or Events
Trauma typically begins with exposure to a distressing or life-threatening event. This could be a one-time occurrence, such as a motoring accident or prolonged exposure, such as ongoing abuse or neglect [18].

Perception of Threat
The perception of an event as threatening is crucial in the development of trauma. Even if the event itself is objectively dangerous, individual factors such as prior experiences, coping mechanisms and support systems can influence how a person perceives and responds to the event [19].

Physiological Response
When faced with a traumatic event, the body's natural stress response system, often referred to as the 'fight or flight' response, is activated. Prolonged exposure to trauma, and the associated physiological response of the release of stress hormones such as adrenaline and cortisol, can lead to chronic stress, altered brain functioning, hypervigilance and hyperarousal, dysregulation of the autonomic immune system and immune system suppression [20].

Psychological Impact
Traumatic events can have profound psychological effects on individuals. Common reactions include shock, disbelief, fear, anxiety, anger, guilt and sadness. These emotions can be intense and overwhelming and may persist long after the event has occurred [21].

Cognitive Processing
Following a traumatic event, individuals may struggle to make sense of what has happened. They may experience intrusive thoughts, flashbacks and nightmares. Some may also engage in avoidance behaviours, such as avoiding reminders of the event or numbing their emotions [22].

Social and Environmental Factors
The social and environmental context in which a traumatic event occurs can significantly impact its development and aftermath [23]. Factors such as social support, cultural beliefs, socioeconomic status and access to resources can influence an individual's ability to cope with and recover from trauma.

Resilience and Coping
Not everyone who experiences a traumatic event will develop trauma-related symptoms [24]. Many factors contribute to resilience, including individual coping skills, social support networks and access to appropriate mental healthcare. Recovery within mental health services often requires a comprehensive assessment and approach that addresses the biological, psychological, social and environmental dimensions of the individual's experience [25].

TRAUMA-INFORMED CARE

Trauma-informed care (TIC) should be the foundation of healthcare services. TIC is an approach based in the understanding that trauma exposure can impact an individual's neurological, biological, psychological and social development [26]. TIC can be directly related to advanced practice in mental health in relation to the developed awareness of how to create organisational change and environments that promote patient recovery and prevent re-traumatisation [5].

TABLE 7.2 The four assumptions: the four R's.

Realisation	Staff's realisation of trauma and knowledge. How it can impact individuals, families, groups and communities and influence all areas of a person's life.
Recognise	The signs of trauma and how these can manifest in individuals accessing services.
Response	The organisation adjusts every aspect of their care through staff training, language and policies, providing a physically and psychologically safe environment.
Resist re-traumatisation	Of patients and staff. Organisations take steps to reduce toxic cultures and environments that may interfere with the recovery of clients. There is an awareness of how organisational practices may trigger painful memories for patients.

Adapted from SAMHSA Concept of Trauma and Guidance for a Trauma-Informed Approach [3].

TABLE 7.3 The six principles of trauma-informed care.

Safety	Patients and staff feel psychologically safe.
Trustworthiness and transparency	Decisions are made with transparency; staff explain what they are going to do and why; following through on agreements building a trusting relationship.
Peer support	People with a shared experience are integrated into the organisation and contribute to service delivery.
Collaboration	Patients and staff work together without power imbalance, to support shared decision-making.
Empowerment	Patients and staff strengths are recognised and built on to further support recovery or develop services.
Humility and responsiveness	Biases and stereotypes are recognised and addressed ensuring processes are responsive to the needs of the patients.

Adapted from SAMHSA Concept of Trauma and Guidance for a Trauma-Informed Approach [3].

TIC is based on four assumptions and six key principles [3] (see Tables 7.2 and 7.3).

TIC can improve patient engagement, treatment adherence, health outcomes and staff well-being, resulting in reduced costs for health and social care services [3].

Re-traumatisation Risks

Traumatic experiences can impact someone's behaviour later in life in many ways, including attachment styles, avoiding experiences that remind them of the trauma and so on. Using TI principles can help to navigate these behaviours and support service users.

Iatrogenic Harm

When medical care results in harm or injury to a patient, such as adverse effects from pharmacological treatment or hospital-acquired infections, it is known as *iatrogenic harm*. Mental health services can cause iatrogenic harm and the terms 'sanctuary harm' and 'institutional betrayal' have been used to capture this concept [27]. One source of this can be staff members and/or the clinical environment re-traumatising service users. This is more likely to happen when staff are not aware of the person's trauma history and what might be triggering for them. Research indicates that when trauma is inflicted by an institution which should be relied upon for safety and support it can be more harmful than trauma from services without such expectations, cause more distress and higher severity of symptoms of PTSD and anxiety, as well as being more likely to prevent people from seeking out help in the future [28].

Restrictive practices such as restraint, seclusion and a general loss of control are examples of systemic processes that can be re-traumatising for people in mental health services. Research and service user feedback have established that when these are not fully understood by patients, it can lead to a reluctance to seek help again [29].

An example of this effect is CCTV cameras or Oxevision. Oxevision is a monitoring system introduced into inpatient National Health Services (NHS) in 2020 to detect vital signs and alert staff if there are concerns in order to provide safe and efficient care [30]. However, concerns have been raised by individuals and charity organisations that the prospect of being constantly monitored can be traumatising for people especially when consent is not sought and has resulted in reports of service users not being able to sleep, having increased anxiety and even an increase in thoughts of self-harm [31, 32]. It is therefore vital that services use patient involvement and feedback when reviewing processes.

Implementing a Trauma-Informed Service

Implementing a TI service can help mitigate some of the risks of re-traumatisation and support patients to recover holistically. The NHS Long-Term Plan [33] proposed recommendations for implementing TI approaches to healthcare over a period of 10 years, especially for high-risk, vulnerable children and young people. However, there is no single strategy on how to implement this or any official funding commitment to do so [8]. One of the most frequently referenced frameworks for establishing a TI system is that of SAMHSA which identifies six key principles, as detailed earlier on in this chapter. When organisations try to implement TIC there are various factors that affect how quickly and how successfully this occurs, including organisational support, policy changes and local leadership [8]. APMHs are in a prime position to act as local leaders in implementing TIC by role modelling the principles in their clinical practice, examples for this could include reviewing a patient's history prior to meeting to establish any sensitive topics and avoid retriggering traumatic memories. By keeping the six principles of TIC in mind the APMH can then weave these approaches into every intervention, ensuring transparency and empowerment with the patient throughout their treatment.

APMHs can use their roles in leadership and education to support and teach members of their team to adapt their own practice to include TI approaches by sharing case studies of good practice or helping to create assessment templates that consider the principles. APMHs can also use their senior position within teams to support co-production and encourage the involvement of experts by experience when making changes to services and updating protocols.

One of the key changes suggested by SAMHSA [3] is the introduction of team formulations. This could be based on the 5 Ps (detailed further in the chapter) or other locally accepted frameworks. Nikopaschos et al. [34] suggests that team formulation helps bring a change in culture and a movement towards TIC and understanding patient distress. It also holds space for shared understanding and collaborative care planning. Implementing a formulation framework can significantly reduce episodes of self-harm, seclusion and restraint, which can be causes of both further trauma and re-traumatising. However, other services with shorter involvements with patients may need to adopt other ideas. Greenwald et al. [35] found that working in a busy emergency department didn't allow for working in a fully TI way; however, the introduction of a universal TI screening tool was able to provide information about follow-up support options.

Implementing TIC onto wards has been shown to have positive outcomes in its' immediate mental health impact but also in more complex ways such as increasing levels of trust in the staff and improvements in patients' wider health. One example is a forensic mental health ward where, after implementing TIC principles, including team formulations, the staff were able to increase cervical smear compliance rates from 13% to 47% in a group of women with high rates of sexual assault in their histories [36]. Previous research [37, 38] has found that women who have experienced sexual abuse are less likely to attend cervical screenings by up to 72%, despite women with mental ill health having a 22% higher chance of abnormal results.

Case Study 7.1

Francesca is a 38-year-old woman recently admitted to a forensic mental health service. She grew up with military parents and lived in several countries. She found it difficult to make friends, was bullied and preferred to spend time with adults rather than children of her own age.

When Francesca was 16, her parents split up and she moved to the United Kingdom with her mother and new stepfather. Her stepfather was sexually abusive, and she moved out of the family home aged 17, leading to poor choices in peer groups and subsequent drug addiction, including crack cocaine. She was previously arrested for assault while trying to get money to buy drugs and suffered some physical injuries due to a traffic accident while evading police.

Francesca has a diagnosis of schizoaffective disorder, which was not diagnosed until she was in the prison system. She was later arrested after fatally wounding her partner during an argument; she claimed he had 'come at her' and she 'reacted without thinking'. It was during this prison sentence she was noticed to have bizarre behaviours and was referred to the mental health team.

After being transferred to the forensic mental health inpatient ward, staff reported that Francesca was aggressive and hostile, wouldn't follow the rules of the ward and was verbally threatening when the team try to enforce boundaries.

- What might be a risk of re-traumatisation for Francesca with inpatient services?
- What kinds of trauma has Francesca been exposed to?
- Are there any adaptions the team could make to help build trust with Francesca?

CLINICAL INVESTIGATIONS

Due to the multiple types of trauma a person may endure, trauma presentations may include a wide range of developmental, physical, behavioural and emotional difficulties. The complicated presentation can often lead to multiple diagnoses and misdiagnoses. It is important to complete a comprehensive assessment using a variety of methods and perspectives to capture traumatic incidents [6].

Screening Tools

To determine if a person has trauma-related symptoms, clinicians can use a screening tool to indicate whether further trauma assessment is beneficial and for use in the evaluation and planning of treatment [39].

TABLE 7.4 Examples of trauma-screening tools, listed alphabetically.

Tool	Age range	Suitability/domains
ACE-Q Child (parent questionnaire)	Age 0–12	For use in paediatric settings for children at risk of chronic health, mental or behavioural difficulties due to changes in brain architecture brought on by extreme stress.
ACE-Q Teen (self and parent questionnaires)	Age 13–19	For use in paediatric settings for children at risk of chronic health, mental or behavioural difficulties due to changes in brain architecture brought on by extreme stress.
The Children's Revised Impact of Events Scale (CRIES) (either 8 or 13 question tool)	Age 8–18	Children at risk of post-traumatic stress disorder (PTSD)
Clinician Administered PTSD Scale for DSM 5 (CAPS-5)	Age 18+	The CAPS-5 is based on the DSM5 and considered the benchmark tool for PTSD assessment. Clinicians should have a working knowledge of PTSD. 45–60 minute interview
Clinician Administered PTSD Scale for DSM 5 – Child/Adolescent Version (CAPS-CA-5)	Age 7–18	A 30-item clinician-administered PTSD scale based upon DSM-5 criteria for children and adolescents. It is a modified version of the CAPS-5 that includes age-appropriate items and picture-response options.
Original Adverse Childhood Experiences (ACE) Questionnaire	Age 18+	Assesses exposure to a variety of childhood adversities: physical, sexual and emotional abuse, emotional and physical neglect, domestic violence, parental substance abuse, mental illness and incarceration.
Primary Care PTSD Screen for DSM 5 (PC-PTSD-5)	Age 18+	A five-item screening designed for identification of probable PTSD in primary care settings.
Trauma-Screening Questionnaire (TSQ)	Age 18+	Good for use in primary care to explore PTSD. 10 questions to assess reactions and arousal to trauma.

There are a variety of recommended trauma screening tools [40–42]; however, it is worth thinking about patient experience when using these. Referencing trauma can raise painful memories for people and a patient's experience of health services can be easily shaped by these initial interactions.

Assessment encounters can be viewed as invalidating or 'tick box' exercises by patients if the focus is towards screening tools, so it is worth spending time establishing a good rapport and using screening tools as an addition to your assessment rather than as the assessment itself [43].

The screening tools in Table 7.4 are used to measure different types or the severity of the trauma. If using a screening tool, it is important to consider:

- A person's age, language skills and cognitive capabilities
- Whether the person is part of the populations that the tool has been validated for
- Any factors that might affect the reliability and validity of the tool

Assessment

Trauma can impact on people's health across the lifespan, and its impact is not always evident. APMHs embody a skillset that allows them to autonomously manage an episode of care, which may have previously been considered the domain of medics. Therefore, to be able to assess, manage and treat an episode of care effectively, clinicians need to be thorough in their assessment and truly understand what is beyond a person's presenting behaviour by determining what a person 'needs', rather than 'what is wrong with them' [44].

To consider what has *happened* to a person and understand their emotional distress and behaviours, a five 'P' formulation links theory to practice developing a framework for what care can be provided to meet the person's needs [6].

A five 'P' formulation is a collaborative patient document and used to inform treatment plans and care needs. The five Ps consist of:

- **Presenting issues**: A summary of the current difficulties being experienced by the person that has led to them accessing care or other problems identified during the assessment process.
- **Predisposing factors**: Issues in the persons past that could contribute to them experiencing mental health issues, including family history, significant events, social or cultural issues, ACEs or parental mental health.
- **Precipitating factors**: Events that have contributed or triggered the current access of care, including substance misuse, interpersonal or physical stressors.
- **Perpetuating factors**: Issues that are maintaining the current difficulties, behaviours and beliefs (substance misuse, avoidance or safety behaviours).
- **Protective factors**: Individual and systemic strengths alongside the presenting problem adding to a person's resilience and resources (social support, skills, interests and personal characteristics) [8].

Formulations should be updated when new information arises and treatment plans created to target the presenting issues and maintenance of difficulties.

Clinicians can be reluctant to ask patients about their experiences in fear of causing distress, fear of vicarious traumatisation or a lack of training [5]. Patients should be reassured that they do not have to disclose details of traumatic experiences, but clinicians should remain curious and try to ascertain if the person is currently safe and be aware of how to refer on to trauma-specific support if required.

Diagnosis of Trauma

Symptoms of PTSD can overlap or co-occur with other mental health disorders making diagnosis difficult. Incorrect diagnosis can lead to ineffective treatment; therefore, a diagnosis needs to link formulation to evidence based treatment [45]. Diagnosis should be considered in conjunction with the individual; some people may not want a diagnosis, but for some it can help them understand the context of their difficulties and provide wider validation of their experiences. Despite the stigma attached to mental health diagnosis, research indicates that diagnosis should be made to enable timely and effective treatment [46].

In the United Kingdom, the NHS uses the WHO's International Classification of Diseases (ICD) [47] to make diagnoses. The Diagnostic and Statistical Manual (DSM) [2] is mainly used in the United States, but despite this the DSM is often referred to in scientific literature and some clinical guidelines [48], so it is important to note they have differences in diagnostic criteria. Some children and adults may meet the criteria for diagnosis from one classification but not the other, or present with symptoms that do not meet the threshold for diagnosis but would still benefit from treatment.

PTSD diagnostic criteria ICD-11 [47]:

- Have been exposed to an event/situation of an extremely threatening or horrific nature.
- Experience persistent (over several weeks):
  - Re-experiencing of the traumatic event via flashbacks, vivid memories or recurring dreams or ruminating on the event.
  - Deliberate avoidance of reminders of the traumatic event, such as conversations, places, activities and internal avoidance of thoughts and memories.
  - Persistent arousal and heightened threat displayed by two of the following: sleep difficulties, irritability, anger, poor concentration, hypervigilance or extreme startled response.

PTSD diagnostic criteria DSM5 [2]:

- Exposure to actual or threatened death, serious injury or sexual violence.

Experience for more than 1 month:

- Intrusions
- Avoidance
- Changes in cognitions and mood
- Arousal and reactivity

That causes 'clinically significant distress or impairment of function' and 'due to an event' and not due to 'a substance or medical condition'.

Diagnostic Overlap

PTSD has many symptom and diagnostic overlaps, such as depression, suicidality, self-destructive behaviour, emotional dysregulation, interpersonal problems and dissociation. Individuals may have been under mental health services for many years but have the wrong diagnosis or undiagnosed comorbid trauma conditions that have not been treated due to never having the appropriate trauma screening.

Many individuals with PTSD or complex PTSD (C PTSD) may also meet the diagnostic requirements for emotionally unstable/borderline personality disorder (EUPD/BPD). Cloitre et al. [49] found that up to 54% of those with BPD meet the criteria for C-PTSD, and up to 44% meet criteria for PTSD, although others suggest this could be as high as 70% [50]. The value of assigning an additional diagnosis of personality disorder depends on the clinical situation; diagnosis can bring stigma to an individual and lead to exclusion from treatment or services. It is helpful to discuss with your patient the diagnosis and treatment options; as an EUPD diagnosis can also be validating and lead to appropriate treatment referrals.

Overlaps with Neurodiversity

Assessment in children and adults can be complex, due to developmental variations, but also because trauma can present with other neurodiversities. There is occurrence of trauma being misdiagnosed as attention deficit hyperactivity disorder (ADHD) and/or autism spectrum disorder (ASD) due to the overlap in symptoms. Trauma and neurodevelopmental disorders can also present together further complicating assessment [51, 52].

Trauma can have a significant impact on child development resulting in difficulties in a variety of settings and scenarios, including home or school. It is important to gather information from various sources (child, parents/carers and school – using a range of assessment techniques (interview, assessment tools and behavioural observations).

Tables 7.5 and 7.6 denote common symptom overlap between trauma and alternative or comorbid diagnoses, demonstrating the need for symptom exploration and awareness in care management.

TABLE 7.5 Trauma and ADHD symptom overlap.

Trauma symptoms	Symptom overlap	ADHD symptoms
Feelings of fear, helplessness, uncertainty	Difficulty concentrating and learning	Difficulty sustaining attention
High arousal/nervousness	Easily distracted	Struggle to follow instructions
Avoidance behaviours	Doesn't seem to listen	Difficulty with organisation
Irritability	Disorganised	Fidgety
Guilt/shame	Hyperactive	Difficulty waiting/taking turns
Dissociation	Restless	Talking excessively
Hypervigilance	Difficulty sleeping	Losing/misplacing items
Aggressive, reckless, self-destructive behaviours		Interrupting or intruding upon others

Adapted from The National Child Traumatic Stress Network [7].

TABLE 7.6 Trauma and ASD symptom overlap.

Trauma symptoms	Symptom overlap	ASD symptoms
Prevalence of traumatic event	Phobias	Repetitive behaviour or echolalia
Flashbacks	High anxiety/hypervigilance	Difficulty reading social cues
Intrusive memories/thoughts	Sleeping disturbances	Special interests
Nightmares	Eating disturbance	Impaired functioning in social interaction and communication
	Aggression/agitation	Restricted repertoire of activity/interest
	Self-harm	
	Emotional difficulties	
	Disassociation	
	Fluctuation energy/burnout	
	Over/under active nervous system	
	Chronic pain	

Overlap and Overshadowing with PTSD and Chronic Pain

There is increasing recognition that chronic pain and PTSD frequently co-occur, with pain being one of the most prevalent health concerns reported by people with PTSD [53]. Chronic pain is reported in 20–80% of people with trauma history and 10–50% of individuals with PTSD. There is limited research on the relationship between chronic pain and PTSD, and these have predominantly focused on PTSD and injury-related trauma, whereas the relationship between ACEs and PTSD is seldom explored [54]. See Table 7.7.

There are several theories that explain the comorbidity of chronic pain and PTSD. Admundson et al. [55] proposed a shared vulnerability model suggesting that anxiety sensitivity predisposes the development of both PTSD and pain, further research adds central sensitisation as an underlying mechanism. Central sensitisation has been observed in people with PTSD, who are more likely to experience inhibited pain transmission and increased pain severity [56].

Sharp and Harvey's (cited in Beck [57]) mutual maintenance model suggests that PTSD and chronic pain both maintain and exacerbate each other through:

- Attentional and reasoning biases
- Anxiety sensitivity
- Trauma reminders
- Avoidance
- Depression and reduced activity levels
- Anxiety and pain perception
- Cognitive demand of symptoms limiting adaptive strategies.

APMHs should always consider pain and PTSD comorbidity when screening for PTSD and/or chronic pain to enable effective treatment planning. If pain and PTSD are because of the same traumatic incident, parallel treatment may be required.

TABLE 7.7 Trauma and chronic pain symptom overlap.

Trauma symptoms	Symptom overlap	Chronic pain symptoms
Traumatic exposure	Anxiety	Aching
Intrusive memories/thoughts	Depression	Burning
Avoidance behaviours	Fatigue	Shooting
	Insomnia	Squeezing
	Emotional disturbances	Stiffness
	Restlessness	Stinging
	Poor concentration and memory	Throbbing
	Weight changes	Cramps
	Decreased sex drive/sexual function	

TREATMENT

Therapy

In both the United Kingdom and United States, clinical guidelines [58–60] make similar recommendations for children and adults. The first line of treatment for PTSD should be trauma-focused cognitive behavioural therapy (TF-CBT). For people who present with PTSD more than 3 months after the traumatic event, and who have not responded to TF-CBT, then offer eye movement de-sensitisation and reprocessing (EMDR). For adults, there are further considerations for narrative exposure therapy or prolonged exposure therapy.

TF-CBT

TF-CBT is a short-term intervention between 6 and 25 sessions, using CBT to help challenge the negative thoughts about the experience and develop a healthier narrative. It involves [61, 62]:

- Psychoeducation around trauma/PTSD, normalising the traumatic reactions to help validate and reduce feelings of shame/guilt that are often associated with trauma.
- Develop coping skills, such as mindfulness, relaxation and thought identification.
- Gradual exposure to reintroduce the patient to their memories, reconditioning their response and distress.
- Cognitive processing by developing skills to reconceptualise the experience.
- Caregiver involvement which can include rebuilding trusting relationships or for children, teaching the parent/carer how to be the best resource for their child.

EMDR

EMDR was developed by American Psychologist Francine Shapiro in 1987 based on the adaptive information processing (AIP) model [63]. The AIP model suggests that traumatic memories are unprocessed due to fight and flight response and dysfunctionally stored in the brain. The memories are triggered by our senses and attached meanings about how we view ourselves and the world. EMDR is a cost-effective short intervention (approximately 6 sessions) that has advantages compared to CBT including less sessions needed, no homework element, no detailed verbal description of trauma required or prolonged in vivo exposure. EMDR is used to treat multiple mental health disorders but is mostly recommended for the treatment of PTSD.

EMDR follows an 8-phase protocol based on assessment and developing coping skills before tackling the trauma [64] by:

- Accessing the traumatic memory and identifying where the belief attached to it stems from.
- Stimulating the processing system with bilateral stimulation and *moving* the accessed information to an appropriate resolution.
- Reprocessing the transmuted information through the accessed channels of the memory network resulting in a reduction or elimination of symptoms, changes in behaviour and emotional response.

Pharmacology

In the United Kingdom and American guidance, medication is not recommended as a first line treatment in trauma due to there being a lack of follow-up data for its effectiveness, and medications showing to be less cost-effective than that of EMDR or TF-CBT [58, 60], further highlighting a focus on therapeutic intervention ahead of pharmacological.

In the United Kingdom, guidance [58] recommends the use of sertraline or paroxetine as the only drugs with UK marketing authorisation for PTSD treatment. Serotonin contributes to mood and anxiety disorders due to its impact on the peripheral and central nervous system. Serotonin can be regulated by selective serotonin reuptake inhibitors (SSRIs) or a serotonin and noradrenaline re-uptake inhibitor such as venlafaxine [65]. Venlafaxine is recommended by National Institute of Clinical Excellence (NICE) but is off-label in its' use in PTSD treatment.

Though there is little evidence that medication alone is effective in treatment of PTSD, blocking serotonin could help people 'unlearn' fear more quickly than a control group [66, 67] suggesting that there could be a benefit when combined with exposure-based therapy.

The American Academy of Child and Adolescent Psychiatry (AACAP)/American Psychological Association (APA) [59, 60] and NICE [58] propose alternative treatment with a second-generation antipsychotic if symptoms such as hyperarousal and psychotic symptoms are disabling, not responding to other drug or psychological treatments and the addition of medication may improve engagement in therapy. NICE guidance [58] suggests risperidone, though acknowledges this is off-label use.

Ultimately, there is no medication that can treat trauma maintaining symptoms, such as avoidance and flashbacks, but it is appropriate to consider the severity of anxiety or depressive symptoms and whether medication for these symptoms alongside therapy would improve outcomes for the individual.

RED FLAGS, RISK AND SAFEGUARDING

> ### RED FLAGS
>
> The following red flags of PTSD suggest that urgent intervention and risk management planning are required to ensure the safety of the individual [60, 68]:
>
> - Suicidal thoughts
> - Thoughts of hurting others
> - Self-harm
> - Overwhelming hopelessness
> - Increased substance misuse
> - Risky sexual behaviour
> - Eating disorder behaviour

Risk

A risk management plan must be created to protect individuals and others from harm. It involves developing co-produced strategies and approaches to prevent or minimise harm to themselves or others. It should include a summary of all risks (red flags) identified and actions to be taken by the individual, carers and professionals in such circumstances. Childhood adversity or history of trauma has been found to increase risk of violence and suicide, particularly in males [69].

The Department of Health and Social Care published guidance on assessing and managing risk in mental health services in 2009 [70], and although no further update has occurred, the principles of collaborative care planning and development of risk mitigation strategies remain.

Safeguarding

During the assessment process, you may identify safeguarding concerns. If this happens, you must advise the patient of your safeguarding concern and the need to break confidentiality by way of escalating within your employers' safeguarding processes.

Consider:

- Any immediate risk of harm to the individual or others which may require urgent police assistance.
- Indications of abuse; physical, sexual, psychological, neglect or financial, either to self or others, including dependants (children or other carer responsibilities).
- Indications of female genital mutilation (FGM), forced marriage, domestic abuse, sexual exploitation, hate crimes [71].

Vicarious Trauma in Staff

Many articles and guides about implementing TI services raise the idea of needing to provide TI support for the workforce. There are a variety of terms which refer to the impact on staff working under stress or with a high exposure to trauma, such as vicarious trauma, secondary stress, compassion fatigue and burnout. There exists research that highlights the differences between these in more detail; however, as a general overview, these terms are in relation to when staff start developing symptoms that can impact their cognitive, emotional and behavioural state. This occurs due to significant exposure to distressing situations which could be a one-off or involve extended exposure over a period of time. Evidence suggests that staff who have had their own experiences of trauma are more vulnerable to developing vicarious trauma. Recent research indicates 30% of healthcare staff have themselves been victims of domestic violence and might subsequently need more well-being support [72].

Vicarious trauma can cause a compounding negative affect on the patient as the trauma exposure can cause a change in beliefs and cognitive schemas about self and others [73]. Staff have been found on occasions to develop symptoms of PTSD themselves and mirror the clients' experience; other effects can be desensitisation to trauma, a lack of empathy, depersonalisation and also less satisfaction in aspects of life unrelated to work when staff aren't able to maintain boundaries between work and home [74].

Signs of vicarious trauma are [75]:

- Experiencing ongoing negative feelings about patients' experiences
- Bystander guilt
- Thinking about the patient outside of work
- Horror and/or rescue fantasies
- A sense of hopelessness
- Avoiding listening to the patients' experiences
- Not upholding professional boundaries

Strategies to support teams with vicarious trauma involve interventions such as self-care education, art therapy, psychoeducation about trauma and being aware of the likelihood and symptoms of vicarious trauma. APMHs can provide supervision to staff and talk through complex cases. Research suggests that group reflective discussions show the most positive impact over a long period of time [73]. APMHs can also share their own learning and techniques, thus creating a culture of vicarious resilience in which teams can share between themselves to create an open culture of support. This has been shown to be effective in practice with one ward finding staff turnover reduced from 32% to 5% when improved staff well-being and support initiatives were instated, including a weekly reflective practice session, increased supervision and psychoeducation [76].

These staff support initiatives should be factored in for any organisational developmental plans to make services more TI and will need to be individualised to the requirements of the service.

> ### Case Study 7.2
>
> *Kieron is 15-year-old male admitted to a psychiatric adolescent unit after trying to hang himself at home. He lives at home with his disabled mother and 4 brothers, he is the eldest and the two younger brothers (age 4 and 6) have ADHD and ASD. There is a history of domestic violence between his parents. Kieron recalls witnessing his parents shouting and hitting each other from an early age – they would slam doors and throw things at each other. In one incident, he witnessed his father attempting to strangle his mother, and Kieron thought his mother was going to die. Kieron is not currently in education having been excluded for his behaviour. He attempted suicide as he feels hopeless for the future.*
>
> *While on the ward, Kieron has presented with a fluctuating mental state, at times argumentative, making verbal threats of harm, to elated and hyperactive. He struggles to sleep because of noises on the ward. He feels anxious and has panic attacks; he has started to refuse to sleep in his ward bedroom, and has damaged hospital property. Kieron reports that he is frustrated that some staff are happy to take positive risks with him and others decline his requests with no explanation, such as not letting him go in the kitchen or into the garden. Staff are feeling burned out by Kieron's attitude and threats towards them.*
>
> - Think about Kieron's history and how this may impact and influence his current presentation and put together a 5Ps formulation.
> - Thinking about the staff in relation to vicarious trauma, what is important to consider in this situation when caring for someone with a trauma history?
> - What could be helpful in supporting the staff team caring for Kieron?

LEARNING EVENT

NHS England has created a collaborative 'trauma-informed care training' to support clinicians in deepening their understanding on the importance of becoming more trauma-sensitive in the care they deliver.

You can access the e-learning here:

https://www.e-lfh.org.uk/programmes/trauma-informed-care/

CONCLUSION

Advanced practice in mental health, grounded in TIC principles and approaches, represents a critical evolution in the treatment and management of patients. By understanding how trauma impacts individuals, APMHs can significantly enhance the quality of care they provide. This approach improves diagnostic accuracy and treatment efficacy and fosters therapeutic relationships built on empathy, trust and respect.

TIC ensures that interventions are sensitive to the needs of trauma survivors, preventing re-traumatisation and promoting a safe, empowering environment for recovery. Through individualised treatment planning and holistic care, APMHs can address both the psychological and physical health consequences of trauma, offering comprehensive support to patients. APMHs can use clinical knowledge and leadership skills to implement strategies to protect their own, and colleagues', well-being in relation to vicarious trauma. By advocating for systemic changes and engaging in continuous professional development, APMHs contribute to the advancement of mental health practices and the broader healthcare system.

FURTHER READING

Forkey, H., Szilagyi, M., Kelly, E.T., and Duffee, J. (2021). Trauma-informed care. *Pediatrics* 148 (2): e2021052580.

Kallivayalil, D. (2019). *Group Trauma Treatment in Early Recovery: Promotinog Safety and Self-Care*. Herman JL.

SAMHSA (2014). *A Treatment Improvement Protocol: Trauma-Informed Care in Behavioral Health Services*. SAMHSA. TIP 57. https://library.samhsa.gov/sites/default/files/sma14-4816.pdf

REFERENCES

1. Health Education England (2017). Advanced practice mental health curriculum and capabilities framework. https://www.hee.nhs.uk/sites/default/files/documents/AP-MH%20Curriculum%20and%20Capabilities%20Framework%201.2.pdf
2. American Psychiatric Association (2013). *Diagnostic and Statistical Manual of Mental Disorders*, 5the. Washington, DC: American Psychiatric Publishing.
3. The Substance Abuse and Mental Health Services Administration (2014). SAMHSA Concept of Trauma and Guidance for a Trauma-Informed Approach.
4. Porter, C., Palmier-Claus, J., Branitsky, A. et al. (2020). Childhood adversity and borderline personality disorder: a meta-analysis. *Acta Psychiatrica Scandinavica* 141 (1): 6–20. https://doi.org/10.1111/APs.13118. PMID: 31630389.
5. Sweeney, A., Filson, B., Kennedy, A. et al. (2018). A paradigm shift: relationships in trauma-informed mental health services. *BJPsych Advances.* 24 (5): 319–333. https://doi.org/10.1192/bja.2018.29.

6. Blackie, I.R. (2023). Posttraumatic stress and psychological impacts of human wildlife conflict on victims, their families and caretakers in Botswana. *Human Dimensions of Wildlife* 28 (3): 248–264.
7. The National Child Traumatic Stress Network (2016). *Is it ADHD or Child Traumatic Stress? A Guide for Clinicians*. Los Angeles, CA & Durham, NC: National Centre for Child Traumatic Stress.
8. Benjet, C., Bromet, E., Karam, E.G. et al. (2016). The epidemiology of traumatic event exposure worldwide: results from the World Mental Health Survey Consortium. *Psychological Medicine* 46 (2): 327–343. https://doi.org/10.1017/S0033291715001981.
9. Emsley, E., Smith, J., Martin, D. et al. (2022). Trauma-informed care in the UK: where are we? A qualitative study of health policies and professional perspectives. *BMC Health Services Research* 22: 1164. https://doi.org/10.1186/s12913-022-08461-w.
10. Zarubin, V.C., Gupta, T., and Mittal, V.A. (2023). History of trauma is a critical treatment target for individuals at clinical high-risk for psychosis. *Frontiers in Psychiatry* 13: 1102464. https://doi.org/10.3389/fpsyt.2022.1102464.
11. Sacchi, L., Merzhvynska, M., and Augsburger, M. (2020). Effects of cumulative trauma load on long-term trajectories of life satisfaction and health in a population-based study. *BMC Public Health* 20: 1–1.
12. Downey, C. and Crummy, A. (2022). The impact of childhood trauma on children's wellbeing and adult behavior. *European Journal of Trauma & Dissociation* 6 (1): 100237.
13. Bowlby, J. (1988). *A Secure Base: Parent-Child Attachment and Healthy Human Development*. Basic Books.
14. Shaver, P. and Mikulincer, M. (2002). Attachment related psychodynamics. *Attachment & Human Development* 4 (2): 133–161.
15. Luther, S., Ciccetti, D., and Becker, B. (2000). The construct of resilience: a critical evaluation and guidelines for future work. *Child Development* 71 (3): 543–562.
16. Hughes, K., Bellis, M., Hardcastle, K. et al. (2017). The effect of multiple adverse childhood experiences on health: a systematic review and meta-analysis. *The Lancet Public Health* 2: 356–366.
17. Gilgoff, R., Singh, L., Koita, K. et al. (2020). Adverse childhood experiences, outcomes, and interventions. *Pediatric Clinics* 67 (2): 259–273.
18. Kumari, R. and Mukhopadhyay, A. (2020). Psychological trauma and resulting physical illness: a review. *SIS Journal of Projective Psychology and Mental Health* 27 (2): 98–104.
19. Simms, P. (2022). Psychological trauma. In: *ABC of Major Trauma: Rescue, Resuscitation with Imaging, and Rehabilitation*, 5th ed. (ed. P. Driscoll, D. Skinner, and P. Goode), 259. Wiley-Blackwell.
20. Updegraff, J. and Taylor, S. (2021). From vulnerability to growth: positive and negative effects of stressful life events. In: *Loss and Trauma* (ed. J. Harvey and E. Miller), 3–28. Routledge.
21. Kleshchova, O. and Weierich, M. (2022). The neurobiology of stress. In: *Biopsychosocial Factors of Stress, and Mindfulness for Stress Reduction* (ed. H. Hazlett-Stevens), 17–65. Cham: Springer International Publishing.
22. Spytska, L. (2003). Psychological trauma and its impact on a person's life prospects. *Scientific Bulletin of Mukachevo State University. Series "Pedagogy and Psychology"* 9 (3): 82–90.
23. Ford, J., Grasso, D., Elhai, J., and Courtois, C. (2015). Social, cultural, and other diversity issues in the traumatic stress field. *Posttraumatic Stress Disorder* 503–546. https://doi.org/10.1016/B978.0-12-801288-8.00011-X.
24. Labrague, L.J. (2021). Psychological resilience, coping behaviours and social support among health care workers during the COVID-19 pandemic: a systematic review of quantitative studies. *Journal of Nursing Management* 29 (7): 1893–1905. https://doi.org/10.1111/jonm.13336. PMID: 33843087; PMCID: PMC8250179.

25. Ungar, M. and Theron, L. (2020). Resilience and mental health: how multisystemic processes contribute to positive outcomes. *Lancet Psychiatry* 7 (5): 441–448. https://doi.org/10.1016/S2215-0366(19)30434-1. PMID: 31806473.
26. Office for Health Improvements & Disparities (2022). Working definition of trauma-informed practice. GOV.UK. https://www.gov.uk/government/publications/working-definition-of-trauma-informed-practice/working-definition-of-trauma-informed-practice
27. Jones, N., Gius, B.K., Shields, M. et al. (2021). Investigating the impact of involuntary psychiatric hospitalization on youth and young adult trust and help-seeking in pathways to care. *Social Psychiatry and Psychiatric Epidemiology* 56 (11): 2017–2027.
28. PettyJohn, M., Kynn, J., Anderson, G., and McCauley, H. (2023). Secondary institutional betrayal: implications for observing mistreatment of sexual assault survivors secondhand. *Journal of Interpersonal Violence* 38 (17–18): 10127–10149. https://doi.org/10.1177/08862605231171414.
29. Dewa, L., Broyd, J., Hira, R. et al. (2023). A service evaluation of passive remote monitoring technology for patients in a high-secure forensic psychiatric hospital: a qualitative study. *BMC Psychiatry* 23 (1): 946. https://doi.org/10.1186/s12888-023-05437-w.
30. Malcolm, R., Shore, J., Stainthorpe, A. et al. (2022). Economic evaluation of a vision-based patient monitoring and management system in addition to standard care for adults admitted to psychiatric intensive care units. *England, Journal of Medical Economics* 25 (1): 1101–1109. https://doi.org/10.1080/13696998.2022.2120719.
31. Rethink (2023). https://www.rethink.org/news-and-stories/media-centre/2023/11/our-position-on-oxevision-the-new-monitoring-system-in-mental-health-units/
32. StopOxevision (2024). https://stopoxevision.com/2024/02/27/actions-are-stronger-than-words-we-raised-our-concerns-now-its-time-for-decision-makers-to-take-action/
33. NHS (2019). Long term plan. https://www.longtermplan.nhs.uk/.
34. Nikopaschos, F., Burrell, G., Clark, J., and Salgueiro, A. (2023). Trauma-informed care on mental health wards: the impact of power threat meaning framework team formulation and psychological stabilisation on self-harm and restrictive interventions. *Frontiers in Psychology* 8 (14): 1145100. https://doi.org/10.3389/fpsyg.2023.1145100.
35. Greenwald, A., Kelly, A., and Thomas, L. (2023). Trauma-informed care in the emergency department: concepts and recommendations for integrating practices into emergency medicine. *Medical Education Online* 28 (1): 2178366. https://doi.org/10.1080/10872981.2023.2178366.
36. Hearn, E. (2023). Improving women's health and female equity at a secure unit. *Nursing Times* 119 (12): 40–41.
37. Jo's Cervical Cancer Trust (2018). Three quarters of sexual violence survivors feel unable to go for potentially life-saving test. http://jostrust.org.uk. (accessed 7 November 2023).
38. Manz, C. (2021). Disparities in cancer prevalence, incidence, and mortality for incarcerated and formerly incarcerated patients: a scoping review. *Cancer Medicine* 10 (20): 7277–7288.
39. Center for Substance Abuse Treatment (US). Trauma-Informed Care in Behavioral Health Services. Rockville (MD): Substance Abuse and Mental Health Services Administration (US); 2014. Report No.: (SMA) 14-4816. PMID: 24901203. https://pubmed.ncbi.nlm.nih.gov/24901203/.
40. Tol, W.A., Barbui, C., and van Ommeren, M. (2013). Management of acute stress, PTSD, and bereavement: WHO recommendations. *Journal of the American Medical Association* 310 (5): 477–478. https://doi.org/10.1001/jama.2013.166723.

41. International Society for Traumatic Stress Studies (2024). Clinical resources. https://istss.org/clinical-resources

42. The National Child Traumatic Stress Network (2023). Complex trauma screening and assessments. https://www.nctsn.org/what-is-child-trauma/trauma-types/complex-trauma/screening-and-assessment

43. Marshall, D., Quinn, C., and Child, S. (2016). What IAPT services can learn from those who do not attend. *Journal of Mental Health* 25: 410–415.

44. Newland, R., Lawrence, M., Tyndall, S., and Waterall, J. (2022). Vulnerability and trauma-informed practice: What nurses need to know. *British Journal of Nursing*. Mark Allen Publishing 31 (12): 660–662. https://doi.org/10.12.68/bjon.2022.31.12.660.

45. Rosen, V. and Ayers, G. (2020). An update on the complexity and importance of accurately diagnosing post-traumatic stress disorder and comorbid traumatic brain injury. *Neuroscience Insights* 15. https://doi.org/10.1177/2633105520907895.

46. Campbell, K., Clarke, K., Massey, D., and Lakeman, R. (2020). Borderline personality disorder: to diagnose or not to diagnose? That is the question. *International Journal of Mental Health Nuraing* 29. https://doi.org/10.1111/inm.12737.

47. World Health Organisation (2025). ICD11 – Mortality and morbidity statistics. http://icd.who.int/browse11/I-m/en#/http://id.who.int/icd/entity/207069980

48. NHS England (2023). A national framework to deliver improved outcomes in all-age autism assessment pathways: guidance for integrated care boards. https://www.england.nhs.uk/long-read/a-national-framework-to-deliver-improved-outcomes-in-all-age-autism-assessment-pathways-guidance-for-integrated-care-boards/

49. Cloitre, M., Garvert, D., Weiss, B. et al. (2014). Distinguishing PTSD, complex PTSD, and borderline personality disorder: a latent class analysis. *European Journal of Psychotraumatology* 15: 5. https://doi.org/10.3402/ejpt.v5.25097.

50. Frías, Á. and Palma, C. (2015). Comorbidity between post-traumatic stress disorder and borderline personality disorder: a review. *Psychopathology* 48 (1): 1–10. https://doi.org/10.1159/000363145.

51. Hoover, D.W. (2020). Trauma in children with neurodevelopmental disorders: autism, intellectual disability, and attention-deficit/hyperactivity disorder. In: *Childhood Trauma in Mental Disorders* (ed. G. Spalletta, D. Janiri, F. Piras, and G. Sani). Cham: Springer. https://doi.org/10.1007/978-3-030-49414-8_17.

52. Haruvi-Lamdan, N., Horesh, D., Zohar, S. et al. (2020). Autism spectrum disorder and post-traumatic stress disorder: an unexplored co-occurrence of conditions. *Autism* 24 (4): 884–898. https://doi.org/10.1177/1362361320912143.

53. Ravn, S. and Andersen, T. (2020). Exploring the relationship between post traumatic stress and chronic pain. *Psychiatric Times* 37 (11): 19.

54. Gasperi, M., Afari, N., Goldberg, J. et al. (2021). Pain and trauma: the role of criterion a trauma and stressful life events in the pain and PTSD relationship. *The Journal of Pain* 22 (11): 1506–1517. https://doi.org/10.1016/j.jpain.2021.04.015.

55. Asmundson, G.J., Coons, M.J., Taylor, S., and Katz, J. (2002). PTSD and the experience of pain: research and clinical implications of shared vulnerability and mutual maintenance models. *Canadian Journal of Psychiatry* 47 (10): 930–937. https://doi.org/10.1177/070674370204701004.

56. Murphy, J.L., Driscoll, M.A., Odom, A.S., and Hadlandsmyth, K. (2022). Posttraumatic stress disorder and chronic pain. *PTSD Research Quarterly* 33 (2): ISSN: 1050-1835. https://www.ptsd.va.gov/publications/rq_docs/V33N2.pdf.
57. Beck, J.G. and Clapp, J.D. (2011). A different kind of co-morbidity: understanding posttraumatic stress disorder and chronic pain. *Psychological Trauma* 3 (2): 101–108. https://doi.org/10.1037/a0021263.
58. National Institute of Clinical Excellence (2018). NICE Guideline [NG116]. Post-traumatic stress disorder. https://www.nice.org.uk/guidance/ng116
59. American Academy of Child & Adolescent Psychiatry (2024). Post-traumatic stress disorder (PTSD). https://www.aacap.org/AACAP/Families_and_Youth/Glossary_of_Symptoms_and_Illnesses/Post_Traumatic_Stress_Disorder_PTSD.aspx
60. American Psychological Association (2020). Summary of recommendations of the APA guideline development panel for the treatment of PTSD. https://www.apa.org/ptsd-guideline/treatments
61. Cohen, J.A. and Mannarino, A.P. (2015). Trauma-focused cognitive Behavior therapy for traumatized children and families. *Child Adolescent Psychiatry Clinical North America* 24 (3): 557–570. https://doi.org/10.1016/j.chc.2015.02.005.
62. Smith, P., Perrin, S., Yule, W., and Clark, D. (2010). *Post traumatic stress disorder: cognitive therapy with children and young people*. New York: Routledge.
63. EMDR Centre London (2024). Creation of EMDR. https://emdr-centre-london.org/emdr-method/creation-of-emdr/
64. Shapiro, F. (2018). *Eye Movement Desensitization and Reprocessing Therapy: Basic Principles, Protocols, and Procedures*, 3rd ed. New York, NY: The Guilford Press.
65. Bamalan, O., Moore, M., and Al Khalili, Y. (2024). Physiology, serotonin. In: *StatPearls*. Treasure Island: StatPearls Publishing. https://www.ncbi.nlm.nih.gov/books/NBK545168/.
66. Süß, S.T., Olbricht, L.M., Herlitze, S. et al. (2022). Constitutive 5-HT2C receptor knock-out facilitates fear extinction through altered activity of a dorsal raphe-bed nucleus of the stria terminalis pathway. *Translational Psychiatry* 12: 487. https://doi.org/10.1038/s41398-022-02252-x.
67. Murrough, J., Czermak, C., Henry, S. et al. (2011). The effect of early trauma exposure on serotonin type 1B receptor expression revealed by reduced selective radioligand binding. *Archives of General Psychiatry* 68 (9): 892–900. https://doi.org/10.1001/archgenpsychiatry.2011.91.
68. Smith, L., Bragg-Underwood, T., and Spencer, C.W. (2016). Practice matters: red flags in adults with mental illnesses. *International Journal of Faith Community Nursing* 2 (2): 5. http://digitalcommons.wku.edu/ijfcn/vol2/iss2/5.
69. Björkenstam, C. and Björkenstam, E. (2017). Childhood adversity and risk of suicide: cohort study of 548,721 adolescents and young adults in Sweden. *BMJ* 257: j1334.
70. Department of Health and Social Care (2009). Best practice in managing risk: the assessment and management of risk to self and others in mental health services. GOV.UK.
71. Firmin, C. (2020). *Contextual Safeguarding and Child Protection: Rewriting the Rules*, 1ste. Routledge. https://doi.org/10.4324/9780429283314.
72. Dheensa, S., McLindon, E., Spencer, C. et al. (2023). Healthcare professionals' own experiences of domestic violence and abuse: a meta-analysis of prevalence and systematic review of risk markers and consequences. *Trauma, Violence & Abuse* 24 (3): 1282–1299. https://doi.org/10.1177/152483802110.1771.

73. Kim, J., Chesworth, B., Franchino-Olsen, H., and Macy, R.J. (2022). A scoping review of vicarious trauma interventions for service providers working with people who have experienced traumatic events. *Trauma, Violence & Abuse 23* (5): 1437–1460. https://doi.org/10.1177/1524838021991310.

74. Rauvola, R.S., Vega, D.M., and Lavigne, K.N. (2019). Compassion fatigue, secondary traumatic stress, and vicarious traumatizati: a qualitative review and research agenda. *Occupational Health Science* 3: 297–336. https://doi.org/10.1007/s41542-019-00045-1.

75. British Medical Association (2024). Vicarious trauma: signs and strategies for coping. BMA. https://www.bma.org.uk/advice-and-support/your-wellbeing/vicarious-trauma/vicarious-trauma-signs-and-strategies-for-coping (accessed 8 August 2024).

76. Hearn, E. and Brittin, K. (2023). Trauma-informed care at a forensic mental health ward. *Nursing Times* 119: 12.

CHAPTER 8

Psychopharmacology for Advanced Practice

Diksha Kara[1] and Masuma Tashnim Hussain[2]

[1] East London NHS Foundation Trust, London, UK
[2] Southwest London and St George's Mental Health NHS Trust, London, UK

Aim

This chapter aims to provide advanced mental health practitioners with a thorough understanding of psychopharmacology and evidence-based practice. It covers essential pharmacological principles and practical aspects of prescribing and managing psychotropic medications. By the end of this chapter, practitioners will be better prepared to make informed decisions and enhance patient care.

LEARNING OUTCOMES

After reading this chapter, the reader will be able to:

1. Have an understanding of key principles of pharmacodynamics and pharmacokinetics with emphasis on psychotropic medications.
2. Understand the importance of evidence-based practice and critically appraising sources.
3. Have developed awareness about the impact of psychotropic medications on physical health and health inequalities across different populations.
4. Demonstrate understanding of key principles of prescribing including off-label and unlicensed medication use

This chapter embodies the following competences within the curriculum and capabilities framework of advanced practice in mental health [1] (see Table 8.1):

The Advanced Practitioner in Mental Health, First Edition. Edited by Clare Allabyrne.
© 2026 John Wiley & Sons Ltd. All rights reserved, including rights for text and data mining and training of artificial intelligence technologies or similar technologies. Published 2026 by John Wiley & Sons Ltd.

TABLE 8.1 How this chapter meets the APMH curriculum and capabilities framework.

Pillar of practice	Learning outcomes
Clinical practice	1. Work autonomously within professional, ethical codes and legal frameworks, being responsible and accountable for their decisions, actions and omissions at this level of practice. 2. Demonstrate the underpinning psychological, biological and social knowledge required for advanced practice in mental health. 3. Utilise clinical reasoning and decision-making skills to make a differential diagnosis and provide rationales for person-management plans, through critically reflecting on and evaluating their own role in relation to challenging traditional practices, new ways of working and the impact upon the multidisciplinary team. 4. Initiate, evaluate and modify a range of interventions, which may include therapies, medicines, lifestyle advice and care.
Leadership and management	1. Exercise high-level professional judgement and advanced leadership skills to effectively promote safety in the presence of uncertainty, complexity and unpredictability.
Education	1. Effectively utilise a range of evidence-based educational strategies/interventions to support person-centred care with individuals, their families and carers and other healthcare colleagues.
Research	1. Critically appraise and apply the evidence base in influencing engagement, recovery, shared decision-making, transference and safeguarding.

INTRODUCTION

The term 'psychopharmacology' refers to the study of the effects of substances such as medications and recreational drugs on the mind, emotions and behaviour of individuals [2]. This differs from the term 'pharmacology', in that it focuses particularly on the effect of substances on the mind. However, many terms and concepts are similar to both. Numerous resources focus on the psychopharmacology of individual drugs or classes of drugs. However, there will be an attempt to focus on pharmacology concepts within this chapter that can be useful to readers who do not diagnose or prescribe medications, as well as those who may do so, and for a variety of different scenarios.

History

Though many pharmacological treatment options are available today, in the early days of psychiatry, physical treatments were used with the aim to either directly modify pathophysiological processes or provide symptomatic relief through significant psychological impact [3]. Treatments such as chains, spinning chairs and warm continuous baths were examples of the latter form of treatment and were often based on antiquated theories about the origins of mental illness [3]. Conversely, electroconvulsive therapy (ECT), an example of the former approach of 'physical treatment', is considered an effective intervention today, having first been introduced in 1938 [3].

As early as 4000 BC, references are found to the effects of the poppy plant on a person's mind (euphoria), and in 1832, chloral hydrate (a sedative) was discovered [4]. The first substances discovered, such as opiates, resulted in sedative and seemingly 'calming' effects, as opposed to true treatment of psychiatric illnesses. The insulin coma treatment, developed in 1932, became a widespread intervention despite commonly occurring serious adverse effects [3]. The popularity of this treatment declined due to increasing criticism that insulin coma therapy was no more effective than sedation induced by barbiturates, coupled with the introduction of chlorpromazine in the 1950s [3].

Eventually, substances were found to treat the conditions, rather than solely managing its symptoms. Examples include the discovery of amphetamines in 1941, used to treat hyperactivity in children; lithium in 1949, used to treat mood disorders; and chlorpromazine in 1952, used to treat schizophrenia [3]. We now have an expanded range of medications available to treat various psychiatric conditions. There are different first-line treatments for different conditions based on guidelines from the National Institute of Clinical Excellence (NICE) and other evidence-based sources. To effectively understand these treatment guidelines and their basis, it is essential to be able to interpret the underlying evidence base.

AN OVERVIEW OF PHARMACOLOGY

Pharmacodynamics and Pharmacokinetics

Key concepts discussed when covering pharmacology of medications are its pharmacodynamics and pharmacokinetics. Pharmacodynamics refers to the study of how drugs affect the body – by understanding the mechanisms of action, physiological and biochemical effects and the relationship between dose or concentration and effect [5, 6]. However, to fully comprehend the effects of a drug, it is also crucial to understand its pharmacokinetics, which primarily pertains to how the drug is absorbed, distributed, metabolised and excreted within the body [7]. These topics are very broad, and it is difficult to cover the vast material present on pharmacodynamics and pharmacokinetics; therefore, only key terms and subjects are discussed next.

Within the topic of pharmacodynamics, drug binding within the body is considered and terms such as agonist, antagonist and partial agonist are often used. An agonist drug is a substance that mimics the effects of an endogenous ligand (such as a neurotransmitter or hormone) in the body, and, by binding to a receptor, it triggers a biological response [8]. An example of this is benzodiazepines [5]. This differs from an antagonist, which typically hinders the binding of other ligands by occupying the receptor site without activating it – an example being naloxone [5, 9]. Drugs can also function as partial agonists, meaning they operate in a similar manner to agonists, but their effects are capped, resulting in a partial response at the receptor site [10]. An example of a partial agonist is buprenorphine [5].

There are various types of receptors in the body that facilitate drug binding, along with other target sites such as enzymes and proteins [5]. Once a drug binds, it can elicit a range of effects, including stimulating hormone secretion, decreasing electrical signals or influencing the synthesis of new proteins. Often in practice, we understand that as we increase the dose of a drug, it is likely the effects of the drug will also increase (including side effects). This is commonly studied, and it is understood that drugs will reach a point at which additional increases do not yield further therapeutic benefits and may instead lead to adverse effects for patients. This is often referred to as the E_{max} [5, 11]. The EC_{50} is also often taken into account, referring to the drug concentration at which 50% of the maximum effect is achieved. This measure can be helpful when comparing drugs as a drug with a lower EC_{50} is regarded as more potent [11].

In practice, it is frequently observed that patients exhibit varied responses to medications and require different dosages. This variability may be attributed to differences in pharmacodynamic factors, which can be influenced by genetic makeup and age, and pharmacokinetic factors. Pharmacokinetics first considers how a drug may be absorbed systemically into the body, i.e. how does the drug after it has been taken orally (or inhaled, applied, etc.) make its way through the body and enter into plasma [12]. This process may entail a portion of the drug being 'lost' along the way. For instance, during absorption, the drug may decompose within the gastrointestinal lumen or may be influenced by enzymes present in the gastrointestinal tract [13]. Most psychotropic medications tend to be lipophilic (fat soluble), thus are easy to absorb via the gut [3]. The bioavailability of drugs refers to the extent to which the administered drug is present in systemic circulation. This parameter is influenced by various factors for orally administered medications, including gastric acidity, digestive enzymes and processes involving the gut or liver (commonly referred to as first-pass metabolism). As a result, a portion of the medication may be lost by the time it enters systemic circulation. For medications given intravenously, the bioavailability is assumed to be 100%, i.e. all of the administered medication is available systemically [14]. Other factors affecting bioavailability include age, sex, genetic factors, psychological stress, medical conditions such as malabsorption syndromes, levels of physical activity, interactions with other medications and history of gastrointestinal surgery [15].

Drug distribution refers to the process by which a medication is transported throughout the body, from the circulation to the target tissues. This process is influenced by the properties of the drug; for instance, its molecular structure determines whether it is fat-soluble or water-soluble, which in turn affects its movement from the circulation into tissues. Lipophilic drugs, in particular, diffuse more readily across the blood–brain barrier [16]. As the drug travels to its target site, it can bind to proteins, reducing the quantity of 'free' drug available to exert its intended effects at the target site (e.g. receptors). Therefore, it is crucial to consider conditions that may influence protein binding, such as hypoalbuminemia, renal failure and drug interactions [17]. In instances where protein binding is reduced, there is an increased availability of 'free' drug that can exert its effects at the target site; however, this may also lead to additional adverse effects and toxicity [14]. Textbooks and reference sources frequently refer to a drug's volume of distribution as an indicator of the drug's distribution within the body. This term pertains to the volume of fluid required to dilute the drug at the administered dose in order to achieve the desired plasma concentration [18]. This provides insight into whether the drug tends to remain in plasma or is distributed to other tissues within the body. Consequently, a drug with a high volume of distribution is more likely to disseminate to other tissues, meaning patients may require higher doses of the medication to achieve a sufficient plasma concentration for efficacy [19]. Patient factors, including age and pregnancy, can influence the volume of distribution of drugs. Furthermore, the characteristics of the drug itself can impact its protein binding and thus, its volume of distribution. For instance, more basic drugs, in terms of their pH, such as amphetamines, are absorbed more readily by the body's tissues, resulting in a higher volume of distribution [18]. Once distributed, and following first-pass metabolism, the drug undergoes further metabolism that enhances its water solubility, facilitating detoxification and excretion from the body [20]. Such biotransformation occurs in the liver as part of phase I (modification), phase II (conjugation) or phase III (additional modification and excretion) reactions [21]. In phase I reactions, a water-soluble and often active metabolite is produced, while in phase II, conjugation with endogenous groups may occur, resulting in the formation of soluble inactive compounds to facilitate excretion. Phase III involves further metabolism and excretion as necessary [22]. An example of a psychotropic drug producing active metabolites is diazepam which produces nordiazepam, temazepam and oxazepam through metabolic processes [23]. The cytochrome P450 (CYP450) system comprises a group of enzymes that are frequently engaged in various metabolic processes. The majority of these enzymes are located in the liver, although they can also be found in other tissues, including the intestines and kidneys [24]. Certain medications are known to either inhibit or induce CYP450 enzymes, impacting the metabolism of other substances and leading to drug–drug interactions. For instance, fluoxetine is a strong inhibitor of the CYP2D6 enzyme, which consequently decreases the metabolism of drugs that are processed by this enzyme. This reduction can result in an increased availability of other medications that are substrates of CYP2D6 [25]. Another psychotropic medication, carbamazepine, serves as an inducer of certain CYP enzymes, including CYP3A4. Consequently, it can accelerate the metabolism of any substrates that are processed by this enzyme and diminish the effectiveness of such medications. These interactions can be checked using the British National Formulary (BNF) [26]. It is essential to document any substances the patient may be using, including medications prescribed for physical health conditions and recreational substances, as these may cause inhibition or induction of certain enzymes.

Once drugs are rendered more hydrophilic through metabolic processes, they can be excreted from the body through the kidneys, liver or other pathways, including the lungs and various bodily fluids such as sweat, tears or reproductive fluids [7]. Drug elimination is influenced by both drug-related factors (such as polarity, water solubility and size) and patient-related factors (including comorbidities, genetic variations, etc.) [27]. The liver has the ability to secrete certain drugs into bile, depending on their molecular weight and polarity. This process allows for the potential elimination of the drug in faeces or its reabsorption from the intestine [27, 28]. The kidneys excrete the majority of drugs via either passive (glomerular filtration) or active (tubular secretion) processes, which depend on various factors such as the size of the drug, its protein-binding characteristics and the pH of the urine [29].

The aforementioned describes key processes of absorption, distribution, metabolism and excretion which are often mentioned when discussing pharmacokinetics. Another crucial concept commonly addressed is the half-life ($t_{1/2}$) of a drug, defined as the time taken for the plasma concentration of the drug to decrease by fifty percent. It is essential to acknowledge that the half-life of a medication is also affected by factors such as age, interactions with concomitant medications and comorbidities, including hepatic and renal dysfunction [30]. The half-life of a drug, along with its dosing schedule, both influence the time required to achieve steady state – the point at which the drug concentration remains stable, meaning that the drug's rate of entry into the plasma equals its rate of clearance. For most drugs administered at intervals equal to their half-life, steady state is typically reached after about five half-lives. However, this may not hold true for drugs with extended half-lives, such as diazepam, which is further complicated by the formation of active metabolites, as previously discussed [31].

Special Considerations

Certain patient populations need additional consideration when evaluating treatment options. These groups include paediatric patients, the elderly, individuals who are pregnant or breastfeeding and those with renal or hepatic impairments. Furthermore, specific psychotropic medications are classified as higher risk, including anticholinergic agents in elderly or frail patients, morphine and other opioids, benzodiazepines, lithium, valproate and clozapine [32]. Certain workplaces or trusts may also include additional medications beyond those specified; this may be based on local prescribing practices, data or in response to local error reports.

Children

Children and adolescents are usually defined as being under the age of 18 years old; however, consideration should be given to body weight and licensing when considering medications. Key pharmacokinetic differences exist between children and adults. Firstly, the absorption of medications is influenced by shorter intestinal transit times in young children. In newborns, variations in gastric pH, bile secretion and intestinal permeability further impact medication absorption, thereby affecting drug plasma concentrations. Distribution is also influenced by the fact that children exhibit varying volumes of distribution (which depend on the specific drug) compared to adults, contingent upon factors such as the child's age, protein binding and body composition (including fat and water levels). Depending on the different pathways/enzymes available, metabolism can be affected in children. Children may exhibit increased rates of hepatic clearance due to higher hepatic blood flow compared to adults. Renal excretion is typically reduced in newborns; however, in infants, renal excretion is often comparable to or greater than that of adults. [33]. It is essential to take such factors into account when evaluating treatment options for paediatric patients. Additionally, the formulation of the medication should be considered, as well as the ease of administration for carers, which may be influenced by the drug's palatability [34]. The drug dosages should be verified in accordance with the BNF and the manufacturer's guidelines, taking into consideration factors such as body weight and age. While medications should be prescribed in alignment with their marketing authorisation, it is acknowledged that the informed use of unlicensed medications may be necessary for paediatric patients [35].

Older Adults

There can be some debate regarding at what age patients are defined as older adults, with some services defining this as over 75 years of age. However, pharmacokinetic alterations can be seen earlier such as renal function declining by 35% by the age of 65 [36]. Furthermore, there is reduced first-pass metabolism, decreased renal clearance and reduced hepatic oxidative metabolism, all of which may influence the pharmacological effects of certain medications. Additionally, hepatic clearance may be impaired due to a decrease in liver mass [37, 38]. People in this group often develop additional comorbidities and complexities that can lead to drug–drug and drug–disease interactions. Furthermore, with advancing age, patients typically exhibit an increase in body fat and a decrease in total body water, which can influence the pharmacokinetics of drugs based on their lipid and water solubility profiles. In the elderly population, decreased serum albumin levels are observed, which impacts the protein binding of drugs, consequently elevating the free concentration of drugs that are predominantly protein-bound, such as phenytoin [38]. As individuals age, pharmacodynamic changes can occur due to variations in neurotransmitter concentrations, receptor activity, hormonal changes and increased permeability of the blood–brain barrier. For instance, elderly patients may experience increased sedation or extrapyramidal side effects (EPSEs) from antipsychotic medications, which often leads to recommendations for lower dosages [20]. Patients with dementia are at a higher risk for weight loss, which consequently leads to a decrease in muscle mass and albumin levels, thereby impacting drug protein binding. In this patient cohort, the permeability of the blood–brain barrier is also increased, which can heighten the likelihood of adverse effects, particularly in the context of reduced acetylcholine levels [20]. Numerous tools exist to assess the anticholinergic burden of medications, and some can provide guidance on when clinicians should consider reviewing, switching or discontinuing a medication [39]. Clinicians may utilise tools such as Screening Tool of Older Persons Prescriptions (STOPP)/Screening Tool to Alert to Right Treatment (START) to optimise medication regimens for geriatric patients and should also consider modifying medication formulations in the event of any swallowing difficulties [40].

Pregnancy and Breastfeeding

In patients who may be pregnant, a thorough evaluation of the risk versus benefit of medication prescribing is essential. This assessment should involve detailed discussions with the patient and be informed by the latest evidence. Whenever feasible, it is advisable to avoid the use of medications during the first trimester, as this period is associated with the highest risk of teratogenic effects, including malformations. For certain medications, risks may persist into the second or third trimester, potentially impacting foetal growth. Additionally, some medications can pose risks during labour or shortly before delivery, including neonatal withdrawal effects in the infant [41]. The risks associated with each medication must be evaluated on an individual basis, as their effects can vary depending on the different stages of pregnancy. Whenever feasible, the minimum effective dose should be used, and polypharmacy should be minimised [42]. Certain medications are essential for the development of the baby during pregnancy, such as thyroid medication. Additionally, pregnancy can influence pharmacokinetics; for instance, gastrointestinal transit time may be prolonged, there is a reduction in plasma proteins and an increase in plasma volume, all of which affect the volume of distribution of drugs [43]. Clinicians should also evaluate the risk associated with prescribing medications, such as valproate, in cis gender male patients who may potentially father children [44].

When evaluating pharmacological options for patients who are breastfeeding, it is essential to assess the potential quantity of the medication that may be transferred to the infant and the possible implications for their health. Numerous medications lack specific licensing for administration to breastfeeding patients. Ideally, mothers should be supported in breastfeeding whenever feasible, and a thorough discussion regarding the benefits and risks associated with medication use during lactation should be had with the patient. Critical considerations include the necessity of the medication, the age of the infant, the volume of breastmilk ingested by the infant and the pharmacological properties of the drug. Typically, medications that are highly protein-bound, exhibit a low plasma-to-milk ratio (indicating reduced transfer to breastmilk) and possess a short half-life are favoured for use in breastfeeding women [45].

PHARMACOGENOMICS

Advancements in technology may enable us, in the future, to optimise medication regimens based on an individual's genomic profile. Numerous studies have assessed the outcomes of implementing pharmacogenetic testing in patients. A meta-analysis indicated that patients treated with antidepressants following pharmacogenetic testing exhibited higher remission rates for major depressive disorders compared to those who did not undergo such testing [46]. Pharmacogenetic testing has also helped with reducing adverse effects related to treatment [47]. Through pharmacogenetic testing, patients have been identified to exhibit varying rates of metabolism mediated by different cytochrome (CYP) enzymes. For instance, individuals may be classified as ultra-rapid metabolisers, indicating a significantly elevated rate of drug metabolism, or as poor metabolisers, characterised by a slower metabolic rate. The rate of metabolism can influence the therapeutic efficacy of medications, potentially leading to suboptimal drug responses, or it may increase the risk of adverse effects. Numerous psychotropic medications are subject to these genetic variations, including antipsychotics such as aripiprazole, antidepressants such as citalopram and other pharmacological agents such as atomoxetine, which is a non-stimulant medication used to treat attention deficit hyperactivity disorder (ADHD) [48]. Although such testing is currently not accessible via the NHS, it is essential to ensure that clinicians are aware about the variations in medication response and tolerability due to genetic differences.

A Quick Summary of Receptor Sites and Their Actions

Table 8.2 serves as a guide, identifying certain neurotransmitters (receptor sites) that may be targeted by medications, which can include agonists, antagonists or partial agonists. It is important to note that this table is not exhaustive. Additionally, some drugs may influence multiple receptor sites, and the neurotransmitter they affect may, in turn, impact the levels of other neurotransmitters within the

TABLE 8.2 Summary of function and adverse effects of neurotransmitters [49–63].

Neurotransmitter	Possible therapeutic benefit	Possible associated adverse effects
Serotonin	Regulation of mood, anxiety, emotions and sleep cycles, with effects on blood pressure and gastrointestinal function.	Excessive serotonin levels may lead to symptoms such as nausea or vomiting, appetite suppression, sleep disturbances, sexual dysfunction and headaches. Conversely, insufficient serotonin levels may impact mood, resulting in low mood, and can also lead to poor sleep quality.
Noradrenaline	Regulation of sleep, concentration, emotion and motivation, with an impact on blood pressure, heart rate and respiration.	Excessive levels of noradrenaline may lead to symptoms such as jitteriness, anxiety, chest pain, increased sweating, irritability and poor sleep quality. Additionally, it can elevate blood pressure and heart rate. Conversely, insufficient levels of noradrenaline may result in dizziness, drowsiness and low mood.
Dopamine	Functions across various pathways in the brain, influencing muscle movement, emotions, reward, behaviour, pleasure, appetite, motivation, planning and prolactin levels.	Insufficient dopamine in one pathway may lead to muscle stiffness, as observed in Parkinson's disease. In another pathway, a reduction of dopamine can result in an increase in prolactin, which impacts menstruation and lactation. Conversely, excessive dopamine in another pathway can lead to alterations in perception, such as those seen with positive symptoms of schizophrenia or hallucinations associated with mania or psychosis. High levels of dopamine may also induce feelings of euphoria in some patients. Additionally, in yet another pathway, a deficiency of dopamine can result in negative symptoms, including apathy, anhedonia and cognitive impairments.
Acetylcholine	Regulation of memory and arousal with an impact on the muscles of the body.	Anticholinergics have the ability to inhibit acetylcholine, potentially leading to symptoms such as dry mouth, blurred vision, constipation, urinary retention, fatigue, impaired concentration and confusion.
Histamine	Regulates sleep and exerts an influence on the immune system.	Excessive histamine levels can lead to sedation and may contribute to weight gain in certain patients. Additionally, it is associated with inflammation within the body.
Glutamate	This is an excitatory neurotransmitter in the brain that can influence memory, cognition and mood.	An excess of glutamate in certain networks may lead to anxiety, psychosis or seizures, while a deficiency of glutamate may result in excessive sedation.
GABA	This is an inhibitory neurotransmitter that may induce a calming or relaxing effect.	Excessive amounts may lead to oversedation or forgetfulness, while insufficient amounts could result in restlessness and anxiety.

body (for example, dopamine and prolactin). Therefore, for the mechanism of action, adverse effects and indications of specific medications, it is advised to consult the manufacturer's information, BNF or other relevant resources.

Interpreting the Evidence Base

It is important to recognise that the evidence presented in journal articles can take various forms, including personal expert opinions, case studies, observational studies, randomised controlled trials and systematic reviews, among others. Figure 8.1 illustrates this concept using a pyramid structure, with systematic reviews positioned at the apex, signifying the superior reliability and quality of evidence [54, 55]. Such evidence is accessible through numerous databases, including the Cochrane Database of Systematic Reviews, EMBASE, MEDLINE/PubMed, CINAHL and prominent medical journals such as the *British Medical Journal* and *JAMA Psychiatry*, among others [56–61].

It is important to conduct a thorough appraisal of the evidence, when conducting literature searches. Different types of studies, such as qualitative research, randomised controlled trials and systematic reviews, necessitate distinct critical appraisal techniques. Many colleagues have found the use of Critical Appraisal Skills Programme (CASP) checklists to be beneficial, as these tools offer valuable questions and prompts for evaluating research [63]. After establishing that an intervention is reliable, cost-effective, feasible, effective and validated through critical analysis, it is essential to determine how to implement this intervention within your practice and promote its adoption within your workplace. This process may involve the development of local policies and operating procedures that are grounded in evidence, while also considering potential barriers and facilitators to translating this evidence into practice.

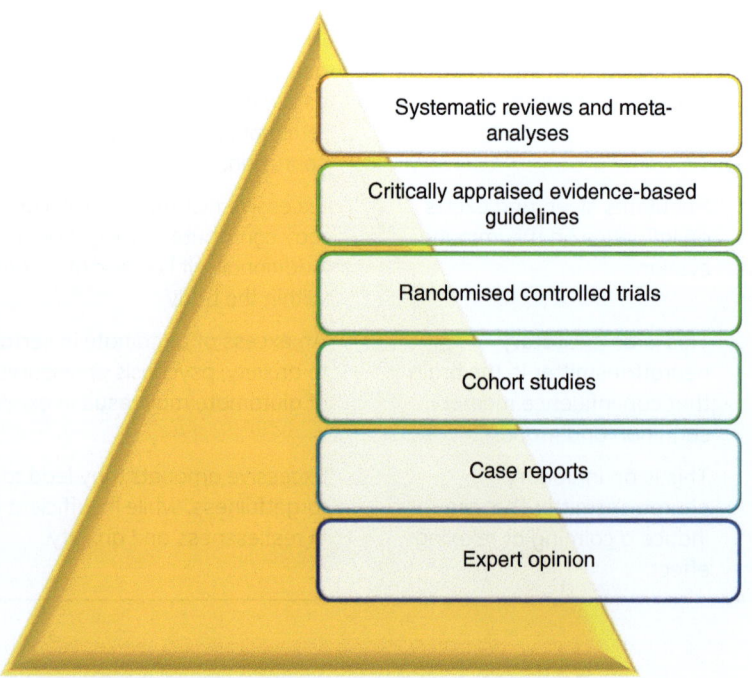

FIGURE 8.1 Hierarchy of evidence. Source: [61] / with permission of CASP UK.

PRESCRIBING

Licensing Considerations

If prescribing within your practice as an advanced practitioner, it is essential to consider both medication licensing and evidence-based guidelines. See later in the chapter for more on this. A medication is classified as 'licensed' when it has undergone assessment and is deemed to meet the standards established by the Medicines and Healthcare products Regulatory Agency (MHRA). Upon meeting these standards, the product receives a marketing authorisation. In some cases, practitioners may need to prescribe unlicensed medications for patients. Such medications do not possess a marketing authorisation in the United Kingdom and must be prescribed based on an assessment of the patient's needs [64]. Examples of unlicensed medication use include pirenzepine for clozapine-induced hypersalivation and melperone for treatment-resistant schizophrenia. When prescribing unlicensed medications, practitioners must ensure that there is evidence supporting the safety and efficacy of the medication, effectively manage the patient's care, complete necessary monitoring, document the rationale for prescribing the unlicensed medication in the patient's records and communicate with the patient and/or their carers regarding the use of the unlicensed medication and the reasons behind this decision [65]. Additionally, medications may also be prescribed for 'off-label' use, which permits the use of a medication outside its licensed indications. Prescribers must adhere to their professional guidelines when prescribing both unlicensed and off-label medications [66].

Patient Factors

It is essential to consider the evidence base and licensing requirements, as well as adhere to legal and professional frameworks when making prescribing decisions. Additionally, for practitioners who may or may not engage in prescribing in their practice, understanding the patient factors that influence treatment choice is crucial. These patient factors include [67, 68]:

- Diagnosis and treatment objectives.
- Assessment of the patient's overall health status (including the evaluation of physical and mental health comorbidities, pregnancy, breastfeeding, allergies and the use of other medications and substances).
- Evaluation of the patient's comprehension of prescribed medications and their capacity for adherence, which may influence treatment compliance and patient preferences.
- Pharmacogenomic considerations.
- Analysis of the patient's historical response to treatment, particularly in cases of inadequate response.
- Economic implications of the medication (considering both the cost to the patient and the financial burden on the healthcare service).
- Consideration of pharmacokinetic and pharmacodynamic parameters.

TREATMENT

Treatment choice is determined by the diagnosis and the desired outcome. In general, different types of mental health diagnoses require different treatments and sometimes different strengths of those treatments (for example, higher doses of selective serotonin reuptake inhibitors (SSRIs) are required to treat obsessive compulsive disorder (OCD) in comparison to depression) [69]. When an accurate working diagnosis has been established (after considering differential diagnoses), a more targeted treatment can be prescribed for the patient. Furthermore, it is essential to discuss the service user's treatment goals with them. For example, a patient who suffers from post-traumatic stress disorder (PTSD) may request help reducing nightmares or flashbacks, or they may request support in developing coping mechanisms. Depending on their desired goal, treatment may consist of medication or psychological therapies, or both.

The choice of treatment is also influenced by the person's overall health. While this may complicate the treatment choice, it is important to take into account this factor so as to reduce the risk of harm, improve tolerability and maximise efficacy. As a result, it is important to take into account the mental and physical health of the individual, which can be determined through an effective history taking process. When taking a history, it is essential to ask questions about the person's past medical history, past psychiatric history, drug history, previously attempted treatments and their response to them, allergies, substance use and for cis gender women, whether they may be pregnant or breastfeeding. A person's medical and psychiatric history can be beneficial to document, particularly when prescribing medications, as clinicians are able to identify any contraindications or precautions by utilising the manufacturers' guidance and the BNF, while also taking into account drug–disease interactions. The psychiatric history can additionally assist in screening for comorbid psychiatric conditions and in evaluating treatment options for patients that may provide benefits for both conditions, while also identifying interventions that should be avoided or approached with caution. For example, it would not be appropriate to start stimulant medications for a patient who may be experiencing mania. As an additional example, you might consider the use of an antipsychotic such as quetiapine for a patient diagnosed with schizophrenia who also experiences mood disorders. When assessing past psychiatric history, it is important to ask service users about previous thoughts, plans and actions in relation to suicide and self-harm. This also affects treatment choice when considering past risk of overdose. With regards to drug history (including allergies), it is important to understand what medication the person may be taking currently (including prescribed, over-the-counter, herbal and homeopathic medications). This not only provides information on drug–drug interactions but also allows clinicians to assess previous response to medications (both in terms of tolerability and efficacy). Drug–drug interactions also need to be considered for people using recreational substances. Use of such substances can also affect a person's mental health and as such may be important to consider for diagnostic purposes. Patients may frequently discontinue the use of substances such as nicotine, caffeine and other drugs, which can lead to withdrawal symptoms. These symptoms may be misattributed by patients to their medication or health. It is important to consider this possibility and to discuss it with the patient.

In addition, patient choice should always be considered. A patient should be provided with information on the different treatment options available to them (including pharmacological and non-pharmacological). Where pharmacological treatment is being considered, different options should be presented to the patient.

In addition, patients should be informed on:

- the indication of the medication.
- how it should be administered.
- how long the medication should be taken for and what effects it may have.
- its adverse effects and how these can be managed.
- advice on missed doses.
- advice on interactions with other medications, diet or their other conditions.
- advice on lifestyle changes that may be needed for the treatment or may affect the treatment.

- monitoring advice.
- any special storage requirements [70].

Patients' understanding of this information should be checked with consideration for those with language barriers. This is particularly important when noting specific risks to certain groups of patients, for example the impact of fertility in cis gender males with valproate treatment. In addition, it is important to understand if they have any barriers to accessing the medication (e.g. cost or needing assistance with administration of medication for elderly patients). At times it may be useful to use pictograms or interpreters to communicate with patients. All such conversations should allow the person to ask questions and raise any concerns they may have with regards to the information discussed. Once the patient has the information available to them, they should be offered time to think about their decision and choice of treatment.

In addition, it is important to ascertain what the person may have tried before and how they have previously responded to this. With certain psychotropic medications, it is also important to consider how long the person took the medication for and whether this was a suitable time frame for the person to respond; for example, a patient who deems an SSRI (such as fluoxetine) ineffective in a week may still have a good response to SSRIs when trialled for a longer period of time, with the correct patient counselling. In addition, it may also help to understand what dose the patient trialled of that medication; as explained previously, some conditions may require higher doses.

Case Scenario

Please note this case scenario is not reflective of a real patient and is intended for the sole purpose of focusing on pharmacology and treatment.

Jane is an 82-year-old female with no prior psychiatric history. Following her husband passing away 6 months ago, her daughter has reported Jane has dramatically decreased appetite and has consequently started to lose weight, become increasingly bedbound and has often found evidence of self-neglect when visiting Jane. Jane has a history of COPD and haemorrhagic stroke 5 years ago. She has been diagnosed with major depression.

When considering the treatment options, the following should be considered:

- **Age:** There is an increased risk of developing adverse effects due to multiple factors – a decreased volume of distribution affecting absorption, decline in hepatic and renal function impacting metabolism and clearance alongside increased comorbidities. We would want to avoid treatment options such as tricyclic antidepressants (TCAs) due to increased risk of anticholinergic burden in this group of patients. This would be a concern alongside additive risk of falls due to reduced mobility reported by Jane's daughter.
- **Comorbidities:** This can impact treatment choice either due to drug–drug interactions or due to a contraindication depending on the medical history. In this scenario, a history of haemorrhagic stroke would mean Jane has an increased bleeding risk that would mean SSRI treatment should be avoided.
- **Symptoms:** Consider the loss of appetite, which had resulted in weight loss. While most antidepressants carry some risk of weight gain, this is commonly seen with mirtazapine and is often used due to its ability to stimulate appetite.

> **What would be your treatment of choice here?**
> In this instance, if we assume that patient choice has been considered, mirtazapine would be considered the most suitable treatment when balancing factors described earlier.

PRESCRIBING IN PREGNANCY OR BREASTFEEDING

For cis gender women, it is especially important to discuss whether they are family planning or if they may be pregnant or breastfeeding. Not only are some medications contraindicated in women of childbearing age without special precautions (e.g. sodium valproate), but also other medications may be prescribed after careful consideration of risks and benefits which need to be discussed with the service user. It is also worth noting the risk to foetuses in males with certain treatments, such as valproate. There are many helpful resources to check whether medications may be suitable in pregnancy or breastfeeding such as 'BUMPS – best use of medicines in pregnancy' or the UK Teratology Information Service [71, 72]. These resources often provide more information than the manufacturer's information leaflets on use of medicines in pregnancy or breastfeeding. Understandably, there are less studies (and clinical trials) completed with women who are pregnant and taking medications and therefore less evidence is available until the medication is used in the 'real world'.

> **Case Scenario**
>
> *Please note this case scenario is not reflective of a real patient and is intended for the sole purpose of focusing on pharmacology and treatment.*
>
> Sarah, a 32-year-old mother, is breastfeeding her 4-month-old baby. She has been suffering with significant sleep difficulties and has trouble falling and staying asleep due to the demands of her baby. Sarah and her partner have trialled various non-pharmacological interventions, including her partner supporting her through the night feeds. However, this has now started to impact her mood; she is becoming increasingly anxious and is often tearful through the day. She is concerned about the use of long-term medications on the baby, especially as Sarah is breastfeeding, but she is hoping for something to help her sleep.
>
> **What would be your key considerations here?**
> The key consideration in this scenario would be the pharmacokinetics of medications. Particularly in insomnia, there would be concern with the use of medications that have long elimination half-lives, as this may impact care for the baby. There would also need to be consideration of how much medication passes into breastmilk, causing adverse effects in the infant. In this instance, there would be a concern about increased drowsiness and regardless of choice, baby would need to be monitored. Due to this, medications such as sedative antihistamines (e.g. promethazine) or benzodiazepines are avoided [73]. There would also be a cautious approach for dosing regimen. For acute management of insomnia, zopiclone or zolpidem are preferred in breastfeeding mothers due to their shorter elimination half-lives, and lower amounts of these drugs are passed through the breastmilk [73].

PRESCRIBING FOR CHILDREN AND YOUNG PEOPLE

There are several differences in the approach to prescribing in children and young people. Due to difficulties in diagnosis in this group, treatment is usually initiated with the aim to provide symptomatic relief [36]. A small number of medications are licensed in children and young people, furthermore treatment initiation depends on individual clinician expertise as these would be considered 'off-label' use [36]. Local trusts may have policies as guidance for treatment choices.

The pharmacokinetic differences with treatment in children and young people were highlighted earlier in this chapter (see special considerations). These influence how dosage is calculated, for example as mg/kg per day, depending on age, physical health and medication being considered [36]. Lower initiation doses and increments for dose increases are recommended [36]. Furthermore, longer periods of monitoring are generally required to establish adequate response and tolerability to treatment as presentations in children tend to be more severe [36]. Questionnaires and structured interviews can be used to support with monitoring symptoms.

Treatment choice and indication are factors to consider, and the impact this may have on children or young people. For example, SSRIs have been associated with increased risk of suicidality in this group when used for depression [36]. However, evidence suggests efficacy of SSRIs used at lower doses for indications such as OCD, alongside careful monitoring [36].

Case Scenario

Please note this case scenario is not reflective of a real patient and is intended for the sole purpose of focusing on pharmacology and treatment.

Andrew is a 14-year-old male, with a diagnosis of autism spectrum disorder (ASD). He has been admitted to hospital due to an injury to his foot, but unfortunately it has been challenging for the medical team to conduct any investigations due to increasingly challenging behaviour in the department. The team have already administered three injections of lorazepam 0.5 mg IM and are requesting a plan for further management.

What would you need to consider in a management plan going forward?

The key considerations in this scenario are the following [36]:

- **Non-pharmacological approach:** while it is considered first line to optimise environment, in this specific case this may be difficult given being in a hospital setting. However, an attempt should be made to consult the patient's Health Passport and to optimise their environment wherever possible.
- **Pharmacokinetics:** as highlighted earlier, lower doses of medications are usually required for treatment. There is also an associated increased risk of side-effects therefore this needs to be considered before further treatment.
- **Prescribing in ASD:** clinicians may use the STOMP (Stopping the Over-Medication of People with a learning disability or autism or both)/STAMP criteria (Supporting Treatment and Medications in Paediatrics) to support with prescribing and reviewing treatment [74].

> These are NHS initiatives to promote review and ensure treatment is appropriate and reduce polypharmacy [74]. This is especially when considering starting antipsychotic medications (there is more detailed information on STOMP/STAMP in Chapter 16).
>
> In this scenario, once non-pharmacological options have been exhausted and where necessary, a low dose antipsychotic may be considered to facilitate investigations and treatment, especially whilst in a hospital setting. Psychotropic medications may need to be considered when considering risk of injury to self or others. Evidence supports the use of risperidone or aripiprazole to manage challenging behaviour in ASD – the recommendation remaining to start at low doses and optimise cautiously [36].

Cost Factors

As a practitioner, it is important to consider cost of treatment to the service. Where possible it is important to consider a medication's economic/cost burden. NICE guidance assesses the cost-effectiveness of treatments by comparing the cost per quality-adjusted life year (QALY) of the proposed treatment to that of the most effective alternative [75]. This is calculated as a ratio and is referred to as the incremental cost-effectiveness ratio (ICER) [75]. Treatment options that are considered cost effective are generally less than £20,000 per QALY and above £30,000 per QALY gained, a stronger case is needed for the intervention to be used in the NHS [76]. There are many ways in which we can reduce prescribing costs such as prescribing generically where possible, regularly reviewing repeat prescriptions to reduce waste and exploring other options for treatment with the patient (aside from medication prescribing) [75, 76].

Physical Health Monitoring

For clinicians operating within mental health services, discussions surrounding parity of esteem – defined as assigning equal importance to an individual's physical health and mental health – are prevalent. Research indicates that patients with severe mental illnesses can experience a reduction in life expectancy by 10–20 years compared to the general population, primarily due to poor physical health. This disparity is associated with various factors, including stigma and inadequate resources, and can be further aggravated by adverse effects of psychotropic medications, such as cardiometabolic side effects from antipsychotics. Consequently, there is a critical need to prioritise physical health monitoring in the care of mental health patients [77]. NICE, BNF and pharmaceutical companies will provide guidance on the parameters that should be monitored during pharmacotherapy. Additionally, workplaces may offer recommendations based on local shared care agreements and protocols established with primary and secondary care services. Monitoring of physical health may encompass vital signs (e.g. blood pressure, pulse), blood tests (including renal and liver function tests) and electrocardiograms (ECGs), depending on the specific medication used. High-risk medications previously mentioned, such as lithium and clozapine, may necessitate more frequent and stringent monitoring protocols due to their associated risks and narrow therapeutic index.

In the assessment of patients' physical health, it is essential to incorporate dietary and lifestyle recommendations, which may include guidance on nutrition, physical activity, smoking cessation and the management of substance use, including both drugs and alcohol. Whenever feasible, the implementation of strategies such as motivational interviewing and the integration of additional support services is advantageous.

CONCLUSION

An understanding of psychopharmacology has significant relevance to advanced practice in mental health, regardless of whether the APMH is involved in prescribing medications. Specifically, in the context of the clinical practice pillar, this knowledge directly aligns with learning outcomes 1, 2, 4 and 5 outlined in the Advanced Practice Mental Health Curriculum and Capabilities Framework [1]. Knowledge of psychopharmacology equips APMHs with a deeper understanding of the potential effects of various treatments on patients, as well as the influence of individual patient factors on treatment efficacy and tolerability. This knowledge empowers APMHs to operate more independently and take responsibility for their decisions. Furthermore, it enables APMHs to demonstrate their understanding of the biological and psychological foundations of care while also considering social factors in their practice. Consequently, APMHs are better positioned to create individualised care plans for patients, utilising their clinical reasoning skills to incorporate interventions ranging from psychotropic medications to psychosocial support.

In relation to the leadership and management pillar, an understanding of psychopharmacology is relevant to learning objective 2 of the framework [1]. This knowledge enables clinicians to evaluate safe treatment interventions, taking into account the complexities associated with patient care. It also empowers clinicians to lead effectively within their multidisciplinary teams and to exemplify best practices while considering safe and effective treatment for patients with complexities.

Furthermore, within the education pillar, an understanding of psychopharmacology can help with achievement of learning outcome 3 [1]. Clinicians can utilise the latest evidence-based guidelines and resources to deliver care to patients and to train colleagues within the team. They can also apply their knowledge of psychopharmacology to educate and counsel patients and carers about their medications, including a discussion of the associated risks and benefits, while giving consideration to individual patient factors.

Lastly, possessing knowledge of psychopharmacology enables clinicians to integrate this understanding with the skills they have developed within the research pillar to effectively achieve learning objective 1 [1]. This enables them to critically assess the current evidence base to make informed decisions about an individual's care, while also understanding the fundamental principles of pharmacology.

FURTHER READING

The references provided next may be useful for further reading on this topic:

Bazire, S. (2018). *Psychotropic Drug Directory 2018: the professionals' Pocket Handbook and Aide memoire.* Lloyd-Reinhold Publications.

Gee, S. and Taylor, D.M. (2023). *The Maudsley Prescribing Guidelines for Mental Health Conditions in Physical Illness.* Wiley-Blackwell.

Royal College of Psychiatrists (2022). Psychopharmacology resources. www.rcpsych.ac.uk. https://www.rcpsych.ac.uk/about-us/our-people-and-how-we-make-decisions/committees-of-council/psychopharmacology-committee/resources

Stahl, S.M. (2021). *Prescriber's guide: Stahl's essential psychopharmacology*, 7th ed. Cambridge: Cambridge University Press.

Taylor, D.M. (2021). *Maudsley Prescribing Guidelines In Psychiatry*, 14th ed. S.L.: Wiley-Blackwell.

The British Association for Psychopharmacology BAP consensus guidelines (2025). www.bap.org.uk. https://www.bap.org.uk/guidelines

REFERENCES

1. NHS England (2025). *Mental Health Advanced Practice Area Specific Capability and Curriculum Framework*. London: NHS England. https://advanced-practice.hee.nhs.uk/wp-content/uploads/sites/28/2025/01/Mental-health-advanced-practice-area-specific-capability-and-curriculum-framework-NHSE.pdf
2. American Psychological Association (2018). APA Dictionary of Psychology. dictionary.apa.org. https://dictionary.apa.org/psychopharmacology
3. Harrison, P., Cowen, P., Burns, T., and Fazel, M. (2018). *Shorter Oxford Textbook of Psychiatry*, 7th ed. Oxford University Press: Oxford University Press eBooks.
4. Semple, D. and Smyth, R. (2013). *Oxford Handbook of Psychiatry*, 3rd ed. Oxford: Oxford University Press.
5. Maxwell, S.R. (2024). Pharmacodynamics and pharmacokinetics for the prescriber. *Medicine* 52 (1): 1–10. https://www.sciencedirect.com/science/article/pii/S1357303923002487
6. Marino, M. and Zito, P.M. (2023). *Pharmacodynamics*. PubMed. Treasure Island (FL): StatPearls Publishing https://www.ncbi.nlm.nih.gov/books/NBK507791/
7. Ernstmeyer, K. and Christman, E. (2023). *Chapter 1 Pharmacokinetics & Pharmacodynamics*. Chippewa Valley Technical College: National Library of Medicine. https://www.ncbi.nlm.nih.gov/books/NBK595006/
8. Health Research Board (2024). Glossary www.drugsandalcohol.ie. https://www.drugsandalcohol.ie/glossary/info/agonist
9. Bristow, S., Singh, V., and Ballantyne, J. (2014). Opioids. In: *Encyclopedia of the Neurological Sciences* (ed. M.J. Aminoff and R.B. Daroff), 653–657. Elsevier.
10. Waller, D.G. and Sampson, A.P. (2018). Principles of pharmacology and mechanisms of drug action. Medical. *Pharmacology and Therapeutics* 3–31.
11. Southwood, R., Fleming, V., and Huckaby, G. (2018). *Concepts in Clinical Pharmacokinetics*, 7th ed. ASHP Publications. https://publications.ashp.org/display/book/9781585285921/front-1.xml (accessed 8 November 2024).
12. Mayor, S. (2017). Pharmacokinetics: optimising safe and effective prescribing. *The Prescriber* 28 (3): 45–48.
13. Derendorf, H., Schmidt, S., and Rowland, M. (2019). *Rowland and Tozer's Clinical Pharmacokinetics and Pharmacodynamics: Concepts and Applications*. Wolters Kluwer Health.
14. Grogan, S. and Preuss, C. (2023). *Pharmacokinetics*. PubMed. Treasure Island (FL): StatPearls Publishing https://www.ncbi.nlm.nih.gov/books/NBK557744/
15. Le J. (2022). Drug bioavailability. MSD Manual Professional Edition. MSD Manuals. https://www.msdmanuals.com/professional/clinical-pharmacology/pharmacokinetics/drug-bioavailability
16. Onetto, A.J. and Sharif, S. (2023). *Drug Distribution*. PubMed. Treasure Island (FL): StatPearls Publishing https://www.ncbi.nlm.nih.gov/books/NBK567736/
17. McLeod, H.L. and He, Y. (2012). Pharmacokinetics for the prescriber. *Medicine* 40 (7): 357–361.
18. Le J. (2022). Drug distribution to tissues – clinical pharmacology. MSD Manual Professional Edition. https://www.msdmanuals.com/professional/clinical-pharmacology/pharmacokinetics/drug-distribution-to-tissues
19. Mansoor, A. and Mahabadi, N. (2023). *Volume of Distribution*. *StatPearls*. StatPearls Publishing. https://www.ncbi.nlm.nih.gov/books/NBK545280/
20. Maanen, A.C.D., Wilting, I., and Jansen, P.A.F. (2020). Prescribing medicines to older people – how to consider the impact of ageing on human organ and body functions. *British Journal of Clinical Pharmacology* 86 (10): 1921–1930. https://bpspubs.onlinelibrary.wiley.com/doi/10.1111/bcp.14094.

21. Susa, S.T., Hussain, A., and Preuss, C.V. (2023). *Drug Metabolism*. Nih.gov. StatPearls Publishing. https://www.ncbi.nlm.nih.gov/books/NBK442023/
22. Phang-Lyn, S. and Llerena, V.A. (2020). *Biochemistry, Biotransformation*. PubMed. Treasure Island (FL): StatPearls Publishing. https://www.ncbi.nlm.nih.gov/books/NBK544353/
23. Gunn, J. (2012). Understanding the toxicology of diazepam. *Practical Pain Management* 12 (1). https://www.medcentral.com/pain/chronic/understanding-toxicology-diazepam.
24. Gilani, B. and Cassagnol, M. (2023). *Biochemistry, Cytochrome P450*. PubMed. Treasure Island (FL): StatPearls Publishing. https://www.ncbi.nlm.nih.gov/books/NBK557698/
25. Lynch, T. and Price, A. (2007). The effect of cytochrome P450 metabolism on drug response, interactions, and adverse effects. *American Family Physician* 76. https://www.aafp.org/pubs/afp/issues/2007/0801/p391.pdf.
26. British National Formulary (2023). Interactions A to Z. National Institute for Health and Care Excellence. https://bnf.nice.org.uk/interactions/
27. Garza, A.Z., Park, S.B., and Kocz, R. (2023). *Drug Elimination*. PubMed. Treasure Island (FL): StatPearls Publishing. https://www.ncbi.nlm.nih.gov/books/NBK547662/
28. Susla, G.M. and Lertora, J.J.L. (2012). Effect of liver disease on pharmacokinetics. In: *Principles of Clinical Pharmacology* (ed. S.P. Markey, R.L. Dedrick, C.E. Daniels, et al.), 81–96. Elsevier. https://www.sciencedirect.com/topics/immunology-and-microbiology/enterohepatic-circulation (accessed 30 September 2024).
29. Maddison, J.E., Page, S.W., and Dyke, T.M. (2008). Clinical pharmacokinetics. In: *Small Animal Clinical Pharmacology* (ed. J.E. Maddison, S.W. Page, and D.B. Church), 27–40. Elsevier Saunders.
30. Andrade, C. (2022). The practical importance of half-life in psychopharmacology. *The Journal of Clinical Psychiatry* 83 (4): 22f14584. https://doi.org/10.4088/JCP.22f14584. PMID: 35900254.
31. Davies, S.J.C. and Nutt, D. (2007). Pharmacokinetics for psychiatrists. *Psychiatry* 6 (7): 268–272.
32. Healthcare Improvement Scotland (2017). High risk medicine. Improvement Hub. https://ihub.scot/media/1300/20171016-examples-of-drug-related-deterioration-v20.pdf (accessed 2 January 2025).
33. Batchelor, H.K. and Marriott, J.F. (2015). Paediatric pharmacokinetics: key considerations. *British Journal of Clinical Pharmacology* 79 (3): 395–404. https://doi.org/10.1111/bcp.12267.
34. Ferro, A. (2015). Paediatric prescribing: why children are not small adults. *British Journal of Clinical Pharmacology* 79 (3): 351–353. https://doi.org/10.1111/bcp.12540.
35. National Institute for Health and Care Excellence. (2023). Prescribing in children. NICE. https://bnf.nice.org.uk/medicines-guidance/prescribing-in-children/
36. Taylor, D.M. (2021). *Maudsley Prescribing Guidelines In Psychiatry*, 14th ed. S.L.: Wiley-Blackwell.
37. McKearney, K. and Coleman, J.J. (2020). Prescribing medicines for elderly patients. *Medicine* 48 (7): 463–467.
38. Holbeach E, Yates P. Prescribing in the elderly. https://www.racgp.org.au/getattachment/383b0d8d-c01f-42e5-9da0-2d567b60b2da/Prescribing-in-the-elderly.aspx
39. Delia Bishara, Justin Sauer, Christoph Mueller, Robert Stewart, David M Taylor (2017). Medichec. www.medichec.com. http://www.medichec.com/
40. National Institute of Health and Clinical Excellence (2022). BNF – prescribing in the elderly. NICE. https://bnf.nice.org.uk/medicines-guidance/prescribing-in-the-elderly/
41. National Institute of Health and Clinical Excellence (2024). BNF – prescribing in pregnancy. NICE. https://bnf.nice.org.uk/medicines-guidance/prescribing-in-pregnancy/
42. SPS – Specialist Pharmacy Service (2021). The principles of prescribing in pregnancy. https://www.sps.nhs.uk/articles/the-principles-of-prescribing-in-pregnancy/

43. El Shamy, T. and Tamizian, O. (2018). Principles of prescribing in pregnancy. *Obstetrics, Gynaecology and Reproductive Medicine* 28 (5): 136–140. https://www.sciencedirect.com/science/article/abs/pii/S1751721418300393.
44. Medicines and Healthcare products Regulatory Agency (2024). Valproate use in men: as a precaution, men and their partners should use effective contraception. GOV.UK. https://www.gov.uk/drug-safety-update/valproate-use-in-men-as-a-precaution-men-and-their-partners-should-use-effective-contraception
45. The Breastfeeding Network. (2019). Introduction to the safety of drugs passing through breastmilk. https://www.breastfeedingnetwork.org.uk/dibm-intro/
46. Wang, X., Wang, C., Zhang, Y., and An, Z. (2023). Effect of pharmacogenomics testing guiding on clinical outcomes in major depressive disorder: a systematic review and meta-analysis of RCT. *BMC Psychiatry* 23 (1). https://www.ncbi.nlm.nih.gov/pmc/articles/PMC10176803/
47. Han, C., Wang, S.M., Bahk, W.M. et al. (2018). A pharmacogenomic-based antidepressant treatment for patients with major depressive disorder: results from an 8-week, randomized, single-blinded clinical trial. *Clinical Psychopharmacology and Neuroscience* 16 (4): 469–480.
48. Baldacci, A., Saguin, E., Balcerac, A. et al. (2023). Pharmacogenetic guidelines for psychotropic drugs: optimizing prescriptions in clinical practice. *Pharmaceutics*. 15 (11): 2540.
49. Choice and Medication (2022). Learn more about your medicines. https://www.choiceandmedication.org/ (accessed 5 January 2025).
50. Choice and Medication (2023). Handy fact sheet – anticholinergic side effects. https://www.choiceandmedication.org/ (accessed 5 January 2025).
51. Choice and Medication (2023). How we think antidepressants help. https://www.choiceandmedication.org/ (accessed 5 January 2025).
52. Pal, M.M. (2021). Glutamate: the master neurotransmitter and its implications in chronic stress and mood disorders. *Frontiers in Human Neuroscience* 15 (15): 722323. https://www.ncbi.nlm.nih.gov/pmc/articles/PMC8586693/#:~:text=Glutamate%20is%20an%20excitatory%20neurotransmitter,%2C%20cognition%2C%20and%20mood%20regulation.
53. Jewett, B.E. and Sharma, S. (2020). *Physiology, GABA*. PubMed. Treasure Island (FL): StatPearls Publishing https://www.ncbi.nlm.nih.gov/books/NBK513311/
54. Minkow, D. (2023). The evidence-based medicine pyramid! – students 4 best evidence. Students 4 Best Evidence. https://s4be.cochrane.org/blog/2014/04/29/the-evidence-based-medicine-pyramid/
55. Cochrane Library (2024). Cochrane Reviews | Cochrane Library. https://www.cochranelibrary.com/
56. Embase. (2025). Embase Search Engine for Research Papers. https://www.embase.com/landing?status=grey
57. PubMed (2024). PubMed – National library of medicine. https://pubmed.ncbi.nlm.nih.gov/ (accessed 14 September 2024).
58. CINAHL Database | EBSCO. (2025). EBSCO Information Services, Inc. | www.ebsco.com. https://www.ebsco.com/products/research-databases/cinahl-database
59. BMJ Journal (2024). BMJ Journals. https://journals.bmj.com/home
60. JAMA (2024). Psychiatry – the science of mental health and the brain. https://jamanetwork.com/journals/jamapsychiatry
61. Critical Appraisal Skills Programme (2024). PICO search strategy tips & examples. https://casp-uk.net/news/pico-search-strategy/ (accessed 19 September 2024).
62. Walden University Library (2025). Evidence pyramid. https://academicguides.waldenu.edu/library/healthevidence/evidencepyramid

63. Critical Appraisal Skills Programme (2024). CASP checklists – critical appraisal skills programme. https://casp-uk.net/casp-tools-checklists/ (accessed 19 September 2024).
64. Specialist Pharmacy Service (2023). Explaining the licensed status of medicines. https://www.sps.nhs.uk/articles/explaining-the-licensed-status-of-medicines/ (accessed 19 September 2024).
65. General Medical Council (2024). Prescribing unlicensed medicines – professional standards – GMC. https://www.gmc-uk.org/professional-standards/professional-standards-for-doctors/good-practice-in-prescribing-and-managing-medicines-and-devices/prescribing-unlicensed-medicines (accessed 19 September 2024).
66. National Institute for Health and Care Excellence (2024). Information for the public on medicines. https://www.nice.org.uk/about/nice-communities/nice-and-the-public/making-decisions-about-your-care/information-for-the-public-on-medicines#:~:text=Unlicensed%20medicines%20and%20'off%2Dlabel,that%20stated%20in%20its%20licence (accessed 19 September 2024).
67. Davari, M., Khorasani, E., and Tigabu, B.M. (2018). Factors influencing prescribing decisions of physicians: a review. *Ethiopian Journal of Health Sciences* 28 (6): 795–804. https://www.ncbi.nlm.nih.gov/pubmed/30607097.
68. Maxwell, S.R. (2016). Rational prescribing: the principles of drug selection. *Clinical Medicine* 16 (5): 459–464. https://www.ncbi.nlm.nih.gov/pmc/articles/PMC6297291/
69. Bloch, M.H., McGuire, J., Landeros-Weisenberger, A. et al. (2009). Meta-analysis of the dose-response relationship of SSRI in obsessive-compulsive disorder. *Molecular Psychiatry* 15 (8): 850–855.
70. Royal Pharmaceutical Society (2011). Counselling patients on medicines – a quick reference guide. Royal Pharmaceutical Society. https://www.rpharms.com/resources/pharmacy-guides/counselling-people-on-the-use-of-medicines (28 September 2024).
71. Bumps (2020). Best use of medicine in pregnancy. Medicinesinpregnancy.org. https://www.medicinesinpregnancy.org/
72. UKTIS (2024) Evidence-based safety information about medication, vaccine, chemical and radiological exposures in pregnancy. https://uktis.org/
73. SPS – Specialist Pharmacist Service (2024). Treating insomnia during breastfeeding. https://www.sps.nhs.uk/articles/treating-insomnia-during-breastfeeding/
74. NHS England. (2022) Stopping over medication of people with a learning disability and autistic people (STOMP) and supporting treatment and appropriate medication in paediatrics (STAMP). https://www.england.nhs.uk/learning-disabilities/improving-health/stomp-stamp/
75. National Institute for Health and Care Excellence (NICE) (2012). Assessing cost effectiveness | The guidelines manual | Guidance | NICE. Nice.org.uk. NICE. https://www.nice.org.uk/process/pmg6/chapter/assessing-cost-effectiveness
76. GP Online (2007). Prescribing the cost-effective way. Gponline.com. GP Online. https://www.gponline.com/prescribing-cost-effective/article/662699
77. Mitchell, A.J., Hardy, S., and Shiers, D. (2017). Parity of esteem: addressing the Inequalities between Mental and Physical Healthcare. *BJPsych Advances* 23 (3): 196–205. https://www.cambridge.org/core/journals/bjpsych-advances/article/parity-of-esteem-addressing-the-inequalities-between-mental-and-physical-healthcare/A54DB7D5D18F28E6DAE1E2152291EF9C

CHAPTER 9

Mental Health and Legal Issues

Christine Hutchinson[1] and Steve Hardy[2]

[1] School of Nursing and Midwifery, Faculty of Health, Social Care and Medicine, Edge Hill University, Ormskirk, Lancashire, UK
[2] Oxleas NHS Foundation Trust, London, Kent and the South West of England, UK

Aim

This chapter will focus on the law as it applies to those in England. There are aspects of legislation covered which do apply in other parts of the United Kingdom; where this is the case, it will be noted in the narrative. The chapter focuses on the law utilised within services delivered to those aged 18 and above, and therefore, it does not cover legislation specific to children and young people, which is discussed briefly in Chapter 14. The depth, breadth and complexity of the law in this field means that this chapter can only touch on the salient points for practice.

LEARNING OUTCOMES

After reading this chapter, the reader will be able to:

- Have both a revision of and an elevated understanding of the complexity of the legal frameworks advanced practice in mental health operates within.
- Understand some of the key legal issues impacting advanced practice in mental health.
- Explore the application of the law in clinical scenarios.
- Be aware of where additional help and support can be found for practice situations.

The Advanced Practitioner in Mental Health, First Edition. Edited by Clare Allabyrne.
© 2026 John Wiley & Sons Ltd. All rights reserved, including rights for text and data mining and training of artificial intelligence technologies or similar technologies. Published 2026 by John Wiley & Sons Ltd.

MAPPING TO THE FOUR PILLARS OF ADVANCED PRACTICE AND THE ADVANCED PRACTICE IN MENTAL HEALTH CURRICULUM AND CAPABILITIES FRAMEWORK [1]

This specific area of practice is relevant to all four pillars of advanced practice, not least in the areas of clinical practice and leadership.

Given the level of seniority of advanced practitioners, they are often involved in cases where there is a complexity of legal and ethical issues at play. Additionally, they are often central to the education of patients, their families and other staff in relation to the law; it is, therefore, important that it and its' application in practice are well understood.

Some advanced practitioners in mental health (APMHs), after consolidating their learning and role development, might consider progressing to consultant level practice and to developing as a Mental Health Act Approved Clinician, a Mental Health Act Approved Mental Health Professional, a Deprivation of Liberty Safeguards Best Interests Assessor or becoming an expert witness for Tribunals and the Courts. These roles require a good depth of clinical and practice understanding, coupled with in-depth knowledge of statute law, case law and ethics of direct relevance to practice. This includes consideration of the enablers and tensions that arise from these legal frameworks.

The Advanced Practice in Mental Health Curriculum and Capabilities Framework [1] developed to standardise advanced practice education and development and has aspects that map directly and specifically with the clinical and leadership pillars as follows:

Clinical

- 1 Work autonomously within professional, ethical codes and legal frameworks, being responsible and accountable for their decisions, actions and omissions at this level of practice.
- 2.4 Demonstrate knowledge and application of local, statutory and legal obligations related to the care and treatment of those with mental ill health.
- 2.9 Critically assess and determine a person's capacity to make choices and decisions.

Leadership and Management

- 6.5 Negotiate an individual scope of practice within legal, ethical, professional and organisational policies, governance and procedures, with a focus on mitigating risk and upholding safety.
- 6.7 Act as a professional role model and educator in understanding and practice, in accordance with evidence-based practice and statutory responsibilities, including legislation, guidance, standards and regulatory requirements.

STATUTE THAT SETS THE FOUNDATION FOR MENTAL HEALTHCARE

There are two pieces of statute that set out the foundations for health and social care in the United Kingdom. This section will look at each of those in addition to the provisions of the Mental Capacity Act (for England and Wales) [2] that promotes planning ahead.

The Human Rights Act 1998 [3]: brought into UK domestic law the European Convention on Human Rights and providing a common platform for all UK health and social care services and has been in force since October 2000. This statute sets out how public bodies, which includes health and social care services, are obligated on two fronts. Firstly, to refrain from breaching a person's human rights, sometimes referred to as a 'negative obligation'; and secondly a 'positive obligation' to take proactive steps to protect people from human rights abuses. There are further obligations, including the 'interpretive obligation' that requires us to consider human rights in the application of any other laws such as the Mental Health Act [4] and Mental Capacity Act [2].

Mahdanian et al. [5] undertook a global review of human rights in the context of mental health services citing the drive from inpatient to community-based care as a model for reducing human rights violations. However, there continue to be concerns over the care and treatment of people accessing mental health services [6], in particular inpatient settings, and there is ongoing discourse in relation to how certain practices such as segregation should be perceived [7].

It is important therefore that all staff, but particularly APMHs, understand the Article rights, which ones are absolute and cannot be breached in any event and which are limited or qualified and allow for a breach in specific circumstances (see Figure 9.1).

In mental healthcare, we need to consider our actions and responses through the lens of the Human Rights Act [3] when working with people who pose a risk to themselves or others. Examples would include considering Article 2 where there is suicidal ideation or attempts to take their own life; Article 3 when considering the use of seclusion, segregation and restrictive practices; Articles 5 and 8 when considering how to support people and Article 6 when ensuring that people know of their rights to a Tribunal or application to the Court.

> Schedule 1 of our HRA [3] lists the rights that have been brought over from the European Convention on Human Rights.
>
> Article 2: Right to life (absolute)
> Article 3: Freedom from torture and inhuman or degrading treatment (absolute)
> Article 4: Freedom from slavery and forced labour (absolute)
> Article 5: Right to liberty and security (limited)
> Article 6: Right to a fair trial (absolute)
> Article 7: No punishment without law (absolute)
> Article 8: Respect for your private and family life, home and correspondence (qualified)
> Article 9: Freedom of thought, belief and religion (qualified)
> Article 10: Freedom of expression (qualified)
> Article 11: Freedom of assembly and association (qualified)
> Article 12: Right to marry and start a family (limited)
> Article 14: Protection from discrimination in respect of these rights and freedoms (limited)

FIGURE 9.1 The Article rights [3].

The Equality Act 2010 [8] which applies to England, Scotland and Wales provides detail on the application of Article 14 for specific groups. It requires public authorities, which include health and social care services to eliminate unlawful discrimination.

The Equality Act [8] sets out nine protected characteristics: age, disability, gender reassignment, marriage and civil partnership, pregnancy and maternity, race, religion or belief, sex, and sexual orientation.

It's important to consider that there are different ways in which discrimination can occur.

- 'Direct discrimination' is where one person is treated different to another because of a protected characteristic.
- 'Indirect discrimination' is where a policy or way of doing things applies in the same way for everybody, but in some way disadvantages a group of people who share a protected characteristic.

This could include, for example, where service eligibility criteria specifically exclude a group in the population that has a certain protected characteristic.

- 'Failure to make reasonable adjustments' – this is where an organisation doesn't make reasonable changes to (a) the way they usually offer a service or to their procedures, (b) to the environments or (c) to provide aids so that a person covered under the act is no longer substantially disadvantaged.

Mental health, learning disability and autism come within the definition of disability. *A person has a disability for the purposes of the Equality Act if he or she has a physical or mental impairment and the impairment has a substantial and long-term adverse effect on his or her ability to carry out normal day-to-day activities* [8 – Section 6(1)].

The cause of the impairment is of no relevance in deciding if the aspect of the definition is met, and it is not necessary to have a diagnosis (this is particularly important for the autistic population). There are some issues which mental health staff will work with which are excluded from the definition of impairment, including addictions and certain offences such as fire setting, theft and sexual offences. Whilst these aspects are excluded, if the person undertaking these acts has a mental impairment as defined in the Equality Act, then that impairment is subject to the public sector duty.

The aspect of whether the impairment has a substantial and long-term adverse effect needs to be considered. A substantial effect is one that is *more than a minor or trivial effect* and can be determined by considering how long it takes for the person to complete a day-to-day task in comparison to their non-disabled peers or by considering the cumulative effect of the impact of the impairment. Long term is defined as 12 months or more [9]. If an APMH is working to determine whether a person's mental impairment is included within the Equality Act definition of disability, there is extensive guidance available on the Government Equalities Office website:

https://www.gov.uk/government/organisations/government-equalities-office.

In the main, all people accessing mental health, learning disability or specialist autism services are highly likely to meet the requirements of the Equality Act's disability definition [8]. As such the Act's requirements should be core to the practice of all staff. This will ensure they meet the public sector duties to eliminate any discrimination and to make reasonable adjustments in their policies, procedures and ways of providing services.

Reasonable adjustments in mental healthcare are a statutory duty, once you become aware that the person has one of the nine protected characteristics. Whilst this is not an 'anticipatory duty' if working in mental health, learning disability or specialist autism services, it is likely known that anyone referred to those services will fall within the Equality Act duties [8]. As such all policies, procedures, systems and ways of working should be reasonably adjusted to reduce or eliminate any inequality in access or provision of services. Person or patient centred services contribute significantly to ensuring reasonable adjustments are in place for those accessing services.

If you fail to make a reasonable adjustment when you are under a duty to do so, the Equality Act [8] treats that as discrimination (set out in sections 13–19A of the Act). This means you could become liable to pay damages should a successful claim to be brought.

The Act does not specify or list what adjustments are required, sometimes these can be identified for large population groups (such as ramps for those who rely on wheelchairs for mobility), but more often the adjustment is more person centred or bespoke.

Reasonable adjustment does not require significant finance or resources, more popular reasonable adjustments include matters such as quiet space, shorter waiting, more time to process information or communicate and information in more easily understood formats. The National Development Team for Inclusion has developed resources specific to mental health services on reasonable adjustments [10, 11] that contain a range of reasonable adjustment examples. They also developed a toolkit for auditing services and their accessibility [12]; whilst this is specific to two population groups, much of the content is applicable to many others with protected characteristics.

> **Scenario Pablo**
>
> Pablo is a 19-year-old autistic man in a category A prison for attempted murder. He has struggled to transition to the prison setting. The wing staff have sought support from the advanced practitioner to make reasonable adjustments.
>
> Pablo was finding the morning routines difficult, if his day didn't start well, he struggled to manage the demands of the remainder of the day, experiencing significant symptoms of anxiety and depression. Shower and breakfast time were important times, Pablo and the advanced practitioner identified that he needed a quieter routine in the morning to set the day up and subsequently minimise his symptoms. Exploring options with the prison staff they identified that if he worked to clean the bathrooms he could shower alone before everyone else was released from their cell. This then allowed for him to eat his breakfast whilst others were showering.
>
> *Note:* Pseudonyms are used to protect the anonymity of the person, and some details have been changed. Confidentiality has been fully maintained in line with ethical and professional standards [13].
>
> **Considerations:**
>
> What are the reasonable adjustments seeking to achieve? What other reasonable adjustments could have been considered? How would the impact of a reasonable adjustment be measured?

Mental Capacity Act 2005

The Mental Capacity Act 2005 [2], fully enacted in October 2008, applies in England and Wales. It concerns people aged 16 and over, although some provisions are only available to those aged 18 and over.

It contains 5 statutory principles that must be followed along with provisions for planning for a time when you might lack capacity (Lasting Powers of Attorney, advanced statements, advanced care planning and Advanced Decisions to Refuse Treatment) and an outline of how to make decisions where someone lacks the necessary mental capacity to do so, whether this be through a statutory best interests process, the decision of a Court Appointed Deputy or a Court of Protection decision/order.

The Statutory Principles provide a logical order for approaching decision-making with people: approach the situation with the presumption of capacity (principle 1) and if there is cause for doubt or concern about capacity, take practicable steps to enable that person's capacity (principle 2). Where a person has mental capacity, they have the right to make decision others may consider unwise (principle 3). Where a person lacks mental capacity, any decision made must be in their best interests (principle 4) and be the least restrictive alternative available (principle 5).

It is important that we promote the proactive arrangements provided through the Mental Capacity Act with all people that we have contact with.

Lasting Powers of Attorney (LPAs) can be made by people aged 18 or over, who have the mental capacity to do so, for either a) property and finance or b) health and welfare or both. These do not require solicitors, and the forms are available on the Office of the Public Guardian website (see here https://www.gov.uk/power-of-attorney/make-lasting-power). A fee must be paid for them to be registered, once registered they are legally binding. In practice if someone states that they hold a Lasting Power of Attorney (LPA), then a copy of this document must be received and retained on file to evidence the approach you will take to decision-making for a person who lacks mental capacity, namely that where the LPA's power provides authority you will seek a decision from them.

Advanced Decision to Refuse Treatment (ADRT) is a means of recording in advance refusal of treatment and nothing else; it cannot include refusal of care and support or refusal of accommodation. For most decisions, the ADRT can be communicated verbally; in these circumstances, it would be helpful to formally record the conversation in a location that others would be able to access. Where the ADRT is refusing life-sustaining treatment, it must be in writing and witnessed. The ADRT is legally binding for the decisions covered by it, unless there have been advances in treatments since it was made or there is concern about the person's mental capacity or free will when it was made.

For anyone aged 16 and over, whether they have mental capacity or not, advanced statements and advanced care planning are available as a means of communicating with others their preferences and wishes. These can be provided verbally or in writing and whilst they are not legally binding, any best interests decision-making process must take account of them. It is therefore helpful if any advanced statements are incorporated into care plans and documented where others who may be required to have contact with the person can access them.

How we approach each decision-making situation is critical. The need to integrate the Mental Capacity Act [2], Human Rights Act [3] and Equality Act [8] in almost all situations with some also requiring the integration of the Mental Health Act [4] and Care Act [14].

Determining a lack of mental capacity requires a clear transparent process and good documentation. It is not uncommon to see statements such as 'lacks capacity'; this is unhelpful and leads to further questions such as does the person lack physical capacity, lack resource capacity or some other form of capacity. If this is referring to mental capacity, be explicit. Another question might be lacks mental capacity for what? What is the decision that was under consideration. This is important to prevent assumptions and so that yourself or others can consider if reframing the decision might enable a person's capacity (principle 2).

It is not necessary in every situation to complete a formal assessment of mental capacity. The code of practice at paragraph 6.5 [15] sets out a wide range of matters that can be completed on the basis of a 'reasonable belief' of a lack of mental capacity and a reasonable belief of best interests as described in paragraphs 6.31 [15] and 6.32 [15]. Whilst reasonable belief does not require formal assessment or extensive processes, it does require some evidence to underpin it which must be documented.

For decisions which are more significant for the person or involve the use of restrictive practices to action, there should be a formal process fully documented. The Mental Capacity resources at 39 Essex Chambers (see further reading/useful resources for link) are extremely helpful and are regularly updated as case law is issued. They have a specific guide relating to assessing mental capacity and another on the salient points for specific decisions considered by the Courts.

Case law reading is particularly helpful in understanding how the Courts have applied the law in specific cases, particularly where the circumstances are very similar to situations an APMH might find themselves in. A monthly newsletter is also published by 39 Essex Chambers highlighting case law, its meaning for practice and with links to the public judgment where available. They also have a searchable database of caselaw specific to mental capacity on their website.

For significant decisions, where there are conflicting views on whether the person has mental capacity, it may be necessary to apply to the Court of Protection for a determination on mental capacity.

When people lack mental capacity, there are additional aspects of the Mental Capacity Act [2] that must be followed. The statutory best interests checklist set out in the Mental Capacity Act [2] is often not well understood, for example people presume that the law requires a best interests meeting to be held, when in fact the statutory checklist requires that people interested in the person's welfare be consulted, this consultation can be done by any means. It is important that meetings are not used to coerce or overpower people who may have different views about the person's best interests.

It is important for advanced practitioners to have clarity on what types of situations require legal advice and those where the process and resolution of differing opinions can be managed through local processes. Each statutory organisation will have a process for accessing legal advice, in some cases just one organisation's legal team might progress a matter or legal support might be shared.

As a result of the Mental Capacity Act [2] and the development of case law many more practitioners are finding themselves involved in cases before the Court of Protection. There are a number of training providers that offer training in understanding how the Court of Protection operates and how best to present yourself.

> ### Case Study 9.1 Alfie and the Relationship Between Safeguarding and the MCA
>
> Alfie is a 77-year-old man who lives with his wife in a council flat. He is in the early stages of Alzheimer's dementia and has periods of depression followed by periods of being well.
>
> He is seen by a psychiatrist every six months and visited at home by a community mental health nurse (CMHN) once a month. Alfie also has a chronic pressure ulcer which is seen by the district nursing (DN) team. The psychiatrist, DN team and CMHN have all seen Alfie recently and have deemed him to have mental capacity in relation to his health and well-being and have capacity in relation to the care he is receiving from the psychiatrist, DN team and CMHN. He is also under review by Social Services and known to local workers from Alzheimer's UK and Age Concern. Alfie is accepting of care and allows nurses and others to provide the required treatment for pressure ulcer care and monitor his mental state.
>
> The DN and CMHN have raised concerns about the state of his flat, his self-neglect of personal hygiene and bed bugs in his mattress, bedding and clothing. Alfie and his wife do not wash or change their clothes; the flat is dirty and very unpleasant with rubbish and excrement covered with news papers. Flies and maggots are noticeable.
>
> A year ago, Alfie and his wife agreed to stay elsewhere enabling a deep clean of their flat. It has come to the point this is required again; however, they are both refusing to move out temporarily and refusing to cover the cost of the clean. Recognising their vulnerabilities and needs, supported living accommodation has also been offered and refused by them.
>
> It is becoming extremely difficult to provide them the planned care in the current conditions. The relationship with social services has broken down. The two charities are offering extra support with advice, new clothing and attempts to clean but with limited success.
>
> *Note:* Pseudonyms are used to protect the anonymity of the person, and some details have been changed. Confidentiality has been fully maintained in line with ethical and professional standards [13].
>
> ### Legal and Practice Considerations:
>
> ***Human Rights Act:*** Which Article rights are engaged in this scenario?
>
> ***Equality Act:*** Does Alfie have a protected characteristic? If yes, how might you reasonably adjust how you deliver health and care interventions? How do you prevent discrimination?
>
> ***Mental Capacity:*** How would you frame the decision to assess mental capacity? How would you approach the assessment? How would you discern if an unwise, capacitated decision is being made by Alfie or if he lacks the ability to use and weigh information and put it into practice?

> ***Care Act:*** Consider the statutory assessment of need, promotion of self-determination and safeguarding adult aspects, where does this statute support the situation? Where might there be conflicts in the legal framework?
>
> Learning Points:
>
> Person-centred approaches are central to protecting Alfie's Article rights; however, under the circumstances, there are also his wife's Article rights to consider.
>
> Safeguarding adults requires both proactive and reactive approaches, safeguarding alerts can often support proactive steps such as engagement of broader services; increased support and monitoring or offers of enhanced care and changes of accommodation.
>
> Mental capacity is important to self-determination; however, it is not the sole factor. Alfie's choices about his home are impacting on the health and safety of others, including his wife and the health and social care staff entering the property. Comprehensive risk assessments will help to determine the extent of risk for each party involved.

Mental Health Act

The Mental Health Act for England and Wales dates back to 1983 [4]. It did receive some updating in 2007; however, large parts remained the same. A new Code of Practice and Reference Guide were issued in 2015 [16, 17] which helped to further progress practice in implementing the Mental Health Act [4]; however, this has not been enough to keep pace with societal change and expectation. There has been extensive lobbying and work to draft out a Mental Health Bill which has received parliamentary scrutiny. It is possible that a new Mental Health Act for England and Wales may be seen before the end of 2025 or soon after.

The Mental Health Act [4] has guiding principles set out in the Code of Practice [16]; these guiding principles would apply to anyone who has a mental disorder, defined in the Act as any disorder or disability of the mind. However, often staff are unable to share what these guiding principles are. APMHs should reinforce these principles in discussions, multidisciplinary team conversations and in recording contacts and decisions. They also provide a useful structure for reflective practice and for considering those more complex situations.

The Mental Health Act [4] sets out rules and processes so that anyone being treated using provisions from within the Act will know what their legal rights are and what they can expect to experience. It covers a wide range of eventualities and is split into aspects for those living in the community, those being dealt with in the court system and those who are in prison. There are particular sections for those whose movement through health services is monitored and restricted by the Ministry of Justice. Mental Health Law Online is a great resource for all aspects of the Mental Health Act [4] and related case law with searchable content to get you quickly to the information you need (see further reading and resources).

Mental Health Units (Use of Force) Act [18]

The Mental Health Units (Use of Force) Act [18] became law in England and Wales in November 2018. There is statutory guidance [19] that accompanies the Act specific to NHS and Independent sector hospitals. The Act aims to put in place measures to prevent the inappropriate use of force and ensure accountability and transparency about the use of force within mental health units.

The statutory guidance outlines that force includes the use of physical, mechanical or chemical restraint and the isolation of a patient, including seclusion and segregation.

Scenario: Anita

The APMH has been seeing patients in clinic including Anita, a young woman diagnosed with personality disorder. The APMH is leaving the community health centre heading towards the car park. Anita suddenly ran towards her, pushing her up against the wall, put her arms around her neck and began to strangle her. The APMH hit Anita in the face and pushed her away then ran back towards the health centre shouting for help.

Note: Pseudonyms are used to protect the anonymity of the person, and some details have been changed. Confidentiality has been fully maintained in line with ethical and professional standards [13].

Considerations:

Would this be considered a use of force? Is it necessary and proportionate to the anticipated harm likely to be caused by the strangulation? What other reflections do you have about this scenario?

The use of force can be a frightening, traumatising and humiliating experience that can have a lasting impact. Often those subject to the use of force within mental health, learning disability and autism services are very vulnerable. Further there is a need and expectation for the delivery of person-centred and trauma-informed care (which is explored in more detail in Chapter 7), with an emphasis on prevention and understanding the person's needs.

Force has been seen in use where a person is self-harming and placing themselves at significant risk; making attempts to assault or harm others; to prevent someone absconding and in some cases to deliver treatment. In these situations, there is a trigger of the Human Rights Act Article 2, 3 and 5 rights [3] for those involved and the potential for other statutes to be considered in determining the best course of action. Often culture, ethics and morals come into play, and this is where some staff may act differently to others. The Use of Force Act [18] seeks to reduce the variation of staff's actions, and the need to ensure any use of force is necessary and is proportionate to the harm likely.

As a result there has been specific focus on reducing the use of restrictive practices within health and social care, many of which would fall under the statutory definition of restraint contained within the Mental Capacity Act [2] at section 6(4) *'when someone uses force (or threatens to) to make someone do something they are resisting, and when someone's freedom of movement is restricted, whether or not they are resisting'*.

HOW CLINICAL INVESTIGATION AND EXAMINATION UNDERPINS LEGAL PROCESSES

Other than clinical leadership and facilitation of understanding and decision-making in more complex situations, the APMH has a further role to play in the implementation of the various statute outlined. The clinical assessment of an individual by the APMH will collect information that will underpin statutory assessments of matters such as 'unsound mind' and 'mental disorder'.

Unsound mind is a term used within the European Convention of Human Rights in relation to the Article 5 right to liberty [20]. Case law in England, specifically Stockport Metropolitan Borough Council v KB & Ors [2023] EWCOP 58, directs us to understand the term 'unsound mind' as meaning 'mental disorder'. Mental disorder is defined in the Mental Health Act [4].

This Article right to liberty can be infringed where a person is of unsound mind. Burdzik [21] raises concern regarding this term given it is not in keeping with current medical terminology and calls for it to be changed. The procedures prescribed in law for the deprivation of someone's right to liberty within mental health, learning disability and autism health and social care environments are covered by the Mental Health Act amendments that created the Deprivation of Liberty Safeguards [4, 22] and the Court of Protection Procedures [23], each of these applies to defined populations. It is not possible to have more than one procedure authorising the infringement of the deprivation of liberty, also called confinement, detention and custody.

Mental disorder is the term used within the Mental Health Act [4]; this is the term which Burdzik [21] suggests should replace unsound mind.

Current UK law requires the evidence of unsound mind and mental disorder to come from medical evidence; however, case law is bringing a broader view of the scope of what constitutes medical evidence which could include evidence from advanced practitioners.

THE LAW RELATING TO TREATMENT

Medical treatment is defined in the Mental Health Act [4] at section 145 as *treatment the purpose of which is to alleviate, or prevent a worsening of, the disorder or one or more of its symptoms or manifestations*. It progresses to outline that *medical treatment includes nursing, psychological intervention and specialist mental health habilitation, rehabilitation and care*.

However, any treatment falling outside of this definition, namely treatment not for mental disorder is covered by other statute.

The term consent to treatment remains parlance and is the current wording in much statute. However, there is discourse relating to the binary nature of 'consent to', effectively either agreeing to or refusing, when in fact these events include the consideration of multiple options in the process of making a decision. Case law and practice in the Mental Capacity Act [2] arena is progressing to using the term 'making a decision about' the issue.

Consent to treatment Mental Health Act

Consent to treatment is covered by Mental Health Act (MHA) [4] Part 4 for inpatients and Part 4A for Community Treatment Order (CTO) patients. The details within MHA section 58 permits a period of three months prior to any certificate of consent (such as a T2 form or a CTO12 form) being required. These MHA sections also outline the requirement for a CQC Second Opinion Appointed Doctor for situations where the person either lacks mental capacity to consent to treatment or is refusing necessary treatment (such as T3 form or CTO11 form). There are provisions in MHA section 62 for giving people detained, treatment in an urgent situation where it is immediately necessary to save life, to prevent a serious deterioration of their condition, to alleviate serious suffering or to prevent violence or being a danger to themself or others. In the latter three of these urgent situations, the treatment should not be irreversible or hazardous.

The MHA Code of Practice [16] is clear on the need to implement both MCA [2] and MHA [4] simultaneously, leading to expectations of clear and documented assessments of mental capacity where there is reason to doubt the person's ability to consent to mental health treatment and a rationale underpinning best interest decisions in these situations.

Consent to Treatment Outside MHA

Any treatment that is not for mental disorder falls outside of the MHA provisions. The Mental Capacity Act [2] principles and processes apply, with the person being considered to have mental capacity unless there is reason to doubt this, and a lack of mental capacity has been evidenced by the assessing professional.

The earlier section on determining mental capacity provides detail on the processes to be implemented by advanced practitioners and others.

> **Case Study 9.2   Leo and the Relationship Between the MHA and MCA in 'Rapid Cycling Treatment Resistant Bipolar Disorder'**
>
> **Leo:** Leo is a 22-year-old man with severe learning disability, autism and treatment-resistant rapid cycling bipolar disorder. He is currently an inpatient on a specialist ward.
>
> Leo has limited verbal communication and echolalia. He has very repetitive behaviours and will self-stimulate through these and other behaviours. Leo progressed well in the structured environment of a specialist residential school until the age of 15 when he was seen to experience periods of low mood which responded to antidepressants. Six months later he was noted to have manic behaviours, he rarely slept and was jumping continuously, and despite an increased appetite, he had lost weight. As a result of repeated episodes of depression and mania, he was diagnosed with bipolar disorder and prescribed Lithium which affected kidney function. He was therefore changed to Sodium Valproate which had a good initial effect.
>
> At the age of 18 it was noted that despite treatment, he was having increased episodes of mania, the intensity and severity also increased and manic behaviours were coupled with self-injury and physical aggression towards staff and other pupils, on occasion causing them to need hospital treatment for their injuries.
>
> He was admitted to a specialist acute ward, his detention was lengthy and after a year the severity of his physical aggression increased further, coupled with significant damage to property. Staff were often being injured necessitating lengthy periods of absence from work. Leo was experiencing frequent physical restraint, rapid tranquillisation and use of seclusion. Periods of mental stability and depression were outweighed by the duration of mania.
>
> There is a suggestion that Leo may need to be admitted to a secure hospital. However, on review of case studies reporting success in the use of Clozapine, this was to be considered.
>
> *Note:* Pseudonyms are used to protect the anonymity of the person, and some details have been changed. Confidentiality has been fully maintained in line with ethical and professional standards [13].
>
> **Legal and Practice Considerations:**
>
> ***Human Rights Act:*** Which Article rights are engaged in this scenario?

> ***Equality Act:*** Does Leo have a protected characteristic? Could the use of Clozapine off licence be a reasonable adjustment? How do you prevent discrimination in the consideration of this?
>
> ***Mental Health Act:*** Is the treatment covered by the provision in the Mental Health Act? Will a CQC Second Opinion Appointed Doctor (SOAD) be required?
>
> ***Mental Capacity:*** Would you undertake a formal assessment of mental capacity, or would a 'reasonable belief' suffice? If using a reasonable belief what evidence would support your decision? Does the best interests checklist and process offer a helpful structure for considering and documenting Clozapine off licence?
>
> ### Key Learning Points:
>
> There is a requirement to consider all relevant legal frameworks, whilst Leo is detained under the Mental Health Act, the Mental Capacity Act and other legislation must be integrated into its implementation. The consent processes of the Mental Health Act can be enhanced through the use of the capacity assessment and best interests checklist and process from the Mental Capacity Act.

Covert Administration of Medications

The area of covert administration of medications has received focused attention in recent years. This is considered to be a very restrictive practice given the person is unaware that they are taking medications hidden/disguised in their food, drink or feeds given through tubes. England's regulator the Care Quality Commission [24] has set out guidance on this matter and many Safeguarding Adult Boards have provided guidance also.

This restrictive practice can only be used where:

- a person actively refuses their medicine and
- that person is assessed not to have the mental capacity to understand the consequences of their refusal. Such mental capacity is determined by the Mental Capacity Act 2005 [2] and
- the medicine is deemed essential to the person's health and well-being.

As such, all other options for the administration of the medication should have been explored along with the review of which medications are essential. In these circumstances, the discussions and actions are seeking to reduce the numbers of medications required to those which are essential; being clear about which medications must be given covertly and which could be missed without major concern and considering if the refusal could be ameliorated by the medication being given in a different form such as orodispersible or liquid preparations or less frequent depot injections. APMHs who have successfully completed independent and supplementary prescriber training may become involved in the review of a person's treatment plan as part of a process that is progressing towards a possible covert administration plan. It is essential that they are cognisant of regulator guidance in addition to local and organisational guidance, policy and procedure. Partnership work with pharmacists and medical colleagues in these instances will be required.

Where there is the involvement of the First Tier Tribunal for Mental Health, it must be understood that their procedures may require the disclosure of the use of covert administration.

SOCIAL WORKERS, NURSES AND OCCUPATIONAL THERAPISTS TAKING ON STATUTORY ROLES

Since 1972 there has been consideration of Nurses extending or expanding their scope of practice carrying out tasks not included in their normal training for registration [25]. Over time this has provided several opportunities including taking on statutory roles. There is also the opportunity for Social Workers and Occupational Therapists to take on these statutory roles as we see greater embedding of medico-legal practice into practitioners dealing with cases that present with ethical and legal dilemmas.

Within these areas of law there are three key roles explored here, all require additional training and education, and all require an approvals process.

The Mental Health Act Amendments of 2007 [4] implemented in 2008 brought new role titles and a broadening of the professions who can fulfil such roles, offering opportunities beyond the previous psychiatry and social work statutory roles to include these responsibilities for psychology, mental health and learning disability nursing and occupational therapy. These combined with other initiatives such as independent and supplementary prescribing for nurses further extends the areas of practice as they progress in advanced and consultant level roles.

Mental Health Act Approved Mental Health Professional (AMHP)

Previously reserved to social workers who had been approved (Approved Social Worker/ASW); the role definition of an Approved Mental Health Professional (AMHP) was refreshed allowing other professions to undertake this role and updating the competencies and process required to obtain approval.

The key competencies set out in greater detail in the AMHP Regulations for England 2008 [26] cover the application of the values to the AMHP role, knowledge of the legal and policy framework, knowledge of mental disorder, skills for working in partnership and skills for making and communicating informed decisions.

It is necessary to successfully complete a Social Work England approved course to prepare as an AMHP. Appointment of AMHPs is made by a Local Social Services Authority who will keep a record of each AMHP approved to act on behalf of their Local Authority.

There are challenges to the AMHP role and impact, not least due to the demand for inpatient services and pressures in community mental healthcare. Others hold a view that the role of the AMHP has become politicised with Fish [27] stating that *the genericism movement and the adoption of New Public Management has limited the professionalisation of AMHPs and therefore adequate implementation of 'the social perspective'*.

Deprivation of Liberty Safeguards (DoLS) Best Interests Assessor

DoLS Best Interests Assessors, as described in the Code of Practice [22], are central to the implementation of DoLS. They have a range of duties within the Safeguards and in many authorities are employed full time to undertake these duties. The primary duty is in the completion of a number of statutory assessments required by DoLS in collaboration with the DoLS Mental Health Assessor which is usually a psychiatrist.

The regulations set out the process for approval as a DoLS Best Interests Assessor. It requires that the person to be approved has the skills and experience appropriate to the assessments to be carried out, an applied knowledge of the Mental Capacity Act 2005 [2] and related Code of Practice [15] and the ability to keep appropriate records and to provide clear and reasoned reports in accordance with legal requirements and good practice.

DoLS Best Interests Assessors will have completed an approved preparation course; they will be selected by the 'Supervisory Body' which will be a local authority social services department. They may be required by that local authority to undertake a minimum number of assessments or specific update training annually.

With more adults deprived of their liberty using DoLS than those detained under the Mental Health Act [28], this role is critical in the current health and social care system. However, there has been critique and redefinition of the law, the Mental Capacity (Amendment) Act 2019 [29] covering England and Wales replaces DoLS with the Liberty Protection Safeguards (LPS), statutory guidance relating to this planned change is available [30]. At this time the amendments creating the LPS have not been implemented.

Mental Health Act Approved Clinician

Previously the Responsible Medical Officer/RMO, the Mental Health Act Approved Clinician was redefined through the Mental Health Act 2007 amendments [4] extending the role to other professions who have completed a portfolio demonstrating their competence to undertake this senior role. When acting for a person detained under the Mental Health Act or subject to a Community Order the Approved Clinician (AC) is known as the person's 'Responsible Clinician' (RC). It is important to be clear when the AC is acting as an RC ensuring the appropriate use of the relevant role title. Both roles are different to the section 12 approved doctor whose role is limited to examination and assessment of a person thought to require detention under this Act.

The competencies required to be approved as an AC are detailed within the Secretary of State's instructions and appended schedules [31], they fall within the areas of the AC/RC roles; legal frameworks policy and guidance; clinical assessment; treatment; multi-professional/agency care planning; clinical leadership and multi disciplinary team working; communication, equality and diversity.

To become approved, a portfolio covering the competencies and the mandated content is required necessitating those developing their skills to have both a breadth of experience of the range of mental disorders and the range of settings in which mental healthcare is delivered coupled with a depth of experience in the field and service where they will be deployed as an AC. There is also the requirement to complete a Panel-approved AC induction course.

Where the AC is not able to independently prescribe as a result of either current legislation on prescribing (for psychologists, social workers and occupational therapists) or for nurses, not having completed the nurse prescriber training, they will require an independently prescribing AC to be involved in a person's care where treatment is being provided under the Mental Health Act [4].

CONCLUSION

The skilful integration of law and practice is an integral part of advanced practice in mental health. It is an area where APMHs need to demonstrate capability and leadership.

This chapter has provided an overview of key legislation of direct relevance to mental healthcare at an advanced level and provided key information about specific statutory roles that APMHs could extend into.

FURTHER READING/USEFUL RESOURCES

Mental Health Law online. https://www.mentalhealthlaw.co.uk/Main_Page
39 Essex Chambers. https://www.39essex.com/our-thinking/mental-capacity-resource-centre/
Neil Allen's website. https://www.lpslaw.co.uk/
Alex Rook Keene's website. https://www.mentalcapacitylawandpolicy.org.uk/
Social Care Institute for Excellence. www.scie.org.uk/mca-directory/index.asp
Essex Autonomy Project. https://autonomy.essex.ac.uk/
Equality and Human Rights commission. https://www.equalityhumanrights.com/en/human-rights/human-rights-act

REFERENCES

1. Health Education England (2022). Advanced practice mental health curriculum and capabilities framework. https://www.hee.nhs.uk/sites/default/files/documents/AP-MH%20Curriculum%20and%20Capabilities%20Framework%201.2.pdf
2. England and Wales Mental Capacity Act (2005). https://www.legislation.gov.uk/ukpga/2005/9/contents
3. United Kingdom Human Rights Act (1998). https://www.legislation.gov.uk/ukpga/1998/42/contents
4. England & Wales Mental Health Act 1983 as amended 2007. https://www.legislation.gov.uk/ukpga/1983/20/contents
5. Mahdanian, A.A., Laporta, M., Drew Bold, N. et al. (2023). Human rights in mental healthcare; a review of current global situation. *International Review of Psychiatry* 35 (2): 150–162. https://doi.org/10.1080/09540261.2022.2027348.
6. Mind (2023). Mind reveals true extent of crisis in mental healthcare with more than 17,000 reports of serious incidents in past year alone. www.mind.org.uk/news-campaigns/news/mind-reveals-true-extent-of-crisis-in-mental-healthcare-with-more-than-17-000-reports-of-serious-incidents-in-past-year-alone
7. Hollins, S. (2023). Baroness Hollins' final report: My heart breaks - solitary confinement in hospital has no therapeutic benefit for people with a learning disability and autistic people. https://www.gov.uk/government/publications/independent-care-education-and-treatment-reviews-final-report-2023/baroness-hollins-final-report-my-heart-breaks-solitary-confinement-in-hospital-has-no-therapeutic-benefit-for-people-with-a-learning-disability-an
8. England Scotland & Wales Equality Act (2010). https://www.legislation.gov.uk/ukpga/2010/15/contents
9. Government Equalities Office (2013). Disability: Equality Act 2010 – Guidance on matters to be taken into account in determining questions relating to the definition of disability. https://www.gov.uk/government/publications/equality-act-guidance/disability-equality-act-2010-guidance-on-matters-to-be-taken-into-account-in-determining-questions-relating-to-the-definition-of-disability-html
10. National Development Team for Inclusion (2012). Reasonably adjusted? mental health services and support for people with autism and people with learning disabilities. www.ndti.org.uk/assets/files/Reasonably-adjusted.pdf
11. National Development Team for Inclusion (2020). "It's Not Rocket Science" Considering and meeting the sensory needs of autistic children and young people in CAMHS inpatient services. www.ndti.org.uk/assets/files/Its-Not-Rocket-Science-v.2.pdf
12. National Development Team for Inclusion (2022). Green light toolkit. www.ndti.org.uk/resources/green-light-toolkit (this page contains various documents and resources)

13. Nursing and Midwifery Council (NMC) (2018). The Code: Professional standards of practice and behaviour for nurses, midwives and nursing associates. www.nmc.org.uk/globalassets/sitedocuments/nmc-publications/nmc-code.pdf
14. England Care Act (2014). www.legislation.gov.uk/ukpga/2014/23/contents
15. Department for Constitutional Affairs (2007). Mental Capacity Act Code of Practice. https://www.gov.uk/government/publications/mental-capacity-act-code-of-practice
16. DHSC (2015a). Code of Practice: Mental Health Act 1983. https://www.gov.uk/government/publications/code-of-practice-mental-health-act-1983
17. DHSC (2015b). Mental Health Act 1983: Reference Guide. https://www.gov.uk/government/publications/mental-health-act-1983-reference-guide
18. England & Wales Mental Health Units (Use of Force) Act (2018). https://www.legislation.gov.uk/ukpga/2018/27/enacted
19. Mental Health Units (Use of Force) Act (2018). https://www.gov.uk/government/publications/mental-health-units-use-of-force-act-2018
20. Council of Europe (2021). European Convention on Human Rights, as amended by Protocols Nos. 11, 14 and 15 and supplemented by protocols 1, 4, 6, 7, 12, 13 and 16. https://www.echr.coe.int/documents/d/echr.convention_ENG
21. Burdzik, M. (2023). Who is 'the person of unsound mind'? The problem of terminological incompatibility in law and medical sciences in the context of the proper legal protection of people with mental disorders subjected to penal coercive measures. *European Psychiatry* 66 (Suppl 1): S166. https://doi.org/10.1192/j.eurpsy.2023.403.
22. Ministry of Justice (MoJ) (2008). Mental Capacity Act 2005: Deprivation of Liberty Safeguards – Code of Practice to Supplement the Main Mental Capacity Act 2005 Code of Practice: Department of Health – Publications. https://webarchive.nationalarchives.gov.uk/ukgwa/20130104224411/http://www.dh.gov.uk/en/Publicationsandstatistics/Publications/PublicationsPolicyAndGuidance/DH_085476
23. The Court of Protection Rules (2017). Statutory Instrument 2017 No 1035 (L.16) England & Wales. www.legislation.gov.uk/uksi/2017/1035/contents
24. Care Quality Commission (CQC) (2022). Covert administration of medicines. www.cqc.org.uk/guidance-providers/adult-social-care/covert-administration-medicines
25. Wright, S.G. (1995). The role of the nurse: extended or expanded? *Nursing Standard (Royal College of Nursing (Great Britain))* 9 (33): 25–29. https://doi.org/10.7748/ns.9.33.25.s28.
26. The Mental Health (Approved Mental Health Professionals) (Approval) (England) Regulations 2008 UK SI 2008/1206. www.legislation.gov.uk/uksi/2008/1206/contents/made
27. Fish, J.L.H. (2022). Genericism and managerialism: the limits to AMHP professionalisation and expertise. *International Journal of Law and Psychiatry* 83: 101818. https://doi.org/10.1016/j.ijlp.2022.101818.
28. Edge Training Ltd. (2024). Detention/supervision of people with mental disorder in England. www.edgetraining.org.uk/post/detention-supervision-of-people-with-mental-disorder-in-england-1
29. England & Wales. Mental Capacity (Amendment) Act 2019. www.legislation.gov.uk/ukpga/2019/18
30. Department of Health and Social Care (2021). Liberty protection safeguards: what they. https://www.gov.uk/government/publications/liberty-protection-safeguards-factsheets/liberty-protection-safeguards-what-they-are
31. Statutory Instrument England & Wales Mental Health Act (1983). Instructions with respect to the exercise of an approval function in relation to approved clinicians 2015 https://assets.publishing.service.gov.uk/media/5a7f38e4e5274a2e87db48a8/2015_AC_Instructions.pdf

CHAPTER 10

Collaborative Care Planning and Shared Decision-Making

Ann Cox[1] and Jan McAdam[2]

[1]*Derbyshire Healthcare NHS Foundation Trust, Derby, UK*
[2]*Tees, Esk and Wear Valleys NHS Trust, North Yorkshire, UK*

Aim

This chapter will briefly explore collaborative care planning and the use of shared decision-making in the care planning process. It is not intended to be a comprehensive study in this area but rather an overview to relate directly to practice. As this chapter is intended for advanced practitioners in mental health (APMHs), it will be expected that knowledge and skills in care planning will already have been achieved. This chapter will consider differences in practice and legal frameworks across the lifespan in relation to care planning and the involvement of the patient and their families and/or care givers. Shared decision-making is an important aspect of care planning that ensures the patient is central to the process. It is where the experts in health and the patient collaborate to ensure the care plan is achievable, transparent and progressive [1]. We will consider key challenges in care planning and how these can be overcome by the APMH.

LEARNING OUTCOMES

After reading this chapter, the reader will be able to:

1. Have a revised understanding of care planning theoretical underpinnings.
2. Be reminded about efficiently utilising the multidisciplinary team (MDT) to meet the needs of the patient from an APMH perspective.
3. Have an elevated understanding of the theoretical underpinnings of shared decision-making and advanced care planning.
4. Have an advanced understanding on how to develop, evaluate and achieve collaborative care plans.

The Advanced Practitioner in Mental Health, First Edition. Edited by Clare Allabyrne.
© 2026 John Wiley & Sons Ltd. All rights reserved, including rights for text and data mining and training of artificial intelligence technologies or similar technologies. Published 2026 by John Wiley & Sons Ltd.

This chapter will embody the following competencies within the Advanced Practice Mental Health Curriculum and Capabilities Framework in mental health [2] (see Table 10.1).

TABLE 10.1 How this chapter meets the APMH curriculum and capabilities framework.

Clinical practice pillar

1. Work autonomously within professional, ethical codes and legal frameworks, being responsible and accountable for their decisions, actions and omissions at this level of practice.
2. Demonstrate the underpinning psychological, biological and social knowledge required for advanced practice in mental health.
3. Demonstrate comprehensive knowledge of, and skills in, systematic history taking and clinical examination of patients who are culturally diverse and/or have complex needs in challenging circumstances, to develop a coproduced management plan.
4. Utilise clinical reasoning and decision-making skills to make a differential diagnosis and provide rationales for person-management plans, through critically reflecting on and evaluating their own role in relation to challenging traditional practices, new ways of working and the impact upon the multidisciplinary team.
5. Initiate, evaluate and modify a range of interventions, which may include therapies, medicines, lifestyle advice and care.

Leadership and management pillar

1. Identify, critically evaluate and reformulate understanding of professional boundaries to support new ways of working within the context of organisational and service need.
2. Exercise professional judgement and leadership to effectively promote safety in the presence of complexity and unpredictability.
3. Demonstrate teamworking, leadership, resilience and determination, managing situations that are unfamiliar, complex or unpredictable.

Education pillar

1. Facilitate collaboration of the wider team to support individual or interprofessional learning and development.
2. Critically assess and address individual learning needs that reflect the breadth of ongoing professional development across the four pillars of advanced clinical practice.
3. Effectively utilise a range of evidence-based educational strategies/interventions to support person-centred care with individuals, their families and carers and other healthcare colleagues.

Research pillar

1. Critically appraise and apply the evidence base in influencing engagement, recovery, shared decision-making, transference and safeguarding.
2. Develop and implement robust governance systems and systematic documentation processes, keeping the need for modifications under critical review.
3. Demonstrate the application of quality improvement methodologies in improving service.

FOUNDATION FOR COLLABORATIVE CARE PLANNING

Care Planning Theory in Mental Healthcare

There are many theoretical approaches to care planning in mental healthcare. Person-centred care and goal-based outcome-centred approaches were developed from the seminal psychologist theorist Carl Rogers in the 1940s [3]. Rogers developed the concept of person-centred therapy and associated goal development which considered each person as an individual and therefore having individual needs [3]. Principles of holistic care planning can be traced back to the 1700s; this theoretical approach included key considerations for the whole person including their environment and is inclusive of the recovery model of care [4]. The medical model of care planning, which was initially termed as such by the Scottish psychiatrist and psychoanalyst R.D Laing, involved the assessment and identification of ill health and its diagnoses predicated on the behaviours that are presented because of them and treatment identified thereafter [5]. Laing rejected this as a helpful model of care when working with severe and enduring mental health difficulties and explored a development of this model which considered social development alongside the medical model to expand the focus of the care planning model. Laing was considered 'anti-psychiatry'; however, he always promoted the need for treating mental distress.

There are many models of care planning; however, many are derived from these detailed earlier. As an advanced practitioner, having a collective understanding and implementation of these models will ensure informed care planning. It is important that care planning involves a holistic perspective of the patient and includes their mental and physical health, their personal and spiritual needs related to the treatment and recovery care plan. This should be facilitated by a variety of professionals in a multidisciplinary team (MDT) approach to best meet the needs of the patient. By using a holistic approach, it will ensure that all of the patient needs are identified for the recovery of their mental distress. This approach will include aspects of person-centred care planning, the patient's holistic needs, medical approaches to care and the inclusion of the patients social and emotional needs culminating in a biopsychosocial and spiritual approach [6]. The biopsychosocial framework and holism are discussed in detail in Chapter 3. Care planning should also include information about risk assessment and safety plans, so all information is in one document, in an accessible format that works best for the patient.

Multidisciplinary Team (MDT) Working

As an APMH, you will be working with patients from assessment, through to discharge and ensuring the care planned intervention being provided for the patient is the most efficient and evidenced based for the patient to achieve recovery or be able to manage their condition. Understanding the role and function of MDT working is key to ensuring an efficient and positive outcome for the patient. The APMH should utilise interdisciplinary working to best address the patients' needs [7]. Whilst the APMH may have a higher level of skills and knowledge, it is important that the practitioner remains practising within their scope of practice and utilises other professionals from the MDT to provide intervention for the patient where professional remits determine as per the APMH competencies [2].

Mental health teams can be set up very differently depending on geographic area and needs for the local demographics. The patients' clinical team will be different depending on the needs of the patient and the MDT will work together in achieving the care plan goals for the patient [8]. Health Education England produced an MDT toolkit to help teams maximise their output for the patient which will support the best delivery of care for a patient [8].

Mental health teams may include professionals, such as nurses, doctors, psychotherapists, pharmacists, general practitioners (GP), paediatricians, social workers, occupational therapists and psychologists. The role and responsibility of each of the professions within the MDT should be specific in the care planning, so there is not any duplication or merging of roles as this can cause confusion for the patient. It is also useful in relation to accountability and risk.

Shared Decision-Making

Shared decision-making is the process where all people who are part of the care planning decision-making process contribute to the overall decision in a collaborative way [1]. It can be helpful to think about the 'experts' coming together to make the decision about what the care plan should include and what is important for the patient. The patient should be considered being the expert about themselves, the clinician and other professionals as part of the MDT and skill mix can bring their specialist clinical expertise about what care can be offered from a healthcare practice perspective. The carer/family member/parent should be considered as being an expert in the patients' life from a different perspective and being someone that can support the patient in adhering to the care plan if required. The NHS constitution outlines that all patients, families and their carers should be involved in decisions about their care where appropriate and possible [9].

Care planning will require different decisions to be made around the care for a patient. The focus of care planning decisions must be collaboratively decided where possible. Who is included in the shared decision-making process will depend on the part of the plan being discussed; this may include different members of the MDT and should always include the patient and the clinician responsible for the patient's care. It should wherever possible include partners and carers (if adults) or parents or guardians if children, or this can include any person that can help and inform the shared decision that would be helpful to the patient. They may be included in a variety of ways, depending on whether the patient is agreeable to this and whether there are any safeguarding issues present. The triangle of care framework promotes family being involved in care planning to improve outcomes and also offers a network for carers, professionals and organisations [10].

At times there may be a need to include professionals that have more knowledge and skills to better inform the decision-making process, such as a therapist or someone who has a good understanding of medications such as a pharmacist [11], if these roles have not been within the scope of practice of the APMH. Where a decision could be burdensome to the patient, then it will be important to ensure that the patient is supported to contribute to the decision to the point where they feel happy to do so and it does not negatively impact on their well-being [12]. At times, it may be necessary for the shared decision to be made in the best interests of the patient should there be a concern around the burden of the weight of the decision, capacity, competence or levels of distress. The associated legal frameworks will have to be followed should this need occur, such as the Mental Capacity Act (2005) [13] including best interest decisions and the Children Act (1989) [14] in reference to parental consent.

Legal Frameworks and Associated Considerations

There are many legal frameworks that may need to be referenced when considering care planning across the lifespan and some key considerations in different age groups in respect of mental healthcare. For example, the role of parental consent for the competent/capacitous child and how to manage differences in care planning decisions [15]. Other key frameworks will include Gillick competency [16]; the Mental Capacity Act, which also includes deprivation of liberty safeguards (DOLs) and lasting power of attorney [13] including best interest decision-making; the Mental Health Act (1983) [17] and the Children Act in relation to those children in care and who needs to be involved in the decision-making about care planning [14]. Legal issues in the adult population are discussed in more detail in Chapter 9 and in the Child and Young Person population in Chapter 14.

Advanced Care Planning

Advanced care planning is legally only available for people over the age of 18 years. Advanced care planning allows for a person to make a plan of care or some key decisions about their care in the future, in the event that they lose capacity. The advanced care plan allows for these decisions to be carried out. Such decisions that can be made in advance might be about not receiving certain interventions such as medication, life sustaining interventions and being resuscitated. Advanced care plans are a legal document so it will be important that these are known about during any intervention from healthcare providers [18].

KEY CONSIDERATIONS FOR COLLABORATIVE CARE PLANNING

There are some helpful key considerations for care planning that will ensure that you have collaborative and achievable care plans. A great way to develop care plans is by using the SMART metric for setting goals which stands for Specific, Measurable, Achievable, Realistic and Time limited [19]. Developing care plans using this method ensures that the care plan is clear and objective and it is understood what is to be achieved and by whom. A good example of a goal on a care plan using SMART objectives could be:

> *Alex has difficulties with anxiety, and over the last few months has become more socially isolated. Alex worked with his clinician and family member and developed the following goal for their care plan:*
> *Alex to go out with his friends to a café for a cup of coffee, for at least one hour each week for four consecutive weeks, and this is to be achieved by September of this year.*

This example is specific in that it is clear what Alex has agreed to achieve to complete this goal, he has agreed to go and meet his friends in a café for one hour a week for a coffee. In terms of the goal being measurable, the measurement should always be objective and not made on subjective feelings, such as feeling better in oneself or feeling less anxious, it should be operationalised so that more than one person can observe the measurement. In Alex's case, his goal can be measured by Alex going out, and how long for by both Alex and his friends. This is also measured by the number of times Alex goes out. Alex agreed that this goal is achievable and realistic for him to achieve. Alex also wanted to achieve the goal by September of this year as he felt that was a realistic time frame for him to complete it by [20].

Other key considerations for care planning are ensuring that the goals set are achievable from the service you work in. Goals and care plans should not be reliant on other people's behaviours or interventions unless you have full agreement that these can be achieved. For example, if there was an agreement for another part of the healthcare service to perform a task, such as taking blood tests or giving a depot injection and it was assured that this service could provide this, then that would be helpful to include in the care plan as it is definite it can be achieved. If, however, there were some difficulties in relationships for the patient that were contributing to their mental distress and it was felt helpful for this relationship difficulty to be resolved, including this in a care plan would potentially create further difficulties in these relationships if there was an expectation on another person in achieving the care plan; particularly if the other person did not have the same vested interest in achieving the care plan goal. It is important for the patient to keep to goals in their care plan that are achievable through their own motivation and actions. By involving other people's actions, this may mean the goal is never met. Whilst this may be part of the distress, the importance might be placed on supporting the patient to manage their responses to the other person rather than including an expectation of others to change their behaviours.

Legal Implications

It is important to be aware of any legal implications that might affect care planning such as advance care plans and any other part of the Mental Capacity Act (2005) [13]. We should avoid making assumptions about what people want and recognise diversity and individual choice whilst acting in the best interests of people, whilst respecting a person's right to accept or refuse treatment [21]. In mental healthcare, this can often result in a dichotomy, especially when a patient is detained to hospital against their wishes and treatment enforced. It is important to be aware of your own scope of practice in care planning and ensure that you involve additional professionals from the MDT with specific skills and knowledge to inform your patient and the care plan where appropriate [11].

Utilising advanced skills in managing conflict or differences in opinion to develop a collaborative care plan will be important as an APMH. As an APMH, there is an expectation that you have highly developed clinical expertise and leadership skills which will support you in managing some of these conflicts that can occur in clinical practice [2]. It is important to remember who you are treating when developing care plans, ensuring that the patients voice is central to the decision-making, whilst also taking on board advice and opinions of the family and carers: though it is of course important to remember that carers may not have capacity themselves or may not fully understand the best interests of the patient. Care plans should be dynamic in nature; they should reflect the patients' needs at that moment in time and will change as their presentation and difficulties change [22].

In mental healthcare, particularly where the patient is detained, the law sets out the legal framework in which we should operate [13, 17, 23]. Developing collaborative care plans within the remit of the law can be a challenging task; however, with a creative and patient-centred approach, this can be possible.

ILLUSTRATIONS OF COLLABORATIVE CARE PLANNING IN PRACTICE

Following are some case examples that demonstrate how this can be achieved. All case studies in this chapter are fictitious and aim to represent real-life scenarios in care planning.

> ### Case Example 10.1   Patient and Family Collaborative Care Planning
>
> *Bob is a 33-year-old male who was admitted to an Adult Mental Health (AMH) ward under section 2 of the Mental Health Act (1983)* [17] *with delusional beliefs and auditory hallucinations, resulting in potential of risk of harm to self and others. At the point of admission, his level of conviction in his beliefs was high. When discussing initiating oral antipsychotic medication, Bob was adamant he did not need this. Bob lacked capacity to consent to medication at that time, and although medical treatment could have been forced under section 63 of the MHA, 1983* [23], *it was however felt this was not necessary and proportionate at the point of admission, as risk was mitigated whilst he was in hospital.*

In all cases, it is important to develop a therapeutic relationship with individuals and work in partnership to promote involvement in decision-making about care provision and recovery [24]. If the patient consents, we should always make every effort to include families and carers in this process [25]. Initial discussions with Bob focused on eliciting his perception of his situation, including validation of his concerns, and an exploration of the impact of beliefs on self and others. Discussions about possible alternative explanations of his perception of his situation were explored at great length on several occasions. This allowed for the healthcare team to also consider possible perpetuating causes of his usual worrying thoughts and perceptual disturbances along with options for care and treatment [25]. The effect of Bob's experiences on him was also explored, to try and understand how these beliefs contributed to associated distress and impacted on his social functioning. In addition, formulation and normalisation of Bob's experiences was undertaken through education and discussion of the Stress Vulnerability Model [26]. The aforementioned interventions supported not only the promotion of a person-centred therapeutic alliance but also the ability to establish this at a time when discussing sensitive information whilst dealing with conflict and distress. This allowed for a construction of a biopsychosocial formulation in collaboration with Bob [2].

The assessment, formulation and treatment process were undertaken in keeping with Bobs' and his wife's wishes that she was involved and contributed to this process. A common complaint from carers has been the lack of inclusion from services, resulting in poor communications and carers' wishes being ignored [27]. In this case Bob's wife was invited to share collateral information and offer her perception of the situation. Bob's wife was able to provide valuable information and insight into how Bob's illness manifested, impacted on his social functioning and caused him distress. The information allowed for a more accurate formulation and risk-benefit analysis which informed decision-making around necessity of treatment with medication. In addition, having discussions with Bob and his wife about remaining in hospital, receiving medical treatment and commencing antipsychotic medication, jointly assisted with Bob's decision to accept treatment as she supported and encouraged Bob to consider this. Bob's wife also provided valuable insight on his treatment response and contributed to the decision-making when optimising treatment with medication. As such she not only was a valuable source of support but also played an important role when formulating and considering the treatment plan [25].

Support for Bob's wife was also considered, and she was offered information regarding her right to a carers' assessment in keeping with the Care Act 2014 [28]; however, she declined this. Further written information was provided on support via third sector and local voluntary support groups and how to access these [25].

Another key intervention was to assess Bob's capacity to consent to proposed medication. This process was undertaken with knowledge of statutory responsibilities and the legal framework in which treatment would be given [2]. Despite treatment being administered under the legal framework of the Mental Health Act, 1983 [17], the process of assessing capacity is conducted as set out under the Mental Capacity Act 2005 [13]. One of the principles of the Mental Capacity Act 2005 [13] stipulates that assumption of capacity should be made until unless proved otherwise. During this process Bob was provided verbal and written information on a second-generation antipsychotic medication for treatment of psychosis when antipsychotic naïve [29]. Information on indication, effects and side effects was provided and discussed. This was in conjunction with application of the test as set out under the Mental Capacity Act, 2005 [13] as a means of assessing whether Bob was able to make a capacitous decision to accept or refuse the proposed antipsychotic medication. The assessment concluded that although Bob was agreeable to accept medication, he lacked capacity to consent to this as *his ability to use or weigh up the information as part of his decision-making was limited. In this case it was possible, however, to negotiate initiating antipsychotic medication; however, authority to treat was under section 63 of the Mental Health Act, 1983 [17].*

Other interventions included physical health screening and monitoring relating to the use of psychotropic medication. On AMH wards all patients are clerked in, most often by a medic, though it is a role that may also be fulfilled by APMHs. Initial physical examination should be carried out. Admission bloods, including full blood count, urea + electrolytes, lipids, thyroid, HBA1c and prolactin levels are taken. In addition, QRisk3, a validated tool to estimate risk of future cardiovascular disease [30], should be undertaken to assess this [31]. The LESTER tool is generally used for patients with a serious mental illness and is a cardiometabolic health resource which supports the recommendations relating to monitoring physical health for people with psychosis or schizophrenia [32]. In addition, an electrocardiogram (ECG) will be taken when certain medication is prescribed; this is not just exclusively for antipsychotic medication, as other routine psychotropic medication can cause ECG changes such as QTc interval prolongation [33]. Assessment and investigations along with the ability to assess physical health issues within scope of practice are key interventions [2], and as the aforementioned illustrates particularly relevant when initiating treatment with some psychotropic medication.

After a period of time, Bob became less preoccupied with his delusional beliefs and no longer felt the need to act on these, a behaviour that could have caused himself and others harm. He was then able to make the link between commencing medication and reduction in preoccupation of worrying thoughts, and associated anxiety, paranoia and agitation. This allowed for Bob to be more open to explore alternative explanations of his psychotic experience, as part of his recovery process. During the pre-discharge meeting with the community mental health team, it was identified that ongoing relapse prevention work should continue post discharge. This should include identifying possible early warning signs of a crisis and the development of adaptive coping enhancement strategies. [25]. Other ongoing interventions should be undertaken when individuals are prescribed psychotropic medication post discharge when in the community. People who experience psychosis or schizophrenia and are prescribed antipsychotic medication should routinely have their physical healthcare monitored and offered health promotional interventions. This should include healthy eating and physical health activities programme and nicotine replacement. Increase in weight gain, abnormal lipid levels, problems with management of glucose levels and cardiovascular indicators should be monitored at least yearly and appropriate interventions offered [29, 34]. When planning for discharge back into the community, it was important to liaise with appropriate services who would support Bob on his journey of recovery. Knowledge of the wider care system and ability to effectively refer is a key intervention [2] to ensure collaboration, planning and delivery of care. In this case this would have included a referral to the Community Mental Health Team and allocation of a care coordinator. The team would continue to prescribe the psychotropic medication, and then transfer this to the GP under shared care arrangements [35]. In addition, psychological therapy such as cognitive behavioural therapy (CBT) and/or family interventions should be offered to support Bob's recovery following an episode of psychosis [29].

The aforementioned illustrates someone suffering with psychosis and who lacked capacity to consent to their care and treatment when initially admitted to a ward. Despite which, the team managed to quickly collaboratively develop care plans, with the support of his wife, which had a positive outcome and supported a speedy recovery.

> ### Case Example 10.2 MDT Collaborative Care Planning
>
> There will be times when acutely unwell patients are admitted to hospital under the Mental Health Act, 1983 [13] who will be presenting with associated risk of harm to self and/or others. It may be at such times the environment coupled with relational interventions alone are insufficient to mitigate risk of harm. Timely interventions are required, including treatment with psychotropic medication, higher levels of staff engagement and observations along with further possible restrictive restrictions. True collaboration in all aspects of care may not be possible at this point, and interventions should be provided with the person's best interests through use application of legal frameworks.
>
> *Sue, a 44-year-old female detained under section 3 of the Mental Health Act, 1983 [17], was experiencing psychosis and mania characterised by disinhibited behaviour, grandiose delusions and auditory hallucinations. Sue was at risk of harm to self, in the form of immediate self-neglect, due to chaotic behaviour and inability to care for herself. In addition, she was presenting in a disinhibited manner, was overfamiliar with others, placing herself in vulnerable situations. Sue also presented with irritability and was verbally hostile towards others including both staff and peers, placing her at risk of retaliation from others. At this point of the admission there was limited success in negotiating care and treatment and due to significant risk, it was imperative interventions commenced. Increased levels of nursing engagement and observations, medication management, including rapid tranquillisation (RT) was deemed necessary. In keeping with guiding principles of the Mental Health Act, 1983 [17], consideration was given to least restrictive interventions [23] to mitigate risk of harm for Sue and others. Sue lacked capacity to consent to the aforementioned interventions, although not assumed, treatment was given under part 4 of the Mental Health Act, 1983 [17].*
>
> *A formulation meeting was held 72 hours after admission. When planning for this meeting, standard practice involved invitations to include members of the inpatient MDT, community mental health services, along with other voluntary and statutory agencies if there is an identified need or if other agencies are already involved. In Sue's case a social worker (SW) from the local authority (LA) child and family services was already working with her and her children who were currently being looked after by her sister. As such it was imperative they were included in the meeting. Should this not have been the case the LA would have been automatically notified on admission through completion of a Parental Adult Mental Health Impact on Child (PAMIC) tool which assesses the impact of parental mental ill health on children [36].*
>
> *The purpose of the formulation meeting, based on the 5Ps model, is to gauge information and develop a collective shared understanding of the patient's needs [37]. Prior to the meeting all members of the MDT routinely carried out initial assessment individually with the patient to allow for a collection of information about the patient's needs which is then discussed and considered during the formulation meeting. This assisted with the identification of the aim of admission and interventions which would be necessary to be completed whilst Sue was an inpatient. It also identified longer term support that would be required for Sue to be safely discharged with follow up care provision. The onus is on individual professionals to assess and share information which then informs care through the identification of goals, professional roles and responsibilities within this. Assessment, formulation and collaborative planning of care are key interventions [2] and a routine practice as part of an AMH inpatient stay.*
>
> *During the meeting, nursing staff, led by the APMH, were keen to discuss some of the restrictions the MDT had placed on Sue. The MDT completed a risk-benefit analysis and considered how necessary and proportionate these were at that time and how these would continue to be reviewed and reduced [38]. It*

was agreed that initial and immediate treatment on the ward would consist of ongoing restrictive interventions such as rapid tranquilisation (RT), enhanced engagements and observations, with no access to leave to mitigate risk of harm to Sue and others. This was necessary medical treatment to prevent further deterioration of Sue's mental state [39].

Nursing staff also reported that early in the admission Sue disclosed she was in an abusive relationship, and with her consent a referral was made to the local Domestic Abuse Service, who agreed to work with her to offer support and counselling. In addition, during the meeting we were made aware of potential issues with Sue's tenancy and there was a risk of her being evicted so another goal was to signpost Sue to the local charity organisation who provide support around housing and tenancy. The ward psychologist also identified Sue had a trauma history and highlighted the risk of complex trauma and the need to consider future psychological interventions with Sue once she was able to do so [29].

During the formulation meeting, medication options for acute mental health symptoms and to manage Sue's mental disorder in the longer term was discussed and agreed. The APMH, an independent prescriber, in collaboration with the ward pharmacist, presented a medication history. This included information on past medications, treatment response and any adverse reactions. When considering a treatment plan, they also took into account physical health conditions and any potential interactions with the proposed plan and existing medications. First line treatment with psychotropic medication was based on a thorough consideration of the aforementioned and in keeping with national guidance and best practice [29].

Following the formulation meeting, Sue was prescribed antipsychotic medication which she accepted, and over the course of the next few weeks, there was a notable reduction in some of her symptoms of bipolar affective disorder. This was evaluated through use of day-to-day engagement and observations, but also through use of a formal assessment using the Brief Psychiatric Rating Scale [40]. It was concluded that despite some reduction in mania and preoccupation with delusional beliefs, antipsychotic medication alone was not having an optimum response and associated risks remained. This was discussed further with her Responsible Clinician (RC), and it was agreed that Sue would more than likely benefit from a mood stabiliser, but due to Sue being of childbearing age, further assessment would be required before prescribing this, in keeping with national guidelines [41]. The assessment was undertaken by two specialist prescribers, a consultant nurse and a consultant psychiatrist who concluded that Sue was able to consent to this medication. Sue reported she was not planning to have another child and understood the implications to the unborn child if she were to fall pregnant when taking this medication. Sue also agreed to take precautionary measures to avoid pregnancy and was agreeable to attend an appointment to have a contraception implant fitted via her GP practice which inpatient staff supported her to attend.

As Sue started to recover so did her ability to have meaningful conversations about her care and treatment. This included her ability to consent to remain in hospital on an informal basis and as such Sue's detention under section 3 of the MHA,1983 was rescinded after a capacity assessment to make an informed decision about this was formally undertaken [13] by her RC. Sue remained in hospital until plans were put in place that would ensure she had the adequate support from other agencies before being discharged back home.

Throughout the admission joint working between inpatient mental health services and the child and family SW remained necessary. The SW regularly attended the ward and also assessed Sue with her children when in her home during periods of section 17 leave [17]. Sue's contact with her children remained supervised for some time, and when initially put in place, she struggled to accept this. A key nursing intervention involved liaising with the SW along with offering Sue support and reassurance regarding her current situation. Planning of leave and contact with her children was done collaboratively with Sue, the *inpatient MDT and her SW as child safeguarding procedures were in place. As such there was a heavy reliance on joint working between mental health professionals and the LA to ensure this was completed in a safe and appropriate manner.*

In this case, immediate interventions on the AMH ward focused on stabilising Sue's mental health and elevating subjective distress and associated risks. However, early formulation based on individual professionals' assessments was paramount to identifying both short term and longer goals for Sue. The MDT formulation highlighted the need for a variety of agencies to be involved beyond mental health services to allow for a safe discharge and recovery for Sue. This highlights that effective MDT and interagency working are necessary to promote collaborative and effective care planning and yield the best outcome for the patient [8].

Case Example 10.3   CAMHS Collaborative Care Planning

Jacob is a 14-year-old boy with chronic obsessive compulsive disorder (OCD), and his OCD is affecting all areas of his life. He has been struggling with OCD for around four years. Jacob has responsibility OCD which means that he has to perform specific tasks or rituals when he is trying to neutralise a distressing thought. Jacob feels that he will be responsible for something bad happening to his friends or family if he does not neutralise these distressing thoughts by way of undertaking a behaviour or ritual to make the thought stop or not be meaningful anymore. Jacob involves his parents, sibling, friends and his dog within the rituals he is performing. Jacob's OCD is impacting his schooling as Jacob is having to avoid certain topics and environments within the school.

As part of his care, the APMH, who was allocated Jacob due to the complexities and severity of his OCD difficulties, was responsible for coordinating this episode of care. It was important to involve Jacob and his parents as part of the MDT in developing the collaborative care plan. Jacob's sibling was included in the formulation meeting to help Jacob and his family have a common understanding of the maintenance cycle of OCD and how the parents and the sibling contributed to Jacob's OCD. The maintenance cycle demonstrated how Jacob's OCD was continuing, in that Jacob would have a thought, Jacob would appraise that thought as being a bad thing that could happen and that he needed to perform a behaviour to neutralise the thought and keep himself or others safe. Jacob believed the behaviours he was doing, such as picking his socks up with his elbows or walking two steps forward, two to the side and four steps backwards would stop the bad thought from happening [42]. NICE Guidance indicates that cognitive behavioural therapy (CBT) should be utilised to support children with OCD [43]. CBT manuals have been developed that help inform how to treat a child with OCD and inform care planning [44]. As part of the care plan, Jacob was referred to a CBT therapist. It was important to include the therapist as part of Jacob's MDT as the therapist would be knowledgeable and skilled using CBT theory and associated manuals and would be best placed to provide Jacob with this aspect of his care plan. The CBT therapist undertook most of the individual work with Jacob.

It was important for Jacob to 'own' his OCD and stop asking his parents, sibling, friends and the dog to be involved as part of the routines and rituals, as this can reinforce the maintenance cycle of OCD [42]

When working with children, it is always important to work with the system around the child (please see the CAMHS Chapter 14 for more detail on this); therefore, as school is such a significant part of children's lives, it is important to include them in the MDT. Jacob and his family had given permission for the APMH and the CBT therapist to contact school to see what support could be put in place to help Jacob. The APMH and the CBT therapist were able to understand from the school how Jacob's difficulties affected him in the classroom and school environment. Jacob's form teacher at school became an important part of Jacob's MDT team in ensuring Jacob's OCD in school was managed appropriately and in line with the work Jacob was being asked to do in his individual therapy. The APMH and the CBT therapist were able to provide some strategies for the staff in school, so they could support Jacob better and therefore contribute to the care plan. The overall care plan included the family and the school working collaboratively to support Jacob with his OCD; namely, by not offering reassurance and supporting Jacob to ride out the anxiety rather than performing a behaviour to neutralise the thought.

Jacob was supported to treat his OCD with exposure response prevention (ERP) within his CBT during this episode of care. However, Jacob struggled to engage in therapy as at times as he found his anxiety to be too high. Jacob was therefore reviewed by the APMH who was also an independent prescriber to consider the commencement of a selective serotonin reuptake inhibitor (SSRI) to help reduce his anxiety and engage better in the CBT work [42]. The discussion about the medication was undertaken by the APMH with Jacob and his parents. The risks and benefits of medication were discussed in the appointment and consideration was given to alternative approaches other than medication. However, given Jacob's level of distress from his OCD and associated anxiety, it was felt that medication was indicated and appropriate at this time. Within the discussion the APMH was able to assess Jacob's ability to consent to the medication, this included him understanding the information that was shared with him, Jacob being able to retain the information that was shared, Jacob was able to weigh up the information and consider different options and he was able to communicate the decision that he wanted to try medication [13]. Jacob was therefore deemed Gillick competent [45]. As Jacob was deemed Gillick competent, he could consent to the medication commencement, Jacob's parents were also included in the discussion and they too agreed with Jacob's decision to commence medication.

Gillick competence is akin to having capacity, except this is the legal framework that is used for under 16 year olds. Whilst the assessment for competence is the same for capacity, in that you would have to determine a child could:

- ✓ Understand the information.
- ✓ Retain the information long enough to make the decision.
- ✓ Weigh up the information, benefits and risk and alternatives.
- ✓ Communicate the decision.

The difference for children under the age of 16 years is that the starting point is one of a presumption of the child not having capacity or competence (Gillick competency), where those aged 16 years and over start with the presumption of having capacity (Mental Capacity Act, 2005) [13, 16]. As an APMH you should be helping children to develop competence in order for a child to be a fully involved in their care as possible [46].

As Jacob was prescribed medication, then physical health reviews were added to his care plan to ensure that his physical health was not impacted by the medication he was taking.

Jacob was able to engage much better with the CBT after being on the medication for a few weeks and with this support he was able to reduce his OCD rituals by 80%. As Jacob had the skills and knowledge of how to overcome his OCD through the episode of CBT intervention, he was able to be discharged from mental health services and continue working on ERP by himself. Jacob's life had significantly improved through completing his care plan.

CONCLUSION

This chapter explores some of the theoretical models of care planning and how these can be helpfully utilised to develop the collaborative care plan with the patient. The use of shared decision-making and full use of the MDT ensure the best care plan can be developed for the patient. This requires the APMH to utilise their advanced skills in ensuring involvement from carers and families, leading the MDT decision-making and providing expert levels of clinical care and intervention throughout the process.

The role of the APMH is key to establish quality and safety for the patient [2] and to ensure that the best possible outcome for the patient is at the heart of the care planning. Legal frameworks and clinical guidance must be adhered to during the care planning process to ensure that all necessary considerations are included and lawful. Collaboratively working through shared decision making will ensure the care plan for the patient will be person centred, outcome driven and achieveable.

REFERENCES

1. NHS England (2019). NHS England: shared decision-making. NHS England. https://www.england.nhs.uk/personalisedcare/shared-decision-making
2. Health Education England (2020). Advanced practice mental health curriculum and capabilities. https://www.hee.nhs.uk/sites/default/files/documents/AP-MH%20Curriculum%20and%20Capabilities%20Framework%201.2.pdf (accessed February 2025).
3. Rogers, C.R. (1946). Significant aspects of client-centered therapy. *American Psychologist* 1 (10): 415–422. https://doi.org/10.1037/h0060866.
4. Thornton, L. (2019). A brief history and overview of holistic nursing. *Integrative Medicine (Encinitas)* 18 (4): 32–33.
5. Clay, J. (1996). *R.D. Laing: A Divided Self*. Stoughton.
6. Van Denend, J., Ford, K., Berg, P. et al. (2022). The body, the mind, and the spirit: including the spiritual domain in mental health care. *Journal of Religion and Health* 61: 3571–3588. https://doi.org/10.1007/s10943-022-01609-2.
7. Open University (2018). Multidisciplinary study: the value and benefits. OpenLearn. https://www.open.edu/openlearn/education-development/multidisciplinary-study-the-value-and-benefits/content-section-2
8. Health Education England (2021). Multi-disciplinary team toolkit. https://www.hee.nhs.uk/sites/default/files/documents/HEE_MDT_Toolkit_V1.1.pdf.
9. Gov.uk (2023). The NHS constitution for England. https://www.gov.uk/government/publications/the-nhs-constitution-for-england/the-nhs-constitution-for-england (accessed 8 February 2025).
10. Carers Trust (2024). The triangle of care, ToC, triangle of care. http://carers.org. https://carers.org/triangle-of-care/the-triangle-of-care
11. Org.uk (2025). Regulation 9: Person-centred care. www.cqc.org.uk/guidance-providers/regulations/regulation-9-person-centred-care (accessed 8 February 2025).
12. Alderson, P. and Montgomery, J. (1996). *Health Care Choices: Making Decisions with Children*. London.
13. Mental Capacity Act (2005). Mental Capacity Act 2005. www.legislation.gov.uk/ukpga/2005/9/contents (accessed 8 February 2025).
14. Children Act (1989). Children Act 1989. www.legislation.gov.uk/ukpga/1989/41/contents (accessed 8 February 2025).
15. Care Quality Commission (2019). http://CQC.Org.uk. www.cqc.org.uk/sites/default/files/Brief_guide_Capacity_and_consent_in_under_18s%20v3.pdf (accessed 8 February 2025).

16. Scarman, L., Harwich LBOF, Oakbrook LBOF, Templeman, L. (1985). Gillick v West Norfolk and Wisbech area health authority and another http://Globalhealthrights.org. https://www.globalhealthrights.org/wp-content/uploads/2013/01/HL-1985-Gillick-v.-West-Norfolk-and-Wisbech-Area-Health-Authority-and-Anr.pdf (accessed 8 February 2025).
17. Mental Capacity Act (1983). Mental Health Act 1983. www.legislation.gov.uk/ukpga/1983/20/contents (accessed 8 February 2025).
18. NHS England, NHS Improvement and Partner Agencies (2022). Nhs.uk. https://www.england.nhs.uk/wp-content/uploads/2022/03/universal-principles-for-advance-care-planning.pdf (accessed 8 February 2025).
19. Care Learning (2025). http://CareLearning.Org.uk. https://carelearning.org.uk/blog/frameworks/what-are-smart-goals-in-health-and-social-care (accessed 8 February 2025).
20. Law, D. and Jacob, J. (2015). *Goals and Goal Based Outcomes (GBOs): Some Useful Information*. London, UK: CAMHS Pres.
21. Nursing and Midwifery Council (2023). Read the code online. http://NMC.Org.UK. Org.uk. www.nmc.org.uk/standards/code/read-the-code-online (accessed 8 February 2025).
22. SCIE. Social Care Institute for Excellence (SCIE) (2023). MCA: Care planning, involvement and person-centred care. www.scie.org.uk/mca/practice/care-planning/person-centred-care (accessed 8 February 2025).
23. Gov.uk (2015). Mental health act code of practice https://assets.publishing.service.gov.uk/media/5a80a774e5274a2e87dbb0f0/MHA_Code_of_Practice.PDF (accessed 8 February 2025).
24. NICE (2016). Overview | Transition between inpatient mental health settings and community or care home settings | Guidance | NICE. www.nice.org.uk/guidance/ng53 (accessed 8 February 2025).
25. NICE (2011). Service user experience in adult mental health: improving the experience of care for people using adult NHS mental health services. http://NICE.Org.UK. www.nice.org.uk/guidance/cg136/resources/service-user-experience-in-adult-mental-health-improving-the-experience-of-care-for-people-using-adult-nhs-mental-health-services-pdf-35109513728197 (accessed 8 February 2025).
26. Rudnick, A. and Lundberg, E. (2012). The stress-vulnerability model of schizophrenia: a conceptual analysis and selective review. *Current Psychiatry Reviews* 8 (4): 337–341. https://doi.org/10.2174/157340012803520450.
27. Worthington, A., Rooney, P., and Hannan, R. (2013). Carers Trust https://carers.org/downloads/resources-pdfs/triangle-of-care-england/the-triangle-of-care-carers-included-second-edition.pdf (accessed 8 February 2025).
28. Care Act (2014). Care Act 2014. www.legislation.gov.uk/ukpga/2014/23/contents (accessed 8 February 2025).
29. NICE (2014). Psychosis and schizophrenia in adults: prevention and management | Guidance | NICE. http://NICE.Org.UK. www.nice.org.uk/Guidance/CG178 (accessed 9 February 2025).
30. Hippisley-Cox, J., Coupland, C., and Brindle, P. (2017). Development and validation of QRISK3 risk prediction algorithms to estimate future risk of cardiovascular disease: prospective cohort study. *BMJ* 357: j2099. https://doi.org/10.1136/bmj.j2099.
31. NICE.Org.UK (2023). Cardiovascular disease: risk assessment and reduction, including lipid modification | Guidance | NICE. www.nice.org.uk/guidance/ng238?UID=383762308202525175512 (accessed 9 February 2025).
32. Perry, B.I., Holt, R. I. G. Chew-Graham, C.A., Tiffin, E., French, P., Pratt, P., Byrne, P., Shiers, D. E. (2023). The lester tool. http://Rcpsych.ac.uk. www.rcpsych.ac.uk/docs/default-source/improving-care/ccqi/national-clinical-audits/ncap-library/eip-2024-ncap-lester-tool-intervention-framework.pdf?sfvrsn=21e45dbd_17 (accessed 9 February 2025).
33. Taylor, D.M., Barnes, T.R.E., and Young, A.H. (2021). *The Maudsley Prescribing Guidelines in Psychiatry*, 14the. Hoboken, NJ: Wiley-Blackwell.

34. NHS (2024). NHS England » 10 key actions: improving the physical health of people living with severe mental illness. Nhs.uk. https://www.england.nhs.uk/long-read/10-key-actions-improving-the-physical-health-of-people-living-with-severe-mental-illness (accessed 9 February 2025).
35. Nhs.uk (2018). Responsibility for prescribing between primary secondary/tertiary care. https://www.england.nhs.uk/wp-content/uploads/2018/03/responsibility-prescribing-between-primary-secondary-care-v2.pdf (accessed 9 February 2025).
36. SaferChildrenYork (2022). PAMIC Tool - 8 June 2022 (accessed 9 February 2025).
37. Sampogna, G., Luciano, M., and Fiorillo, A. (2024). The psychiatric formulation. In: *Tasman's Psychiatry*, vol. 1, 1449–1461. Springer eBooks.
38. Department of Health (2014). Positive and proactive care: reducing the need for restrictive interventions prepared by the department of health. https://assets.publishing.service.gov.uk/media/5a7ee560e5274a2e8ab48e2a/JRA_DoH_Guidance_on_RP_web_accessible.pdf
39. Department of Health (2015). Department of Mental Health Act 1983: code of practice. https://assets.publishing.service.gov.uk/media/5a80a774e5274a2e87dbb0f0/MHA_Code_of_Practice.PDF
40. Horan, W.P., Reise, S.P., Subotnik, K.L. et al. (2008). The validity of psychosis proneness scales as vulnerability indicators in recent-onset schizophrenia patients. *Schizophrenia Research* 100 (1–3): 224–236.
41. H.M. Gov (2025). Valproate – reproductive risks. GOV.UK. https://www.gov.uk/guidance/valproate-reproductive-risks
42. Wells, A., Myers, S., Simons, M., and Fisher, P. (2017). Metacognitive model and treatment of OCD. *The Wiley Handbook of Obsessive Compulsive Disorders* 19: 644–662.
43. NICE (2005). Overview | Obsessive-compulsive disorder and body dysmorphic disorder: treatment | Guidance | NICE. https://www.nice.org.uk/guidance/cg31
44. March, J.S. and Mulle, K. (1998). *OCD in Children and Adolescents: A Cognitive-Behavioral Treatment Manual*. New York: Guilford Press.
45. *Gillick v West Norfolk and Wisbech Area Health Authority* (1985). 2. W.L.R. 143.
46. Cox, A. (2020). Chapter 11. Helping children and young people understand issues of consent to treatment. In: *Nursing Skills for Children and Young People's Mental Health* (ed. L. Baldwin). Cham, Switzerland: Springer.

CHAPTER 11

Digital Technology in Advanced Practice: Mental Health

Emma Taylor
Digital Mentality, London, UK

Aim

This chapter aims to review the fundamental principles of the applications of digital technology in healthcare, to understand the legal landscape of recommending digital tools in the National Health Service (NHS) and to elevate and advance skills in the use of digital technology in the enhancement of patient care, specifically in the field of mental health.

LEARNING OUTCOMES

After reading this chapter, the reader will be able:

1. To understand medical device law and how this applies to practice.
2. To understand clinical safety standards for digital technology and how this applies to practice.
3. To be able to identify key indicators of quality assurance in digital technology.
4. To understand the fundamental principles of how and when to implement digital technology in patient care planning.

INTRODUCTION

Digital technology can be perceived as being a relatively new concept in healthcare, though the use of technology in the NHS started right at the beginning of its' creation, with the introduction of the edge notch card in the late 1940s essentially forming an early concept electronic patient record [1].

The Advanced Practitioner in Mental Health, First Edition. Edited by Clare Allabyrne.
© 2026 John Wiley & Sons Ltd. All rights reserved, including rights for text and data mining and training of artificial intelligence technologies or similar technologies. Published 2026 by John Wiley & Sons Ltd.

The Classification of Digital Health Technology and Medical Devices

From the installation of the first pacemaker in 1958 [2] to the introduction of the Fitbit in the 2000's, digital health technology has had many changing faces. Whilst traditionally we might have considered technology to be something that happened on a larger scale, such as x-ray machines or an ultrasound machine, technology now occurs regularly at an individual patient level. For example. in physical health this can include devices such as wearable insulin pumps and in mental health individual usage of a mobile phone app to manage thoughts of self-harm. Currently, health and well-being technology is the largest growing category in the app store(s) and 40% of adults in the United Kingdom own a wearable fitness tracker [3].

However, there is an important differentiation between digital technology in general and digital health technology, particularly in relation to medical devices. When a digital technology is considered a medical device, it is governed under a different legal framework than other digital technology: Medical Device Regulations 2017 [4]. These regulations are designed to ensure that all digital technologies that are considered to have a medical purpose are regulated to ensure that they are safe and if necessary, appropriately packaged and distributed. These regulations also outline the process for onward monitoring of medical devices and ensure that digital technology providers have appropriate safety procedures and recall measures in place if something goes wrong.

There are five different categories of medical device (Table 11.1) and within each category there are four classifications of medical devices as shown in Table 11.2, and these indicate the risk of the device, taking into account the vulnerability of the human body and the potential risks associated with the device [5].

When determining the risk of harm to the patient, and therefore the classification of the device, there are 22 rules to consider taking into account lots of different factors. These include, whether the device comes into contact with the body? If so, for how long? Does it have any toxic parts? What part of the body is affected by the device? This then helps to classify the risk of harm or death. For digital health technology, the most important rules to consider are Rule 11 and Rule 22 (see Table 11.3).

For example, a closed loop insulin system designed to automatically deliver insulin based on digitally recorded blood sugar levels would be a class III medical device as it is an invasive device with an integrated diagnostic function [5]. In comparison a mobile phone app designed to help a patient complete exercises aimed at improving mental resilience would only be a class I [5].

TABLE 11.1 Categories of medical devices.

Category	Definition	Examples
Non-invasive	Devices which do not enter the body	Plasters, walking sticks, wheelchairs
Invasive	Devices inserted into the body's orifices or surgically invasive devices	Contact lenses, dental braces, cannulas
Surgically invasive	Devices used or inserted in surgery	Scalpels, cardiovascular catheters
Active	Devices that require an external source of power	Ultrasound, TENS devices, mobile phone apps
Implantable	Devices implanted into the body	Breast implants, orthopaedic implants

TABLE 11.2 Classes of medical devices.

Class	Examples
Class I (lowest risk)	Wheelchairs, stethoscopes, self-help mental health apps
Class IIa	Dental fillings, surgical clamps, mobile phone apps that help a clinician to diagnose
Class IIb	Condoms, lung ventilators
Class III (highest risk)	Pacemakers, heart valves

TABLE 11.3 Classification rules.

Classification rules	
Rule 11	Software intended to provide information which is used to take decisions with diagnosis or therapeutic purposes is classified as class IIa, except if such decisions have an impact that may cause: • death or an irreversible deterioration of a person's state of health, in which case it is in class III; or • a serious deterioration of a person's state of health or a surgical intervention, in which case it is classified as class IIb. Software intended to monitor physiological processes is classified as class IIa, except if it is intended for monitoring of vital physiological parameters, where the nature of variations of those parameters is such that it could result in immediate danger to the patient, in which case it is classified as class IIb. All other software is classified as class I.
Rule 22	Active therapeutic devices with an integrated or incorporated diagnostic function which significantly determines the patient management by the device, such as closed loop systems or automated external defibrillators, are classified as class III.

Different classifications have different regulation requirements. However, irrespective of the classification, all medical devices must adhere to the general requirements, including meeting general safety and performance requirements, adhering to reporting requirements, issuing a conformity statement and completing clinical investigations and evaluations [5]. If a technology has registered as a medical device, then they will be searchable on the Medicines and Healthcare products Regulatory Agency (MHRA) at pard.mhra.gov.uk. They will also display either the UK Conformity Assessed (UKCA) or the European Conformity Marking (CE) mark on their product, depending on whether the manufacturer is registered in the UK under post-Brexit guidance, or if the manufacturer has registered in Europe under European Union guidance [6]. A medical device must register before it can be placed on the UK market. Currently, products with either a CE or UKCA mark can be placed on the UK market until July 2025 when transitional arrangements will come into force and technologies must begin to transition to UKCA marking by either December 2027 or June 2028 depending on their classification [7] (see Figure 11.1).

In order to determine if a technology can be considered a medical technology, the Medical Device Regulations 2017 [4 Article 2] have defined a medical device as: '*any instrument, apparatus, appliance, software, material or other article, whether used alone or in combination, together with any accessories, including the software intended by its manufacturer to be used specifically for diagnosis or therapeutic*

FIGURE 11.1 Examples of UKCA and CE marks.

purposes or both and necessary for its proper application, which is intended by the manufacturer to be used for human beings for the purpose of:

- *diagnosis, prevention, monitoring, treatment or alleviation of disease*
- *diagnosis, monitoring, treatment, alleviation of or compensation for an injury or handicap*
- *investigation, replacement or modification of the anatomy or of a physiological process, or*
- *control of conception'.*

Therefore, lots of things we come into contact with during our usual working days can be classed as medical devices. They might be classed as general medical devices, for example dressing packs, glasses, mobile phone apps and computer software; implantable devices such as cochlear implants or catheters and in vitro devices such as pregnancy test kits or Hepatitis B test kits. The main characteristic of a medical device is that it does not achieve its main intended action by pharmacological, immunological or metabolic means, although it can assist. For example, a needle is a medical device, the vaccine it delivers is not. Whilst highlighting there are a wide variety of medical devices available, the remainder of this chapter will focus on medical devices that are digital in nature – this includes mobile apps, computer software, digital applications of health prevention and digitally driven devices such as wearable trackers.

One of the primary challenges for health professionals working in mental health is the lack of consistency in manufacturers approaches to medical device licensing which can create uncertainty and introduce risk into the technology landscape.

Many manufacturers will claim that their technology does not require medical device regulation as the intended purpose is for well-being. However, it is difficult to differentiate a clear boundary between what can be classed as well-being and what can be considered a preventative or treatment intervention for mental health. For example, a number of well-known meditation apps have not registered as medical devices in the past as they have claimed the purpose of the app was to provide access to meditations and mindfulness for well-being only and the app should not be considered a substitute for medical intervention. However, mindfulness and meditation are both recognised as important resilience tools that can be used to prevent mental ill health [8]. The medical device regulations 2017 definition [4] identifies a medical device as a device whose purpose prevents a disease, it could be argued these apps are medical devices, which would assume a requirement to appropriately register a medical device before placing it on the UK market. Currently, app stores and website creation sites do not have the same requirement. With over 41,517 healthcare and medical apps available on the app store, it is almost impossible to strictly regulate the market although the MHRA continue to work closely with the National Institute of Clinical Excellence (NICE), the NHS and manufacturers to try and get more mental health regulators to consider the applicability of their products [9].

Clinical Risk Management Standards

Medical device licensing is not the only legislation to take into account when considering the digital tools which may be applicable to our practice. There are also the clinical risk management standards DCB0129 and DCB0160 [10]. These information standards underpin national healthcare incentives across Department of Health (DoH), NHS England and the Care Quality Commission (CQC), as well as other national health organisations. DCB0129 is designed for manufacturers of health software systems, and DCB0160 is designed to be used by health organisations implementing a new health software. Compliance with DCB0129 and DCB0160 is mandatory under the Health and Social Care Act 2012 [11] and covers all health information technology (IT) systems including stand-alone software such as mobile phone apps with or without a medical device license. The only systems which do not fall under these standards are systems not directly associated with patients such as information governance, financial reporting or statistical reporting tools.

These standards mean that any digital health technology product that is considered for use by NHS patients must be DCB0129 compliant. DCB0129 standards are designed to ensure manufacturers of digital health technology, from apps to websites to wearable devices, are undertaking effective clinical risk management to ensure that the product has been appropriately assessed for risk of harm to patients and that appropriate actions have been taken to mitigate those risks [12]. By predicting foreseeable hazards and documenting these at each life stage of the product, from idea, to prototype, to patient use, we are better able to ensure that the risk of harm has been mitigated as much as possible with procedures in place and ongoing monitoring. In order to be DCB0129 compliant the manufacturer must appoint an appropriate clinical safety officer who must be a suitably qualified and experienced clinician holding a current registration with a professional body, for example a nurse who has completed the clinical safety training and has experience completing risk assessments for implementing innovations. The manufacturers must then maintain a clinical risk management file for their product including a clinical risk management plan, hazard log, clinical safety case and safety incident management log. All manufacturers should be prepared to share their clinical risk management file with commissioning healthcare providers when asked.

These standards also ensure that your healthcare organisation has carried out effective clinical risk management when deploying, using, maintaining or decommissioning a health technology [13]. Each healthcare organisation must also have an equally qualified clinical safety officer who can review the clinical safety management file of the technology they are seeking to deploy and who can maintain their own clinical safety management file. This includes post deployment monitoring and appropriate processes for decommissioning.

USING DIGITAL TECHNOLOGY IN THE MANAGEMENT OF CARE

As advanced practitioners in mental health, it is important to consider the best current evidence base for care, and this includes consideration of digital alternatives to traditional care. Statistically, 94% of adults in the United Kingdom own a smartphone [14]. The NHS app has been downloaded 30 million times and in 1 month alone 1.6 million repeat prescriptions were ordered, 130,000 general practitioner (GP) appointments were booked and 4.8 million GP records were viewed by patients [15]. This high level of use of a digital app to engage in fundamental care indicates that many patients will utilise digital technology options when made available to them. The benefits of digital alternatives to traditional interventions can include [16]:

- Easier to access in terms of both hours of availability and location
- More scalable
- More patient-led engagement
- More engaging

- Shorter waiting time
- Longer support
- More cost-effective

There are many areas of advanced practice in mental health where a digital alternative may be appropriate for some of this client group. This can include psychoeducation, support for mild to moderate anxiety or depression, enhancing exposure therapy, symptom monitoring, medication tracking, mindfulness or discharge support.

The Patient Perspective

When considering digital options for support, it is important first to understand the scope of the issue from the patient's perspective. This is of particular note, as studies reveal that clinicians often over report the inclusion of the patient's perspective and the occurrence of shared decision making which does not necessarily reflect their patients reported experience of the inclusion of their perspective [17]. For example, during a 2022 study exploring the use of artificial intelligence (AI) as a waitlist support tool for adults referred to psychological therapies, focus group interviews with clinicians to understand staff attitudes towards digital interventions found clinicians assumed that patients would not want to use an AI-driven app as they would prefer to speak to a clinician [18]. However, patient and public involvement (PPI) groups found that most patients were happy to use an AI app once they understood what AI was, as these groups felt this was preferable to being on a waiting list with no additional support available. PPI groups or experience-based co-design approaches are an excellent way to understand the scope of the problem from the patient's perspective. There are a number of resources that can used to help facilitate these approaches (see Table 11.4).

Getting Started

Once a better understanding of a patients' experience of the problem/identified issue has been sought, then the process of seeking solutions can begin. The Organisation for the Review of Care and Health Apps (ORCHA) has an app library where the search for apps that may support the issue that has been identified is a good initial starting point.

The apps listed here are ranked based on their clinical safety, user experience and privacy [19]. Journals, conferences and the internet can also be used as resources for exploring what other trusts or services have tried.

Finding the digital technological support depends on the type of solution identified and whether the support required is for a singular patient, group of patients or service wide. If digital care is being planned for a single patient, it may be possible to use a free version of a tool or a low-cost option that a patient can self-fund.

TABLE 11.4 Experience-based co-design approaches.

Resource	Description
Service mapping	Service mapping can be used to help understand the pathway a patient follows and facilitate conversations about where there are challenges or bottlenecks.
Patient stories	Collecting patients' stories can help provide a reflective understanding of multiple patients' experiences of a problem, service or intervention.
Story boarding	A more visual approach – this can be used to highlight patients' journeys or experiences to aid reflection and identify challenges.

Individual patient funding may be available from your trust which can be applied for on a case-by-case basis. If the patient is required to pay anything towards the digital solution, it is important this is discussed with them.

If the ask/decision is to implement a solution on a wider scale, funding may be required to pay for an initial trial of the digital technology. Liasion with the technology provider will assist with understanding costs associated with a trial so funding can be explored. Funding may be available from a trust innovation budget, local service underspend, grant funding or a national initiative programme. Working with local and directorate management can help to build the business case required for a trial period of the digital solution you have identified.

Finally, once the need has been identified, the digital solution agreed and funding secured as necessary, it is important to document the review process in relation to the implementation of the solution and record any learning. Gathering evidence, such as before and after outcome measures, or identifying key performance indicators helps to identify if the digital solution is working and inform any changes that may be needed, for example: adjusting the implementation method or adapting the way the innovation is communicated to staff. Reporting on the findings, via case studies and journals, helps to disseminate the learning to other clinicians.

Clinical Example: Embers the Dragon

Embers the Dragon is a digital innovation aimed at supporting the early years development of emotional mental health and well-being.

The initial issue that had been identified in 2018 that could require a digital solution was the increasing numbers of referrals to Child and Adolescent Mental Health Services (CAMHS) for younger children aged 4–7 years. These referrals were not meeting threshold for service due to a number of reasons, including prioritisation of perceived higher risk cases, limited resources to meet overall demand in CAMHS and the decommissioning of lower priority CAMHS services. During this time period there was also a marked increase in parents reporting behavioural concerns to GPs and an estimated 66% of primary school children experiencing anxiety [20].

As per the NMC Code of Conduct (2018) [21] *information about patients and clients should be treated as confidential and therefore details of the patient have been omitted to protect their identity.*

Parent A experienced many of these challenges. A had growing concerns regarding the behaviour of their 5 year old child (B), particularly B's aggression towards their 7 year old sibling. Parent A had asked for support at school and been referred to CAMHS services; however, the referral had been rejected as being below threshold and A was advised to attend a local Sure Start Family support centre. The only support on offer there was a parenting group. Parent A could not attend this group as it ran during work hours, A worked full time and could not afford the additional time off to attend. During this time B's behaviour continued to escalate and B was excluded from school for biting their teacher.

The parenting group offered to Parent A was a social learning theory based parenting group, the NICE recommended early intervention for emotional and behavioural well-being concerns [22]. These traditional therapeutic programmes in early years are delivered in groups on a face-to-face basis through statutory services at a substantial cost. A systematic review of these therapeutic groups/approaches showed high drop-out rates, with barriers to access for working or single parents as was the case for Parent A [23]. Parents reported feeling judged, and the effectiveness of the intervention varied depending on facilitator style, especially in high-need, low socioeconomic communities [23].

Embers the Dragon was designed as a digital psycho-educative, interactive solution to these issues in a collaboration between Mental Health Nurses, media and creative and education experts. The programme aimed to create a scalable digital platform that encompassed key social learning theory-based practices for parents, that didn't exhibit traditional clinical stereotypes that parents may have previously found judgemental and no use of clinical jargon. It also aimed to provide an entertaining and engaging approach for children to help promote a family approach to the psychoeducation being delivered.

The programme includes:

Audience	Resources
Children	An animated entertainment series following the adventures of Embers and his friends where the story lines focused on emotion identification and resilience skills. The characters in the series also feature in digital games aimed to help children practice what they learn.
Parents	Psychoeducation videos for parents explaining core parenting techniques that can help manage children's behaviour and develop emotional resilience.
Parents and children	Downloadable activities and resources for parents and children to do together.
Teachers	Lesson plans and classroom activities to reinforce the learning.

The team received feasibility funding from the National Institute of Health Research (NIHR) in 2019 to develop the prototype and conduct a feasibility pilot. A total of 129 families from the London and Essex region participated in a mixed method evaluation of the digital programme. After completing online surveys and interviews, the test group was given access to the Embers the Dragon platform for 8 weeks whilst the control group continued as usual. 98% of test group parents showed an improvement in parental response in relation to effective parenting styles. During qualitative interviews, child participants verbally recalled an increased range of emotions and coping strategies highlighted in the programme [24].

The results of the feasibility study resulted in the programme receiving a further grant from NIHR in 2023 to complete a national trial measuring the potential benefits of a digital delivery of children's emotional support and social learning theory based parenting interventions.

APPLICATION OF DIGITAL INNOVATION IN ADVANCED PRACTICE IN MENTAL HEALTH

Advanced Practice Mental Health Curriculum and Capabilities Framework (HEE 2020) [25]

This chapter will meet capabilities from across the four pillars, see the following examples:

Clinical Practice 5	Initiate, evaluate and modify a range of interventions, which may include therapies, medicines, lifestyle advice and care
Leadership and Management 2	Identify, critically evaluate and reformulate understanding of professional boundaries to support new ways of working within the context of organisational and service need
Education 3	Effectively utilise a range of evidence-based educational strategies/interventions to support person-centred care with individuals, their families and carers and other healthcare colleagues.
Research 1	Critically appraise and apply the evidence base in influencing engagement, recovery, shared decision-making, transference and safeguarding.

Clinical Practice

Once aware of the legal and legislative requirements for digital technology, it is important to apply this with regards to clinical practice as advanced practitioners.

The professional regulatory bodies, such as the NMC or HCPC, have standards of practice that require us to promote safe and effective care for patients [22, 26]. In practice this includes showing professional curiosity when patients mention digital support options they may be pursuing and applying professional knowledge to risk assess the appropriateness of these alternatives.

For example, if a patient reported that they were taking St. Johns Wort as an over-the-counter medication, you have a professional duty to consider the contraindications of that on any medication they have been prescribed in order to ensure their care plan remains safe and effective. Equally if a patient reported that they are vaping, using a high nicotine content liquid, as a form of reducing their cigarette use, you have a professional duty to consider any implications of the nicotine concentration and to enquire if they device they are using is safe and CE or UKCA marked. Whilst reducing cigarette use may seem a positive improvement for your patient's physical health, over 300,000 counterfeit vapes were seized in a single raid last year, and these devices can be dangerously manufactured and at risk of combustion [27]. Accidental exposure to high nicotine liquid in a badly made vape can also cause acute nicotine poisoning [28]. Exploring a patient's reported use of a medical device and knowing which safety markers to look for are vital for promoting safe care. Failure to do so can lead to patients experiencing increased psychological distress or even physical harm. For example, a recent study showed that some online support groups, appearing to support mental health recovery, actually perpetuate self-harm behaviours and suicidal ideation [29]. Therefore, if a patient is ever reporting use of a digital device, app or online community, it is important we remain professionally curious and apply an evidence based knowledge of safety in digital health technology to help patients understand their options.

Leadership and Management

Leadership is also important in the effective implementation of digital technology in healthcare. This includes supporting your staff to understand how to safely identify digital technologies that may enhance their patient care planning and supporting staff to explore innovative use of digital technologies.

Research has shown that in order to effectively adopt digital technology into a healthcare environment managers must cultivate a culture of transparency regarding the process and identify people who will be most impacted by the use of technology [30]. This can include early adopters, staff members who have an active interest in technology or innovation and must also include individuals who are more wary of technological advancements. Understanding how staff feel about potential digital innovations, and their own confidence levels, can help to remove barriers to implementation as well as identifying areas for personal development, such as allowing a member of staff the opportunity to act as digital champion or supporting a member of staff to access additional training on digital fundamentals.

Education

There are many ways staff can be better supported to understand appropriate digital tools for their practice. Introducing digital tools at staff meetings and giving basic information about NHS safety standards and looking for a UKCA or CE mark can help staff feel empowered to have those initial conversations. Each trust has a Clinical Safety Officer and inviting them to a team meeting can be an excellent way to facilitate this.

Introducing staff to the ORCHA app library and encouraging them to search for their own digital solutions can also be an excellent way of growing an internal suite of digital tools to recommend when considering patient care. This can make a particularly excellent project for students, preceptees and staff who have a particular area of clinical interest.

Research

Research into digital health technology is vital in ensuring that we understand the benefits and implications of health technology in our ever changing communities. Contributing to that evidence base as practitioners is important in ensuring that digital health advancements are a combined effort between health professionals and technical experts.

Advancing Practice, Digital Technology and Next Steps

Document your own implementation

As with any innovation or change to practice following a quality improvement process when implementing digital technology should be thought about [31]. Consider following the Plan, Do, Study, Act (PDSA) cycle with any innovation, ensuring that each part of a digital implementation is carefully planned and evaluated to understand the benefits and barriers experienced during the process. Documenting and sharing these results can help other services to learn from these experiences and further develops the communal understanding of implementing technology effectively (see Figure 11.2).

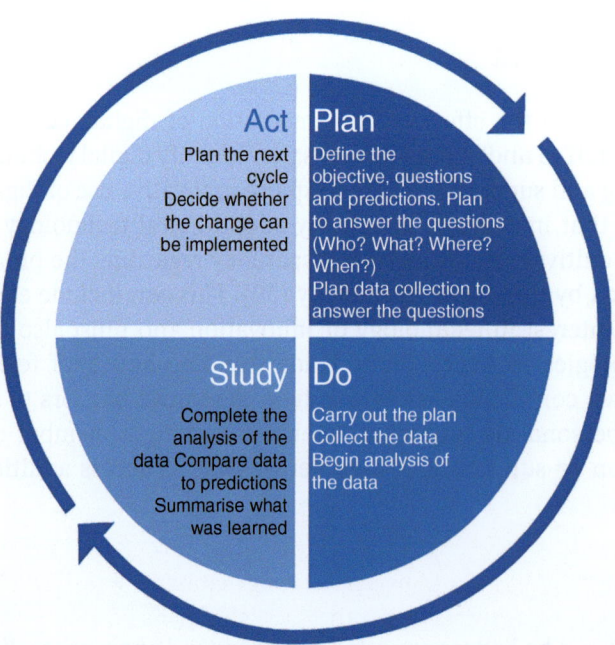

FIGURE 11.2 PDSA cycle.

Approach the Current, New and Emerging Technologies Out There

If a new technology has been identified for trialling, approach the manufacturers directly, as they may be about to run pilots, test beds, trials or feasibility studies in the near future and discussions can be had about the potential for a test site. The medical device regulations require digital technologies to maintain up to date effectiveness of their technology and therefore many are often looking for test sites to work with. Small feasibility studies are often funded through underspend or even trust or integrated care board innovation funding. Alternatively applying for grant funding from bodies such as NIHR, Small Business Research initiative (SBRI) or Innovate UK can be excellent ways to source funding for small to medium projects.

Emerging Technology

There are already many types of digital technologies available to enhance our clinical practice, from apps, to wearables, to machines. However, technology is constantly evolving and being aware of the emerging technologies and how they can be applied to our practice is important in ensuring that clinicians have input into their usage and application in order to ensure the best outcomes for patients.

Virtual reality (VR) is one such emerging technology we are beginning to see have an impact in mental health services. Whilst VR trials have taken place in physical health settings for a few years, including VR games that support children's physiotherapy, VR in mental health is relatively new with companies such as Oxford VR or TEND VR undertaking trials exploring its applications. Oxford VR have developed a number of VR-based programmes for use in a therapeutic clinic under the supervision of a clinician [32]. These include programmes for psychosis, social anxiety and fear of heights that encourage gradual exposure via a VR environment until the patient is able to apply their learning outside of the VR environment. Research showed that an average of 2 hours of VR over a 5 hour period resulted in an average reduction of fear of heights by 68% [33]. Tend VR have created a number of independent VR experiences. This includes a current trial exploring the delivery of VR access to spiritual guidance for inpatients unable to attend traditional faith deliveries [34]. They have also trialled an autonomous Mindfulness Based Cognitive Behaviour Therapy (MCBT) programme, allowing patients to complete an 8 week MBCT course at home in their own time. Their feasibility study showed an average reduction in PHQ-9 scores from 10.8 to 5.5, taking users from moderate depression to low [34].

These emerging findings suggest that VR may be able to address current healthcare challenges such as access, availability and engagement and could become part of care planning in the future.

Another emerging technology now seeing rapid uptake in mental health services is AI. Whilst many clinicians are often sceptical of AI, responses from patients have been generally positive. The majority of AI systems currently being trialled with patients are closed language systems which means the algorithm has been pre-programmed with set responses, rather than generating its own response. This has helped to increase the safety of these systems which are now being explored as a means to improve self-management in the community, support E-triage to services and improve access to support whilst on waiting lists. Companies such as Limbic and WYSA are currently available in a number of NHS and private services and are building the evidence base for the use of AI in mental health. Limbic is an AI designed to support adults to refer to local psychological therapy services [35]. Their studies showed that AI can improve clinical efficiency by reducing the time clinicians spend on mental health assessments and improving other key patient outcome metrics including reduced wait times, reduced dropout rates and improved allocation to accurate treatment pathways [35].

WYSA, which provides a wide suite of tools from population level support, to supported referrals through to waitlist support, have undertaken a number of studies exploring how AI can support users to access mental health resilience tools when they may otherwise not receive a service [36]. A 2018 study showed a significant improvement in PHQ – 9 scores in patients who were higher need using WYSA. This indicates that autonomously enabled self-help can help users to improve their mental health through self-management. A further WYSA study with NHS Scotland in 2023, showed that AI can have particular applicability as a population support tool for young people. Delivered via Schools the trial saw rapid uptake of support with 75% conversion from download to use. 78% of Young people reported that they would rather speak to a Chat bot then a teacher and uptake of tools to support sleep, self esteem and depression were most popular [36].

Whilst the emerging evidence base does not suggest that AI could, or should, replace traditional patient care, it does appear to show that AI can help to augment parts of the care pathway to help increase capacity and support access for service users who would like to explore this route. With adoption already underway in the NHS and further research ongoing exploring autonomous CBT options it is likely to become a wider part of our care planning considerations.

A Special Note on Social Media

An area of digital innovation that currently falls outside the scope of medical device licensing and NHS safety standards is social media. This is because social media platforms position themselves as communication platforms and do not believe they provide a medical purpose as their main function. As a result, social media can often be unregulated and advanced practitioners should be aware of both the positive and negatives associated with social media platforms.

As previously discussed social media platforms can be an excellent tool for the innovative scale of psychoeducation for mental health patients. There are estimated to be 57.1 million users of social media in the United Kingdom [37] highlighting the potential audience reach when platforms are used for the engagement of patients in psychoeducation information. However, there is guidance that should be followed when considering social media as a communication platform for your team or service. Most NHS Trusts and Private Providers will have their own policy on social media usage and NHS England also provide a policy which states that whilst social media can be an excellent resource for communication and engagement it is important that staff are mindful they are representatives of their trusts and professions when engaging with members of the public via this platform [38]. If utilising the platforms for work-related projects, such as a means of psychoeducation or service engagement, then staff should refrain from using personal accounts to interact with users, instead using a central team account where possible. When using social media in a personal capacity clinicians should be aware that the standards of their professional bodies still apply and be mindful of content that they post or share.

Social media often also plays a role in our service users pro-active support mechanisms, although these may not always be positive influences. Social media users will often follow various types of people including celebrities, micro influencers, friends and families as well as joining groups focused on special interests or support. A 2020 qualitative analysis of Facebook showed 154 open access groups aimed at supporting mental health [39]. Many of these groups can be helpful, providing users with quality peer support and opening up access opportunities for minority communities. However, many of these groups are also unregulated and can have negative consequences. For example, some groups have reported incidents of pro-suicidal language, trolling (a term used to described online bullying) or enabling suicidal acts or suicide pacts [40]. New national suicide audit recommendations now include asking about social media use as a routine part of assessment [41]. Encouraging an open discussion with your patients about their use of social media and any groups they are using is an important part of understanding a service users support network and influences on their mental well-being and behaviours.

It is not just the groups service users are part of that can have a significant impact on their mental well-being. Service users can follow individuals who may have a positive or negative opinion on mental health. There are many health influencers on social media who promote positive coping strategies, body confidence and positive body image. There are also many accounts that inadvertently negatively affect a service users' self-esteem. This can occur when comparing their own body image to edited images they see online or experiences of toxic productivity or anxiety when seeing what others appear to be achieving in their online lives [42]. There are also accounts that proactively reinforce negative thinking or behaviours such as dangerous viral trends or hashtags that, when followed, ensure that a user's social media feed is filled with similar negative rhetoric. Social media platforms mean the more certain types of content or hashtags are followed, the more the user will see and hear similar content. This creates an echo chamber where all of the reinforcement received online serves to reinforce any existing thoughts on a topic or experience [43]. This can have significant consequences for service users. A tragic example of this is Molly Russell (14) who sadly died in November 2017 after viewing Instagram content that promoted and encouraged suicide and/or self-harm [44]. During the inquest into Molly's death, concerns were raised that there was no division between adult and child content. The head of health and well-being for Meta, the company owning Facebook and Instagram, reported the majority of the content Molly had viewed prior to her death was considered safe by the platform. Whilst Meta admitted that two of the images were in breach of their guidance, they reported that the platform is intended for freedom of expression and rules for what can be posted are created in consultation with experts. The inquest ruled that more could be done by the platform to protect young people and vulnerable adults. Whilst certain hashtags and terms such as #suicide will breach platform guidance and be prevented from being posted, more abstract terms for self-harm or suicide, not to mention images, can make it on to the platform and are only removed if reported.

As advanced practitioners, it is important to have open conversations with service users about how they feel about their social media use and educate users and care givers as to how to certain types of accounts or hashtags can influence how we feel, encouraging users to unfollow any content that does not positively affect their mood.

CONCLUSION

Digital technology is an increasing part of our service users' lives and is becoming more and more pertinent to their care. As advanced practitioners, it is important to understand how to identify safe, regulated digital products and to promote open and reflective conversations about personal technology and social media use with patients. This enables clinicians to promote safe and effective practice whilst encouraging actively seeking and implementing appropriate digital innovation safely and effectively as necessary to meet current healthcare challenges.

REFERENCES

1. Wyatt, J.C. and Liu, J.L.Y. (2002). Basic concepts in medical informatics. *Journal of Epidemiology & Community Health* 56: 808–812.
2. van Hemel, N.M. and van der Wall, E.E. (2008). D Day for the implantable pacemaker. *Netherlands Heart Journal* 16: S3–S4. https://pmc.ncbi.nlm.nih.gov/articles/PMC2572009/. PMID: 18958267.

3. Statista (2023). Fitness trackers – statistics and facts. https://www.statista.com/topics/4393/fitness-and-activity-tracker/#topicOverview
4. Regulation (EU) 2017/745 of the European Parliament and of the Council of 5 April 2017 on Medical Devices, Amending Directive 2001/83/EC, Regulation (EC) No 178/2002 and Regulation (EC) No 1223/2009 and Repealing Council Directives 90/385/EEC and 93/42/EEC, https://eur-lex.europa.eu/eli/reg/2017/745/oj/eng.
5. Medical Device Coordination Group (2021). MDCG 2021–24. Guidance on classification of medical devices. https://health.ec.europa.eu/system/files/2021-10/mdcg_2021-24_en_0.pdf
6. Department for Business and Trade (2023). Using UKCA marking. https://www.gov.uk/guidance/using-the-ukca-marking
7. BSI Group (2023). UKCA marking. https://www.bsigroup.com/en-AU/medical-devices/global-market-access/ukca-market-access
8. Hofmann, S.G. and Gómez, A.F. (2017). Mindfulness-based interventions for anxiety and depression. *Psychiatric Clinics of North America* 40 (4): 739–749. https://doi.org/10.1016/j.psc.2017.08.008. PMID: 29080597; PMCID: PMC5679245.
9. Statista (2023) Number of mHealth apps available in the Apple App Store from 1st quarter 2015 to 3rd quarter 2022. https://www.statista.com/statistics/779910/health-apps-available-ios-worldwide
10. NHS Digital (2020). Clinical risk management standards. https://digital.nhs.uk/services/clinical-safety/clinical-risk-management-standards
11. Health and Social Care Act 2012, c.7. www.legislation.gov.uk/ukpga/2012/7/contents/enacted
12. NHS Digital (2018). Clinical risk management: its application in the manufacture of health IT systems. https://digital.nhs.uk/services/clinical-safety/clinical-risk-management-standards
13. NHS Digital (2018). Clinical risk management: its application in the deployment and use of health IT systems. https://digital.nhs.uk/services/clinical-safety/clinical-risk-management-standards
14. Statista (2023). Smartphone ownership penetration in the United Kingdom in 2012–2023 by age. https://www.statista.com/statistics/271851/smartphone-owners-in-the-united-kingdom-uk-by-age
15. NHS England (2023). NHS APP. Good practice guidelines for GP electronic patient records. https://www.england.nhs.uk/long-read/nhs-app
16. World Health Organization (2019). Global strategy on digital health 2020–2025. https://www.who.int/docs/default-source/documents/gs4dhdaa2a9f352b0445bafbc79ca799dce4d.pdf
17. Stevenson, F.A., Barry, C.A., Britten, N. et al. (2000). Doctor–patient communication about drugs: the evidence for shared decision making. *Social Science and Medicine* 50 (6): 829–840.
18. Taylor, E., Inkster, B., Tysoe, N., and Paik, A. (2023). Insights from access and adoption – patient and staff views. www.wysa.com
19. ORCHA (2023). App library. https://orchahealth.com
20. Kousoulis, A., McDaid, S., Crepaz-Keay, D. et al. (2020). Coronavirus, the divergence of menta health experienced during the pandemic. Mental Health Foundation. www.mentalhealth.org.uk/sites/default/files/MHF%20The%20COVID-19%20Pandemic%202.pdf
21. Nursing and Midwifery College (2018). NMC code of conduct. www.nmc.org.uk/globalassets/sitedocuments/nmc-publications/nmc-code.pd
22. NICE (2013). Antisocial behaviour and conduct disorders in children and young people: recognition, intervention and management. London: NICE guidelines. www.nice.org.uk/guidance/cg158

23. Clarke, A., Sorgenfrei, M., Mulcahy, J. et al. (2021). Adolescent mental health. A systemic review on the effectiveness of school – based interventions. chrome-extension://efaidnbmnnnibpcajpcglclefindmkaj/viewer.html?pdfurl=https%3A%2F%2Fwww.eif.org.uk%2Ffiles%2Fpdf%2Fadolescent-mental-health-summary.pdf&clen=23504

24. Selby, E., Allabyrne, C., and Keenan, J.R. (2021). Delivering clinical evidence-based child–parent interventions for emotional development through a digital platform: a feasibility trial. *Clinical Child Psychology and Psychiatry.* 26 (4): 1271–1283. https://doi.org/10.1177/135910452110.1580.

25. Health Education England, 2020, Advanced Practice Mental Health Curriculum and Capabilities Framework. https://www.hee.nhs.uk/sites/default/files/documents/AP-MH%20Curriculum%20and%20Capabilities%20Framework%201.2.pdf

26. Health and Care Professions Council (2021). Standards of care – Person centred care. https://www.hcpc-uk.org/standards/meeting-our-standards/person-centred-care

27. BBC News (2022). Vaping: Trading standards detect rise in counterfeit vapes at Channel Ports. www.bbc.co.uk/news/uk-england-kent-64052441

28. Cleveland Clinic (2021). Nicotine poisoning. https://my.clevelandclinic.org/health/diseases/21582-nicotine-poisoning

29. Upadhyaya, M. and Kozman, M. (2022). The blue whale challenge, social media, self-harm, and suicide contagion. *Primary Care Companion for CNS Disorder* 24 (5): 22cr03314.

30. Public Digital (2023). Lessons for implementing digital health technologies. https://public.digital/2023/09/11/lessons-for-implementing-new-digital-health-technologies-in-clinical-settings

31. NHS England and NHS Improvement (2022). Online library of quality service Improvement and redesign tools. https://www.england.nhs.uk/wp-content/uploads/2022/01/qsir-pdsa-cycles-model-for-improvement.pdf

32. Oxford VR (2023). Oxford VR. https://oxfordvr.co

33. Freeman, D., Haselton, P., Freeman, J. et al. Automated psychological therapy using immersive virtual reality for treatment of fear of heights: a single-blind, parallel-group, randomised controlled trial. *The Lancet Psychiatry* 5 (8): 625–632.

34. Tend VR (2023). Tend VR Trial. https://www.tendmentalhealth.com

35. Rollwage, M., Habicht, J., Juchems, K. et al. (2023). Using conversational AI to facilitate mental health assessments and improve clinical efficiencies within psychotherapy services in a large real-world dataset. JMIR Preprints. 16/01/2023:44358

36. WYSA (2023). UK Youth Report. https://www.wysa.com/case-studies-and-reports

37. Statista (2023). Active social media audience in the United Kingdom (UK) in January 2023. https://www.statista.com/statistics/507405/uk-active-social-media-and-mobile-social-media-users/#:~:text=The%20United%20Kingdom%20(UK)%20was,the%20population%20of%20the%20UK

38. NHS England (2013). Social media and attributed digital content policy. https://www.england.nhs.uk/wp-content/uploads/2018/04/social-media-policy.pdf

39. Prescott, J., Rathbone, A.L., and Brown, G. (2020). Online peer to peer support: qualitative analysis of UK and US open mental health Facebook groups. *Digital Health* 2020 (6). https://doi.org/10.1177/2055207620979209.

40. Luxton, D.D., June, J.D., and Fairall, J.M. (2012). Social media and suicide: a public health perspective. *American Journal of Public Health* 102 (Suppl 2): S195–S200. https://doi.org/10.2105/AJPH.2011.300608. PMID: 22401525; PMCID: PMC3477910.

41. Department of Health and Social care (2023). Suicide prevention in England: 5 year cross sector strategy. https://www.gov.uk/government/publications/suicide-prevention-strategy-for-england-2023-to-2028/suicide-prevention-in-england-5-year-cross-sector-strategy
42. Zsila, Á. and Reyes, M.E.S. (2023). Pros & cons: impacts of social media on mental health. *BMC Psychology* 11: 201. https://doi.org/10.1186/s40359-023-01243-x.
43. Terren, L. and Borge-Bravo, R. (2021). Echo chambers on social media: a systematic review of the literature. *Review of Communication Research* 9: 99–118. https://www.rcommunicationr.org/index.php/rcr/article/view/94.
44. The Coroners Service (2022). Regulation 28 Report to prevent future deaths. https://www.judiciary.uk/wp-content/uploads/2022/10/Molly-Russell-Prevention-of-future-deaths-report-2022-0315_Published.pdf

CHAPTER 12

The Role of Experts by Experience (Including Co-production and Co-creation) in Advanced Practice in Mental Health

Narenza Dhanasar
East London NHS Foundation Trust, London, UK

> ### Aim
> The chapter aims to provide an overview for advanced practitioners in mental health (APMHs) of how individuals with lived experience of mental health conditions and/or caring for someone who uses mental health services can meaningfully contribute to the development, design, delivery, evaluation and improvement of mental health services.

LEARNING OUTCOMES

By the end of this chapter, the reader will be able to:

1. Define the concepts of experts by experience, co-production and co-creation within the context of advanced mental health practice.
2. Explain the value and impact of incorporating lived experience in the design, delivery and evaluation of mental health services.
3. Critically examine the ethical, practical and cultural considerations when engaging with experts by experience in practice settings.

The Advanced Practitioner in Mental Health, First Edition. Edited by Clare Allabyrne.
© 2026 John Wiley & Sons Ltd. All rights reserved, including rights for text and data mining and training of artificial intelligence technologies or similar technologies. Published 2026 by John Wiley & Sons Ltd.

4. Identify effective strategies for fostering meaningful partnerships with service users and carers, including shared decision-making and collaborative leadership.
5. Demonstrate how co-production and co-creation can enhance service quality, promote recovery-oriented care and challenge traditional power dynamics in mental health settings.
6. Reflect on the role of the advanced practitioner in mental health as a facilitator and advocate for inclusive, participatory approaches in education, research and clinical innovation.

INTRODUCTION

In the field of mental health, experts by experience (EBEs) play a critical role and are increasingly recognised for their valuable insights and contributions in enabling the provision of more holistic, person-centred care.

EBE can be classified in two parts: – gifted and owned experienced [1].

1. Gifted experience provides insights gained through professional training, education or second-hand exposure. For example, mental health professionals, researchers and policymakers may have gifted knowledge about mental health through academic study or working with people who have lived experience.
2. Owned experience refers to personal, first-hand experiences of mental health challenges, recovery or navigating systems of care. This is most often associated with the concept of being an EBE, where someone has direct, personal knowledge of what it means to live with a mental health condition or other significant life experiences.

The distinction between gifted and owned experience is important in mental health because:

Both perspectives are valuable: Professionals with gifted experience bring theoretical and clinical expertise, while those with owned experience bring real-world, lived insights.

Lived experience is often undervalued: Historically, owned experience has been dismissed or overshadowed by academic and clinical perspectives, but there is growing recognition of its importance.

True collaboration is needed: Mental health services improve when professionals and those with lived experience work together, ensuring that policies and support systems are both evidence-based and experience-informed.

Who Are Experts by Experience?

In the United Kingdom, the involvement of EBEs (individuals with lived experience of mental health conditions) began to gain formal recognition in the 1980s, influenced by the mental health survivor and service user movements that had emerged during the 1970s [2, 3]. These service user-led efforts challenged institutionalised models of care and advocated for improved rights, dignity and meaningful participation in the development of mental health services [4, 5].

By the 1990s, UK mental health policy began to adopt a more structured approach to service user involvement, with organisations such as the National Health Service (NHS) and MIND supporting and promoting user-led initiatives [6, 7]. The term 'experts by experience' gained wider use in the 2000s, reflecting a growing commitment to integrating lived experience into advanced practice, spanning the training of clinicians, co-production of services, quality improvement initiatives and mental health research [8].

DEFINTION OF EBE

For the purposes of this chapter, we will focus on EBE-owned experience in mental health, using the following combined definition.

EBEs are people who have personal experience within the last 8 years [9], who either use or care for someone who uses health, mental health and/or social care services that the Care Quality Commission (CQC) regulates [10]. EBE have personally lived through mental health difficulties and therefore have first-hand experience from a service user's perspective. They have the ability to reflect on, articulate and use these experiences to improve outcomes in healthcare. With this knowledge and insight EBE are equipped to shed light on both positive and negative aspects of care within healthcare interactions, systems and recovery journeys. EBE brings unique perspectives that professional training and experience alone cannot provide [11]; their lived experience adds depth, authenticity and practical insight to mental health services, policymaking and peer support. EBE bridges the gap between reality and theory [12]. EBE can also highlight practical barriers in mental health systems – such as stigma, bureaucracy and accessibility issues – that professionals might overlook [13].

Example: A therapist may understand post-traumatic stress disorder (PTSD) theoretically, but someone who has lived through trauma can explain the day-to-day realities of managing triggers, flashbacks and stigma. While professional expertise is crucial, it becomes truly powerful when combined with lived experience [14].

THE CONTRIBUTIONS OF EBE

In advanced practice in mental health, EBEs contribute across multiple settings including:

Patients/clients: Sharing lived experiences through assessment, intervention, treatment and recovery.
Carers/family members: Offering personal insights from the perspective of supporting someone with mental health issues.
Advocates: Providing a voice for those navigating the system or challenging its inadequacies.

EBE make an invaluable contribution to mental health [15]. Their unique perspectives as individuals who have lived through mental health challenges enable them to impact clinical practice, service design, policy development and patient care in ways that professionals without lived experience might not be able to [16]. Conceptualisation of lived experience is far greater than a textbook [17]. Some examples of EBE contributions to advanced practice in mental health can include:

Enhancing person-centred and recovery-oriented care: Designing individualised care plans that respect patients' lived experiences and self-defined recovery goals. Example: An advanced practitioner in mental health (APMH) co-develops a treatment plan for a patient with bipolar disorder with input from a peer support worker (PSW) who has successfully managed their own condition.

Co-designing and improving mental health services: Collaborating on the co-production of services, ensuring that they are accessible, user-friendly and culturally competent. EBE can provide feedback on treatment protocols, policies and interventions based on their lived experiences. Example: An APMH works alongside a former patient to design a crisis response program that incorporates perspectives on what works best in a mental health crisis.

Enhancing trauma-informed care: EBE can offer insights into the psychological and emotional impact of trauma, informing clinicians about what trauma survivors find helpful or harmful in mental health settings. Also, helping integrate trauma-informed policies in hospital wards, therapy settings and community-based programs. Example: An APMH receives training from an EBE with lived experience of PTSD, learning how certain clinical environments can be triggering and how to create a more trauma-sensitive setting.

Peer support and workforce development: Working alongside clinical staff as PSWs, recovery coaches and mentors. Example: An APMH co-facilitates a psychoeducation group with a PSW who shares personal strategies for managing anxiety and depression.

Reducing stigma and improving cultural competency: Providing first-hand accounts of how stigma affects mental healthcare access. Educating professionals on the unique mental health challenges of marginalised groups (e.g. LGBTQ+, people with disabilities). Example: An LGBTQ+ mental health advocate with lived experience works with an APMH to create a more inclusive therapy framework that addresses minority stress and discrimination.

Informing policy and systemic change: Helping shape policy recommendations that reflect the experiences of patients. Advocating for rights-based approaches in mental healthcare. Example: An EBE who has experienced involuntary hospitalisation provides testimony to a policy committee, advocating for more humane and consent-based treatment options.

Research and evidence-based practice: Assisting in co-producing research by providing lived experience perspectives in study design, implementation and analysis. Ensuring research outcomes are meaningful and applicable to patients. Example: A university research team collaborates with EBEs to develop a study on the impact of peer-led interventions for individuals with schizophrenia.

Crisis response and suicide prevention: Offering insights into what is helpful (or unhelpful) in a crisis from a personal perspective. Assist in designing compassionate crisis care models. Example: A suicide attempt survivor collaborates with an APMH to improve suicide risk assessment tools, ensuring they are non-judgemental and person-centred.

Strengthening holistic and non-medical interventions: Advocating for complementary approaches, such as art therapy, mindfulness and community-based healing. Highlighting the importance of housing, employment and social connection in mental health recovery. Example: An EBE who has recovered from homelessness and addiction collaborates with an APMH and local authority to implement a Housing First initiative, ensuring mental health services prioritise stable housing. Housing First is a strategy for ending homelessness through the provision of housing and support services.

Teaching and training future mental health professionals: Being guest lecturers, workshop facilitators or co-trainers in mental health education. Provide case studies and real-world scenarios to enrich classroom learning. Example: An APMH educator invites an EBE with obsessive compulsive disorder (OCD) to share their experiences with treatment-resistant symptoms, giving students deeper insight into real-life therapy challenges.

By partnering with EBEs, APMHs can create more compassionate, effective and recovery-focused mental health systems.

The Importance of Experts by Experience in Advanced Practice in Mental Health

The role of EBE in advanced mental health practice aligns closely with the four pillars of advanced clinical practice: clinical practice, leadership, education and research [18].

Clinical Practice

APMH deliver high-level clinical care on a day to day basis. In line with the professional bodies such as the Nursing and Midwifery Council (NMC), General Pharmaceutical Council (GPhC) or Health and Care Professions Council (HCPC), APMH must adhere to standards of practice which require them to provide and promote safe and effective care for patients and their families [19, 20]. For many years in mental health there has been EBE involvement through personal valuable insights, tailoring person-centred care. EBE can contribute significantly to the clinical pillar of advanced practice in healthcare settings, particularly in enhancing patient outcomes and supporting APMHs, as highlighted in the following examples.

EBE can support healthcare professionals develop a deeper understanding of the patient experience by promoting empathy and reducing stigma [21]. This leads to more compassionate and patient-centred care, which is crucial for improving patient outcomes [22]. EBE can enhance patient engagement by providing relatable role models who have successfully navigated challenges, this can inspire hope and motivate patients to actively participate in their own recovery [15]. In addition, EBEs advocate for and model recovery-oriented practices, emphasising the importance of personal recovery goals and holistic care which can lead to more individualised and effective treatment plans [23]. Furthermore, they contribute to the education of APMH by creating interactive learning environments and encouraging critical thinking through real-life case studies and reflection and linking theory to practice to enhance clinical understanding. This helps practitioners develop a more nuanced understanding of mental health and recovery in clinical practice. EBEs enhance the application of interpersonal skills among APMHs, fostering better communication and therapeutic relationships with patients [15, 23]. By sharing their lived experiences, EBEs foster greater empathy, model person-centred communication and provide constructive feedback that enables APMHs to reflect on and refine their approach. This collaboration supports culturally sensitive care, encourages shared decision-making and strengthens therapeutic relationships grounded in trust and mutual respect [15]. Integrating EBEs into training and service development also aligns with the principles of advanced practice by promoting reflective, evidence-informed and holistic care that is responsive to individual needs and lived realities [23]. In addition, they bring diverse perspectives that can help APMHs understand and address the cultural needs of different patient populations, leading to more culturally competent care [21]. APMH trainees report that listening to a patient perspective provides a deeper understanding of assessment, risk assessment, care planning and formulation skills [10], which can also lead to more individualised person-centred care.

Clinical effectiveness is informed by evidence-based practice. By integrating the perspectives of EBE, APMH can develop and implement interventions that are more relevant and effective [21] and identify potential risks and barriers to treatment adherence, leading to the development of strategies that mitigate these risks and improve patient outcomes [24]. EBE contribute significantly by providing unique insights in the form of co-design and implementation of services. For instance, a study in Italy called 'All about my ideal mental health service' [25] demonstrated that EBE involvement in service co-design led to strategies that improved user reception, reduced stigma and enhanced the physical and organisational aspects of mental health services [16]. This was done by collating and sharing feedback from the community through structured discussions, interviews and participatory research methods.

The involvement of EBE in recruitment and service development can enhance APMHs working with complex high-risk patients, in several key ways [22]. EBE can provide valuable insights during the recruitment of staff ensuring that candidates possess not only the necessary clinical skills but also the empathy and understanding required to work effectively with high-risk patients. Similarly, their involvement can help identify individuals who are more likely to engage in patient-centred care and who value the contributions of lived experience [26].

Risk management can improve significantly with the perspectives of EBE who provide lived experiences of risk, particularly in the context of APMH working with complex high-risk patients. Patients' involvement in their own risk management, including having agency and autonomy, is crucial for effective risk mitigation [27]. This aligns with the notion that EBE can provide valuable perspectives that enhance the relational and participatory aspects of risk management, thus empowering patients to actively participate in their care which can improve safety and therapeutic outcomes [28].

Leadership

The integration of EBE in leadership promotes a more inclusive, recovery-oriented approach to mental healthcare [10]. EBE can be involved in strategic influencing, planning and decision-making by being a part of steering groups and project meetings on national and local levels. Inclusive partnership working enables collaborative leadership and fosters a model where patient voices are valued. EBE actively contribute to service redesign and improvement initiatives by sharing insights from community listening and feedback, which drives meaningful changes in service delivery. Feedback from EBE drives meaningful changes by highlighting practical and actionable insights that can be directly implemented. For instance, the 'Ask Us!' method adjusted the experience-based co-design process to be more responsive to vulnerable populations, leading to the development of practical tools and strategies to improve care relationships and service delivery [29].

NHS Trusts often focus their feedback on the 'you said we did' motto [11] where posters are left visible for patients to view the feedback provided by them. APMH can use this feedback to be responsive and action the needs of community by:

1. **Identifying key areas for improvement:** APMHs can prioritise these areas to ensure that the most pressing concerns are addressed first [30].
2. **Enhancing patient-centred care:** APMHs can tailor their services to better meet the needs and preferences of their patients [31].
3. **Building trust and engagement:** Displaying 'you said, we did' posters demonstrate to patients that their feedback is valued and acted upon. This transparency can build trust and encourage more patients to provide feedback, creating a continuous loop of improvement [32].
4. **Incorporating feedback into clinical practice:** APMHs can integrate patient feedback into their clinical practice by using it to inform treatment plans, communication strategies and service delivery models. This ensures that care is aligned with patient needs and expectations [33].
5. **Collaborative service development:** Engaging with patient feedback allows APMHs to collaborate with patients in the co-design of services. This collaborative approach can lead to more effective and sustainable service improvements [34].

Communication and stakeholder engagement enables EBE to assist with co-design communication materials and resources for service improvement by utilising frameworks like Experience-Based

Co-Design (EBCD) [35]. EBCD allows EBE to work alongside clinicians and other stakeholders to identify priorities and develop interventions that are both evidence-based and grounded in lived experience [36]. Furthermore, they can help translate complex clinical information into practical, easy-to-understand resources [35]. This can include developing toolkits, brochures and other educational materials that support therapeutic engagement and self-management, as seen in the development of the Let's Talk toolkit [37]. The Let's Talk toolkit is a structured resource designed to facilitate conversations between professionals, clients and their families, particularly in mental health or social care settings [37]. It aims to promote open, age-appropriate discussions about mental illness, emotional well-being and coping strategies. Developed to support both therapeutic engagement and self-management, the toolkit includes a range of materials – such as visual aids, conversation guides and worksheets – that help practitioners engage with children, young people and families in a sensitive and constructive manner [37].

NHS leaders focus on a whole system approach rather than a fixed approach, this allows APMHs and EBEs to look at a system wide perspective [38]. A whole system approach rather than a fixed approach advocates for a model of care that is flexible, integrated and person-centred [38]. This approach recognises that individuals often require support from multiple services such as physical health, mental health, social care and community organisations and seeks to coordinate these elements to deliver seamless, holistic care [39]. Unlike a fixed approach, which relies on standardised, siloed services with rigid pathways, a whole system approach encourages collaboration across sectors, adaptability to local needs and a focus on prevention and early intervention [40]. It places the individual at the centre, aiming to improve outcomes by responding to the complexity of real-life circumstances rather than forcing people to navigate fragmented systems.

Experienced EBEs have mentoring/role modelling roles in the NHS to provide guidance and support in peer support programs. EBEs empower cultural change by disintegrating stigma power differentials between professionals and patients in several transformative ways [12]. By sharing their lived experiences, EBEs help to challenge the stigma often associated with mental illness and foster an environment where open and honest discussions are encouraged [41]. In roles such as mentors or peer leaders, EBEs help shift the traditional hierarchical power structure in healthcare, promoting a more egalitarian approach where patients are seen as equal partners in their care [41]. This shift encourages shared decision-making, where both professionals and patients contribute to care plans, making the process more collaborative and person-centred. Through their example, EBEs teach empathy, resilience and the value of lived experience, helping professionals develop deeper understanding and compassion for their patients. They also advocate for systemic changes that prioritise equity and inclusion, ensuring that patient voices are heard and respected [42]. Ultimately, EBEs empower patients by reducing power imbalances, fostering mutual respect and creating a healthcare environment that values both professional expertise and the insights gained from lived experience.

APMHs and EBE can advocate for recovery-oriented practices, empowerment strategies and resilience. Through their leadership and advocacy, they can help shift the healthcare culture towards a system that values the empowerment, dignity and resilience of individuals.

Education

In education. EBEs complement the teaching process in a variety of ways. EBE are involved in developing, planning and evaluating curriculum and training programs for mental health professionals, including advanced practice programmes, ensuring the training programmes are compassionate, relevant, diverse and effective. EBEs sharing lived experiences in the classroom (lectures, workshops) and in practice (clinical placement) highlights real-world emotive challenges and allows APMH trainees to reflect upon therapeutic relationships. EBE involvement is multifaceted and includes direct participation in educational initiatives, co-production of training modules and providing unique insights from their lived experiences. The viewpoint of a patient provides insight into the level of complexities in mental health practice.

EBE also are involved in continuous professional development (CPD) to ensure APMHs keep up to date with emerging trends in patients' needs.

One effective strategy for engaging EBEs in CPD is through critical reflexivity, which involves systematically challenging assumptions and fostering equitable partnerships [43]. This approach ensures that the perspectives of those with lived experience are meaningfully integrated into professional development programs. This method not only enriches the learning experience but also promotes systemic changes that align with the evolving needs of patients [44]. For example, the development of the Standards for Co-production of Education (Mental Health Nursing) provides a structured framework to support EBE involvement in higher education [15]. Additionally, the involvement of EBE in teaching within nursing and allied health professionals (AHPs) programs has shown significant benefits. The NHS Long Term Plan and the AHP Strategy for England: AHPs Deliver [8] emphasise the need for personalised, recovery-focused care across services. To strengthen the education pillar of APMH, it is recommended that EBE be systematically integrated into educational programmes and professional development pathways [45]. This includes embedding EBE-led teaching sessions in both pre-registration and postgraduate training, involving EBEs in curriculum design and simulation-based learning and incorporating their perspectives into clinical supervision and reflective practice. Their contributions should be formally recognised, adequately resourced and supported by clear governance structures to ensure meaningful, ethical and sustainable involvement [18]. This co-produced approach will enhance the relational and reflective capabilities of APMHs, aligning with the principles of recovery-focused and person-centred mental healthcare.

Furthermore, the establishment of academic positions for EBE in mental health education has been shown to foster positive attitudinal changes among students and professionals [15]. This involvement helps bridge the gap between theoretical knowledge and practical. Support from APMH can enhance the confidence and retention of EBE in academic roles, further enriching the educational experience for all trainees [26]. EBE engagement in academia is facilitated through interactive learning environments, trainees' discussions, role-plays and feedback sessions, promoting critical thinking and empathy [44].

Research

EBE involvement in the research pillar is particularly through co-production and co-creation in mental health research. EBE as co-researchers ensures research studies are more effective, relevant and impactful and directly complementing clinical practice. Involving EBE in study design and planning ensures meaningful questions and approaches that consider patients' perspectives. This improves the quality and application of research findings, making them more useful for improving mental healthcare delivery. EBE can increase research relevance with their input in conceptual development and participant recruitment ensuring that research questions reflect real-life concerns and priorities. Their involvement in participant recruitment helps build trust and improves access to underrepresented groups. Additionally, they enhance research quality by promoting accurate data collection through culturally and contextually appropriate tools and by informing more sensitive methodologies that capture nuanced experiences. This, in turn, strengthens the validity and applicability of the research findings. EBE have recently taken on more research lead roles to conduct research. Furthermore, they also work in collaborative research teams bringing expertise resulting in extensive research outcomes [38].

Research has highlighted the role of PSWs in co-production and co-creation within public mental health and addiction services [46]. PSWs bring valuable insights from their lived experiences, which can influence both the content and quality of services, and drive innovation and systemic change. Other research showed young people as co-researchers in a study on online help-seeking for emotional abuse and neglect. This co-produced research emphasised building capabilities, adapting methodologies and evaluating the impact of involvement, demonstrating the epistemological value of including young people in complex qualitative research [47].

EBE are also involved in communicating findings to the participants and general public and can support trainee researchers in specific projects. Their contribution in research ethics enhances co-production by addressing issues of epistemic injustice, by ensuring that marginalised voices are heard and valued in the research process. This is crucial for developing interventions that are culturally sensitive and responsive to diverse patient populations.

See Figure 12.1 for the key emerging trends.

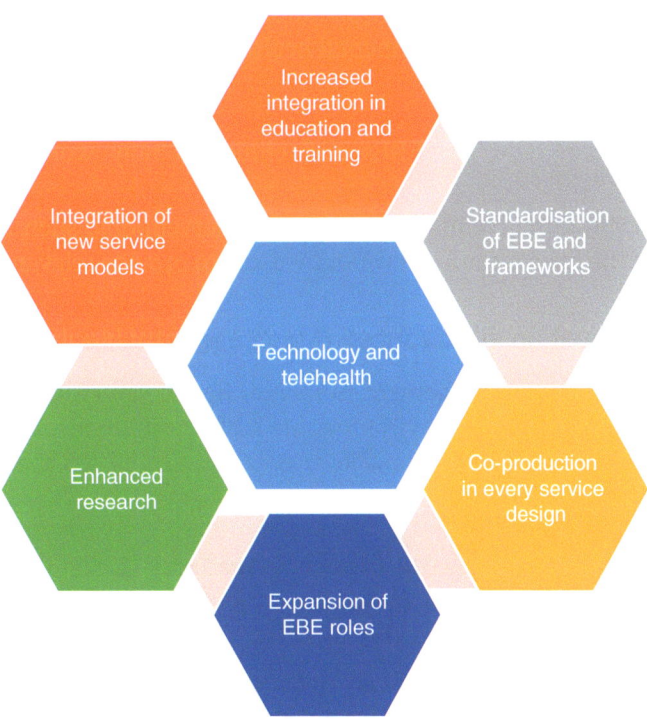

FIGURE 12.1 The key trends of the future in APMH and involvement of EBE.

KEY METHODS OF EBE INTEGRATION

Co-production and Co-creation

Co-production and co-creation are two key methods through which EBE are integrated into mental health practice [48, 49].

Co-production

Co-production refers to the collaborative development of mental health services where EBEs work alongside professionals. This model is based on the principle that service users are equal partners in the design, delivery and evaluation of services.

In co-production:

- The patient is seen as an active agent with expertise.
- Professionals and users share power and responsibility.
- It emphasises collaboration, equality and mutual respect

Co-creation

Co-creation takes this a step further. In co-creation, EBEs are involved from the very beginning of a project or initiative, engaging in idea generation, planning and implementation. Co-creation emphasises shared ownership and creativity in designing mental health solutions.

Examples include:

- Mental Health Service Redesign: EBEs and clinicians may work together to create new service models.
- Developing Therapeutic Interventions: Co-created interventions, such as peer support groups, draw directly from the lived experiences of individuals to provide relevant and accessible care.

Co-production and Co-creation in Advanced Practice Mental Health:

Recovery Colleges enhance patient engagement in mental health services through co-production and co-creation by fostering an empowering environment, enabling different relationships and facilitating personal growth. Here, are some examples of how Recovery Colleges and Advanced Practice roles intersect in real-world settings:

1. **Greater Manchester Mental Health Recovery Academy (UK)** [50]
    - ➤ **How it connects with advanced practice:**
        - APMHs work with the Recovery Academy to co-develop courses on self-management of conditions like anxiety, depression and psychosis.
        - APMHs contribute to workshops on medication management, early warning signs and relapse prevention.
        - They use Recovery College principles to enhance person-centred care in clinical settings.

2. South London and Maudsley (SLaM) NHS Trust Recovery College (UK) [51]
   ➢ **How it connects with advanced practice:**
   - APMHs engage in the co-production of educational programs alongside people with lived experience.
   - Recovery College graduates are sometimes invited to co-facilitate training sessions for healthcare professionals, including APMHs.
   - APMHs use Recovery College strategies to promote shared decision-making in clinical settings.
3. The Recovery College at CAMH (Centre for Addiction and Mental Health) (Canada) [52]
   ➢ **How it connects with advanced practice:**
   - APMHs contribute to peer-led educational programs, integrating the latest evidence-based mental health practices.
   - APMHs help design courses that incorporates clinical knowledge with self-management techniques for conditions like schizophrenia or bipolar disorder.
   - APMHs mentor junior staff and students, incorporating Recovery College approaches into professional training.
4. Western Australia Recovery College [53]
   ➢ **How it connects with advanced practice:**
   - APMHs collaborate with the Recovery College to develop culturally safe mental health programs, particularly for Indigenous communities.
   - They incorporate Recovery College principles into crisis response teams, emphasising self-determination and empowerment.
   - APMHs use insights from Recovery College participants to shape mental health policy and service development.
5. Ireland's National Framework for Recovery in Mental Health [54]
   ➢ **How it connects with advanced practice:**
   - APMHs are key drivers in integrating Recovery Colleges into mainstream healthcare.
   - Recovery-focused training is embedded in APMH roles, ensuring mental health services prioritise empowerment over just symptom management.
   - APMHs support service users transitioning from hospital-based care to community-based self-management programs through Recovery Colleges.

The Recovery Colleges Characterisation and Testing in England (RECOLLECT) program and Recovery Colleges

These contribute to the involvement of EBE through co-production and co-creation in mental health research by actively engaging individuals with lived experience in the design, implementation and evaluation of their programs. The RECOLLECT study aims to evaluate the effectiveness and cost-effectiveness of Recovery Colleges in England, incorporates a Lived Experience Advisory Panel to provide input at all stages of the research process. This ensures that the perspectives of those with lived experience are integral to the study's design and execution, enhancing the relevance and applicability of the findings [55].

Challenges and Considerations for the Inclusion of EBE in Advanced Practice Mental Health

Incorporating EBE into APMH brings many benefits, but it also presents several challenges and considerations that need to be carefully managed. These can be grouped into ethical, professional, emotional, practical and systemic considerations.

1. **Ethical and Professional Challenges** [56, 57]
    A. Boundaries and Scope of Role
        - **Challenge:** EBE may not have clinical training but are sometimes perceived as professionals by patients or colleagues. This can create role confusion, especially in clinical settings.
        - **Consideration:** EBE roles must be clearly defined, ensuring they do not give medical advice or influence treatment decisions beyond their scope.
    B. Confidentiality and Safeguarding Risks
        - **Challenge:** EBE may be exposed to sensitive patient information or may unintentionally share personal experiences that contain confidential details.
        - **Consideration:** APMHs can provide training on confidentiality, safeguarding and data protection to ensure ethical engagement in service development and co-production.
    C. Influence on Service Users' Treatment Choices
        - **Challenge:** Patients may view EBE experiences as recommendations, which could impact medication adherence or treatment choices.
        - **Consideration:** APMHs must ensure discussions about medication or therapy are balanced and encourage shared decision-making with clinicians rather than solely relying on lived experience.
2. **Emotional and Psychological Challenges** [7, 58, 59]
    A. Re-traumatisation and Emotional Burden
        - **Challenge:** Sharing personal mental health experiences can be emotionally taxing and may re-trigger trauma, particularly when discussing difficult past experiences.
        - **Consideration:** APMHs can implement support structures (e.g. supervision, debriefing sessions, peer support) to help EBE manage emotional challenges.
    B. Managing Expectations and Emotional Labour
        - **Challenge:** EBE may feel pressure to 'represent all patients', leading to emotional strain or burnout.
        - **Consideration:** APMHs must acknowledge that one lived experience is not universal and ensure EBE are not burdened with unrealistic expectations.
    C. Power Imbalance and Tokenism
        - **Challenge:** EBE may feel their role is symbolic rather than impactful, leading to feelings of frustration and disengagement.
        - **Consideration:** EBE should be given meaningful roles with real decision-making influence, not just included for representation.
3. **Practical and Logistical Challenges** [60]
    A. Payment, Recognition, and Fair Compensation
        - **Challenge:** Many EBE are unpaid or underpaid, which can lead to financial strain and exploitation of lived experience.
        - **Consideration:** Services must provide fair compensation for EBE contributions, ensuring equal pay for equal work compared to professionals with similar responsibilities.

B. Training and Professional Development
- **Challenge:** Some EBE may lack formal training in areas like public speaking, co-production or service evaluation.
- **Consideration:** APMHs can offer training opportunities to develop skills in professional settings while respecting and valuing their lived experience.

C. Accessibility and Inclusion
- **Challenge:** EBE may face barriers to participation, such as travel costs, digital exclusion or disability-related issues.
- **Consideration:** Services must ensure accessible meeting formats (e.g. hybrid meetings, travel reimbursement) and inclusive communication methods.

4. **Systemic and Organisational Challenges** [14, 26]

   A. Resistance from Professionals and Service Culture
   - **Challenge:** Some mental health professionals may devalue lived experience, seeing it as less valid than clinical knowledge.
   - **Consideration:** Promote a culture shift by integrating EBE perspectives into staff training and leadership structures.

   B. Lack of Clear Policies and Structures
   - **Challenge:** Many organisations lack clear frameworks for integrating EBEs, leading to inconsistent engagement.
   - **Consideration:** Develop structured guidelines, contracts and role descriptions to clarify expectations and responsibilities.

   C. Balancing Subjectivity with Evidence-Based Practice
   - **Challenge:** Lived experience is subjective and may sometimes conflict with evidence-based clinical approaches.
   - **Consideration:** Encourage collaboration between clinicians and EBEs, ensuring that lived experience informs but does not replace clinical expertise.

   See Figure 12.2 for a framework for engagement.

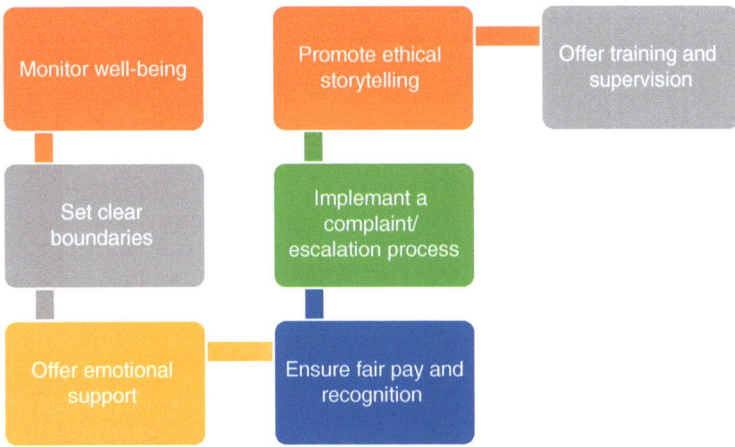

FIGURE 12.2 A Safe and Ethical Framework for EBE Engagement.

Pharmacology Considerations in APMH in Relation to EBE

While EBE provide valuable insight into medication experiences, side effects, adherence challenges and holistic treatment approaches, their involvement in advanced mental health practice raises key pharmacological considerations. These include medication adherence, shared decision-making, polypharmacy risks, patient education and ethical boundaries which are listed in the Table 12.1:

TABLE 12.1 EBE contributions to pharmacology in mental health [61, 62].

EBE contributions to pharmacology in mental health	Consideration	Advanced practice mental health role
Medication Adherence and Service User Experience	EBE offers lived experience on barriers to medication adherence, such as: • Side effects (e.g. weight gain, sedation, cognitive dulling). • Stigma associated with mental health medication. • Personal beliefs about mental health recovery without medication. • Difficulty accessing regular prescriptions or monitoring.	• Use EBE insights to develop adherence strategies that address barriers. • Implement shared decision-making approaches that respect patient autonomy.
Supporting Shared Decision-Making in Prescribing	EBE can bridge the gap between clinicians and service users by advocating for personalised medication plans.	• Encourage service users to express concerns about medications. • Use co-production models to develop psychoeducation resources about medications. • Support clinicians in explaining risks vs. benefits in an accessible way.
Polypharmacy and Complex Cases	Many mental health service users are prescribed multiple psychotropic medications, increasing risks of: • Drug interactions. • Metabolic syndrome (e.g. from antipsychotics). • Over-sedation and reduced quality of life. • Non-compliance due to pill burden.	• Use EBE feedback to refine medication reviews and deprescribing approaches. • Ensure regular medication monitoring includes patient perspectives on burden vs. benefit.
Risks and Safeguarding in Pharmacology with EBE	**Red flag**	**Mitigation**
Risk of EBEs Influencing Medication Decisions Inappropriately	EBEs discouraging service users from taking prescribed medications based on personal negative experiences.	• Train EBEs on the importance of neutral, non-directive discussions. • Emphasise individual responses to medication vary. • Encourage EBE to redirect medical questions to clinicians.

TABLE 12.1 (Continued)

Risks and Safeguarding in Pharmacology with EBE	Red flag	Mitigation
Ethical Boundaries and Non-clinical Roles	EBEs providing advice on dosage changes, medication switches or stopping treatment.	• Define clear role boundaries – EBEs should share experiences, not medical advice. • Ensure advanced practitioners facilitate clinically informed discussions.
Addressing Misinformation About Medications	Service users refusing essential treatment based on misleading or biased EBE experiences.	• Use evidence-based medication education in co-production sessions. • Promote a balanced view of pharmacological and non-pharmacological treatments.
Integrating EBEs into Pharmacology in Advanced Mental Health Practice	EBE Involvement in Medication Education Programs	EBE can co-develop easy-to-understand materials on: • Common side effects and how to manage them. • Importance of gradual withdrawal (to avoid discontinuation syndrome). • Balancing medication with psychological and lifestyle interventions.
	EBE Input in Clinical Training for Advanced Practitioners	EBE can educate staff on: • How service users experience different medication regimes. • The psychosocial impact of long-term medication use. • Supporting patients to make informed choices.
	Co-production of Medication Review Processes	EBE can help reshape medication review strategies, ensuring they: • Focus on quality of life, not just symptom reduction. • Address patients concern proactively. • Encourage collaborative prescribing between service users and clinicians.
Role of EBE in Pharmacovigilance	Raising Awareness Co-producing Medication Information Encouraging Open Conversations	• EBE can help patients identify and report side effects early. • Ensuring accessible, lived-experience-informed materials on managing side effects. • Reducing stigma around reporting medication concerns to clinicians.
Role of EBE in Medication Safety Research	Co-designing Studies Data Peer-Led Surveys and Focus Groups Improving Research Translation	• Ensuring research addresses medication concerns. • Gathering perspectives on medication use in different communities. • Helping make study findings accessible and relevant to patients.

Testimonials from EBE and/or Professionals

1. **Written anonymously by an advanced practitioner pharmacist working in CAMHS:**
   As an advanced pharmacist practitioner, I work with children with neurodevelopmental conditions and prescribe medication for a range of neurodevelopmental conditions. I have also been a part of the parent and young person's forums, such as listening to parental concerns about care and medication and helping develop a video with young people on their experience of attention deficit hyperactivity disorder (ADHD) and the role of medication. Through my involvement with the parent/carer forums, I have been able to have open conversations with parents about what has worked well and how services can be improved.

   The stories and experiences of caregivers and young persons have helped me understand what matters most to those accessing care. This could be help making friends, being able to concentrate at school, improved sleep and appetite or even someone to talk to who understand what they are feeling.

   I have worked on quality improvement projects which have been aimed at improving the experience of care for young persons and their families. This led to changes in the way information was shared and communicated with the young person and families. As a result, there was an improvement in the quality of care.

   The lived experience of young persons and caregivers have been invaluable in shaping my clinical practice and ethos. It has helped me to ensure that I take a holistic approach to care and work collaboratively with young persons and families when thinking about medication and other healthcare interventions.

2. **Written by Laura Pisaneschi (nurse consultant, APMH, NMP and RMN) lead for the ability network for NHS trust:**
   Being a nurse consultant who is neurodivergent is also not easy and has lots of challenges but also strengths. I have always known I was different; I have seen things in my own unique way and at times felt completely overwhelmed and other times in complete control, but I think that might also be about working in an ever-changing NHS! Working in the crisis pathway my strengths and ADHD brain means being able to work with complexity, not being phased by crisis situations and managing competing demands at once which has resulted in me excelling at my job and being promoted to consultant nurse. I have been utilising coaching, tips and tools which have helped ensure I can stay on top of my workload and some non-dopamine-fulfilling tasks. I can also relate to my neurodivergent patients and can see how healthcare can be confusing and overwhelming meaning that hospital environments can be over stimulating and cause sensory overload. However, at times I can also get overwhelmed by simple things like struggling to put together a report and can spend hours writing a paragraph because of my dyslexia and end up feeling like a failure. I found studying to be an APMH difficult, and I often left the coursework to the last minute – submitting at 11.59 pm for a midnight deadline. Training during Covid, with everything online, did not work for me, and I wouldn't have got through the course if it were not for the two close friends and best APMH colleagues you could ask for.

   Being neurodivergent has meant my work life balance has been all over the place, hyper focusing on work and being time blind, which has helped my patients and probably my workload, but it has had an impact on my family and myself. Getting to this stage in my career where I am a consultant nurse, I am now working on work/life balance and realising that just because

I can doesn't mean I have to do it all! I have also been network lead for my trust's disability staff network most of my working life and take joy from helping others and advocating for adjustments and support for staff with disabilities. Although reported numbers of staff with neurodiversity and other disabilities are low, the more staff I speak to the more I realise there are a lot more of us out there and that changes are happening to support staff and ensure they bring their best selves to work. This ultimately means they will help patients which is what I entered healthcare for and where my passion lies.

3. **Written by Stephanie Leighton, people participation worker in CAMHS:**
As a people participation worker at CAMHS, I see first-hand how active participation leads to more effective and person-centred mental health services. When young people and their caregivers are genuinely involved in decision-making, their voices shape services to better meet their needs. For example, our service user consultation directly influences core work streams both locally and on a trust-wide level. Co-production, where young people are equal partners from the start, ensures that services are built with them, not just for them.

Participation also has its challenges. Some professionals used to traditional service models, may be hesitant about sharing decision-making power with young people or those who aren't professionally qualified. For this reason, embedding participation in everyday practice through staff training, reflective spaces and leadership support, all contribute to creating a culture where co-creation is the norm. Making participation accessible is also crucial, i.e. flexible involvement options, valuing lived experience as expertise and ensuring young people see the impact of their contributions.

This is still a work in progress. For participation to truly work and be sustainable, there needs to be a shift towards genuine collaboration where it is meaningful rather than tokenistic. Although it takes time, co-producing services leads to better outcomes and empowers young people as active agents in their care.

4. **Written anonymously by parent of a young person:**
As a young Black mother and nurse practitioner, my journey through the NHS has been both formidable and deeply personal. Growing up in the care system and living independently from the age of 15, I faced many struggles before starting my own family at 19. Much of my life was spent undiagnosed, navigating a world that misunderstood me. I was misdiagnosed with bipolar disorder and emotionally unstable personality disorder (EUPD), carrying the weight of labels that never truly reflected my reality. It wasn't until later that I was correctly diagnosed with autism and ADHD – an experience that was both liberating and painful, highlighting the systemic failures that so many individuals like me endure. Now, as a mother to neurodivergent children, I see these same barriers through a new lens. The very system I work within is the same one that often fails families like mine – where misdiagnosis, inadequate support and a lack of culturally competent care create cycles of harm. Yet, through these challenges, I have persevered, determined to be the change I once needed.

As nurse practitioners, we have a duty to do better – to listen, to advocate and to challenge the biases ingrained in healthcare. We must push for a system that recognises the diversity of neurodivergence, one that provides equitable and accessible care, free from harmful assumptions. By integrating lived experience into best practice, we can transform the way healthcare supports neurodivergent individuals and their families, ensuring that the struggles I have faced do not befall others.

Reflection on Participating in an ADHD Awareness Video with Young People

Written by Narenza Dhanasar

As a nurse consultant and APMH, I recently had the privilege of participating in a video project led by young people with lived experience of ADHD. The purpose of the video was to raise awareness, challenge stigma and offer an authentic insight into what living with ADHD feels like through the voices of those who experience it daily.

The experience was profoundly eye-opening. Uniquely, the project was entirely youth-led: the young people directed the narrative, shaped the messaging and made the final editorial decisions. This reversal of roles was both humbling and inspiring. It reminded me of the immense value that lived experience brings to service development and education. As clinicians, we may unintentionally dominate spaces meant for shared learning, and this project powerfully demonstrated the importance of stepping back and listening.

A key theme that emerged from the young people's stories was the deep sense of being misunderstood by teachers, clinicians, peers and sometimes even family. Many described being labelled as 'lazy', 'difficult' or 'disruptive' when, in reality, they were coping with challenges in attention regulation, emotional intensity and the exhaustion of masking symptoms. These accounts challenged me to re-evaluate how I interpret certain behaviours in clinical settings. What can appear as non-compliance or disinterest is often a manifestation of distress, anxiety or unmet needs.

Equally striking were the young people's reflections on what made a difference. They spoke about the importance of being truly heard, having their strengths acknowledged and being supported in flexible, non-judgemental ways. This highlighted for me how often our systems are shaped around deficit-based models and rigid pathways, rather than neurodiversity-affirming and individualised approaches.

Participating in this project has strengthened my commitment to co-production and to embedding the voices of young people in clinical practice and service design. It has reinforced the need to approach each assessment and interaction with curiosity, empathy and openness making space for narrative, not just symptomatology.

Most of all, this experience reinvigorated my passion for delivering care in a way that makes young people feel seen, heard and genuinely valued. Their insights were not only educational but also transformative.

CONCLUSION

The integration of EBEs in advanced practice mental health has demonstrated significant benefits as evidenced in this chapter. Their involvement has been shown to foster positive attitudinal changes towards mental health, by reducing stigma and promoting a deeper understanding of recovery-oriented practices. As an APMH it is important to understand that continued efforts to support and expand EBE roles are essential for the ongoing improvement of mental health services. This chapter has emphasised that listening to, valuing and working alongside people with lived experience is not just good practice, it is advanced practice.

Reflective Practice

(Use this space to reflect individually or as part of group learning.)

REFLECTIVE QUESTIONS FOR ADVANCED PRACTITIONERS

1. How do I currently use my advanced role to create space for experts by experience in clinical decision-making, service planning or training?
2. Am I role-modelling inclusive, co-productive practice for junior staff or students I supervise?
3. What structural or cultural barriers in my setting limit meaningful co-creation – and how might I influence change?
4. How do my leadership and advocacy skills support the development of trauma-informed, recovery-oriented systems co-designed with service users?
5. What further knowledge or support do I need to deepen my ability to engage with lived experience authentically and effectively?

REFERENCES

1. Transforming (2018). Mental Health 2 3. www.mentalhealth.org.uk/sites/default/files/2022-04/mhf-annual-report-2018.pdf
2. Campbell, P. (2001). Psychiatric survivors and testimonies of self-harm. In: *Madness, Distress and the Politics of Disablement* (ed. H. Spandler, J. Anderson, and B. Sapey), 95–105. Bristol: Policy Press.
3. Beresford, P. (2002). User involvement in research and evaluation: liberation or regulation? *Social Policy & Society* 1 (2): 95–105.
4. Beresford, P. (2013). From 'other' to involved: user involvement in research: an emerging paradigm. *Nordic Social Work Research* 3 (2): 139–148.
5. Department of Health (1999). *National Service Framework for Mental Health: Modern Standards and Service Models*. London: DH.
6. Mind (2020). Service user involvement in mental health. www.mind.org.uk
7. Slay, J. and Stephens, L. (2013). *Co-Production in Mental Health: A Literature Review*. London: New Economics Foundation.
8. NHS England (2019). The NHS long term plan. https://www.longtermplan.nhs.uk
9. CQC (2023). Experts by experience | care quality commission. www.cqc.org.uk. www.cqc.org.uk/about-us/jobs/experts-experience
10. NHS England (2019). Health education England. https://www.hee.nhs.uk
11. Nursing and Midwifery Council (2018). The code: professional standards of practice and behaviour for nurses, midwives and nursing associates. Nursing and Midwifery Council. www.nmc.org.uk/standards/code
12. Health and Care Professions Council. (2021) Standards of care – person centred care. https://www.hcpc-uk.org/standards/meeting-our-standards/person-centred-care
13. Knaak, S., Mantler, E., and Szeto, A. (2017). Mental illness-related stigma in healthcare: barriers to access and care and evidence-based solutions. *Healthcare Management Forum* 30 (2): 111–116. https://www.ncbi.nlm.nih.gov/pmc/articles/PMC5347358
14. Kerry, E., Collett, N., and Gunn, J.R. (2023). The impact of expert by experience involvement in teaching in a DClinPsych programme; for trainees and experts by experience. *Health Expectations* 26 (5): 2098–2108. https://www.ncbi.nlm.nih.gov/pmc/articles/PMC10485345

15. Horgan, A., Manning, F., Donovan, M.O. et al. (2020). Expert by experience involvement in mental health nursing education: the co-production of standards between experts by experience and academics in mental health nursing. *Journal of Psychiatric and Mental Health Nursing* 27 (5): 553–562.
16. Hay, M.C., Weisner, T.S., Subramanian, S. et al. (2008 Oct). Harnessing experience: exploring the gap between evidence-based medicine and clinical practice. *Journal of Evaluation in Clinical Practice* 14 (5): 707–713.
17. BPS (2025). Expert by experience. www.bps.org.uk/member-networks/division-clinical-psychology/expert-experience
18. Health Education England (2017). Multi-professional framework for advanced clinical practice in England. *Health Education England* 1–23. https://www.hee.nhs.uk/sites/default/files/documents/multi-professionalframeworkforadvancedclinicalpracticeinengland.pdf
19. East London NHS Foundation Trust. 2023 You said, we did poster boards | East London NHS foundation trust. [cited 2025 Feb 02]. https://www.elft.nhs.uk/you-said-we-did-poster-boards
20. Ryan, S., Maddison, J., Baxter, K. et al. (2024). Understanding and using experiences of social care to guide service improvements: translating a co-design approach from health to social care. *Health and Social Care Delivery Research.* 28: 1–84.
21. Classen, B., Tudor, K., Johnson, F., and McKenna, B. (2021). Embedding lived experience expertise across the mental health tertiary education sector: an integrative review in the context of Aotearoa New Zealand. *Journal of Psychiatric and Mental Health Nursing* 28 (6): 1140–1152. https://doi.org/10.1111/jpm.12756.
22. Happell, B., Warner, T., Waks, S. et al. (2022). Something special, something unique: perspectives of experts by experience in mental health nursing education on their contribution. *Journal of Psychiatric and Mental Health Nursing* 29 (2): 346–358. https://doi.org/10.1111/jpm.12773.
23. Happell, B., Gordon, S., Hurley, J. et al. (2024). It takes it out of the textbook: benefits of and barriers to expert by experience involvement in pre-registration mental health nursing education. *Journal of Psychiatric and Mental Health Nursing* 31 (5): 945–955. https://doi.org/10.1111/jpm.13042.
24. Schleider, J.L. (2023). The fundamental need for lived experience perspectives in developing and evaluating psychotherapies. *Journal of Consulting and Clinical Psychology* 91 (3): 119–121. https://doi.org/10.1037/ccp0000798.
25. Rocelli, M., Aquili, L., Giovanazzi, P. et al. (2024). All about my ideal mental health service': users, family members and experts by experience discussing a co-designed service. *Health Expectations: An International Journal of Public Participation in Health Care and Health Policy* 27 (2): e13999. https://doi.org/10.1111/hex.13999.
26. Happell, B., Donovan, A.O., Warner, T. et al. (2022). Creating or taking opportunity: strategies for implementing expert by experience positions in mental health academia. *Journal of Psychiatric and Mental Health Nursing* 29 (4): 592–602. https://doi.org/10.1111/jpm.12839.
27. Heerings, M., van de Bovenkamp, H., Cardol, M., and Bal, R. (2022). Ask us! Adjusting experience-based codesign to be responsive to people with intellectual disabilities, serious mental illness or older persons receiving support with independent living. *Health Expectations: An International Journal of Public Participation in Health Care and Health Policy* 25 (5): 2246–2254. https://doi.org/10.1111/hex.13436.
28. Hamilton, C., Filia, K., Lloyd, S. et al. (2022). 'More than just numbers on a page?' a qualitative exploration of the use of data collection and feedback in youth mental health services. *PLoS One* 17 (7): e0271023. https://doi.org/10.1371/journal.pone.0271023.
29. Baines, R., Donovan, J., Regan de Bere, S. et al. (2018). Responding effectively to adult mental health patient feedback in an online environment: a coproduced framework. *Health Expectations: An International Journal of Public Participation in Health Care and Health Policy* 21 (5): 887–898. https://doi.org/10.1111/hex.12682.

30. Sheard, L., Marsh, C., O'Hara, J. et al. (2017). The patient feedback response framework – understanding why UK hospital staff find it difficult to make improvements based on patient feedback: a qualitative study. *Social Science & Medicine (1982)* 178: 19–27. https://doi.org/10.1016/j.socscimed.2017.02.005.
31. Oliver, B.J., Nelson, E.C., and Kerrigan, C.L. (2019). Turning feed-forward and feedback processes on patient-reported data into intelligent action and informed decision-making: case studies and principles. *Medical Care* 57 (Suppl 5 Suppl 1): S31–S37. https://doi.org/10.1097/MLR.0000000000001088.
32. Flott, K., Darzi, A., Gancarczyk, S., and Mayer, E. (2018). Improving the usefulness and use of patient survey programs: National Health Service Interview Study. *Journal of Medical Internet Research* 20 (4): e141. https://doi.org/10.2196/jmir.8806.
33. McAllister, S., Simpson, A., Tsianakas, V. et al. (2021). Developing a theory-informed complex intervention to improve nurse-patient therapeutic engagement employing experience-based co-design and the behaviour change wheel: an acute mental health ward case study. *BMJ Open* 11 (5): e047114. https://doi.org/10.1136/bmjopen-2020-047114.
34. Morley, C., Jose, K., Hall, S.E. et al. (2024). Evidence-informed, experience-based co-design: a novel framework integrating research evidence and lived experience in priority-setting and co-design of health services. *BMJ Open* 14 (8): e084620. https://doi.org/10.1136/bmjopen-2024-084620.
35. Deering, K., Pawson, C., Summers, N., & Williams, J. (2019). Patient perspectives of helpful risk management practices within mental health services. A mixed studies systematic review of primary research. *Journal of Psychiatric and Mental Health Nursing* 26(5–6), 185–197. https://doi.org/10.1111/jpm.12521
36. Rimondini, M., Busch, I.M., Mazzi, M.A. et al. (2019). Patient empowerment in risk management: a mixed-method study to explore mental health professionals' perspective. *BMC Health Services Research* 19 (1): 382. https://doi.org/10.1186/s12913-019-4215-x.
37. Tapsell, A., Martin, K.M., Moxham, L. et al. (2020). Expert by experience involvement in mental Health Research: developing a wellbeing brochure for people with lived experiences of mental illness. *Issues in Mental Health Nursing* 41 (3): 194–200. https://doi.org/10.1080/01612840.2019.1663566.
38. NHS Confederation (2019) Taking a whole-system approach to mental wellbeing | NHS Confederation. www.nhsconfed.org. https://www.nhsconfed.org/case-studies/taking-whole-system-approach-mental-wellbeing
39. Health Education England. (2019). New ways of working in mental health. https://www.hee.nhs.uk/our-work/mental-health/new-roles-mental-health
40. NHS England (2022). Meeting the mental health needs of the population: a whole system approach. https://www.england.nhs.uk/blog/debra-gilderdale
41. Mendon, G.B., Gurung, D., Loganathan, S. et al. (2024). Establishing partnerships with people with lived experience of mental illness for stigma reduction in low- and middle-income settings. *Cambridge Prisms: Global Mental Health* 11: e70. https://doi.org/10.1017/gmh.2024.69.
42. Krendl, A.C. and Perry, B.L. (2023). Stigma toward substance dependence: causes, consequences, and potential interventions. *Psychological Science in the Public Interest* 24 (2): 90–126.
43. Harris, H., Clarkin, C., Rovet, J. et al. (2023). Meaningful engagement through critical reflexivity: engaging people with lived experience in continuing mental health professional development. *Health Expectations: An International Journal of Public Participation in Health Care and Health Policy* 26 (5): 1793–1798. https://doi.org/10.1111/hex.13798.
44. Kerry, E., Collett, N., and Gunn, J. (2023). The impact of expert by experience involvement in teaching in a DClinPsych programme; for trainees and experts by experience. *Health Expectations: An International Journal of Public Participation in Health Care and Health Policy* 26 (5): 2098–2108. https://doi.org/10.1111/hex.13817.

45. Reynolds, L.M., Davies, J.P., Mann, B. et al. (2016). StreetWise: developing a serious game to support forensic mental health service users' preparation for discharge: a feasibility study. *Journal of Psychiatric and Mental Health Nursing* 24 (4): 185–193.
46. Oborn, E., Barrett, M., Gibson, S., and Gillard, S. (2019). Knowledge and expertise in care practices: the role of the peer worker in mental health teams. *Sociology of Health & Illness* 41 (7): 1305–1322. https://doi.org/10.1111/1467-9566.12944.
47. Bennett, V., Gill, C., Miller, P. et al. (2022). Co-production to understand online help-seeking for young people experiencing emotional abuse and neglect: building capabilities, adapting research methodology and evaluating involvement and impact. *Health Expectations: An International Journal of Public Participation in Health Care and Health Policy* 25 (6): 3143–3163. https://doi.org/10.1111/hex.13622.
48. Horgan, A., Manning, F., Bocking, J. et al. (2018). 'To be treated as a human': using co-production to explore experts by experience involvement in mental health nursing education – the COMMUNE project. *International Journal of Mental Health Nursing* 27 (4): 1282–1291.
49. NHS Providers (2024). Co-production and engagement with communities as a solution to reducing health inequalities. https://nhsproviders.org/media/698572/co-production-health-ineq-1e.pdf
50. Newbury G (2013), FT GMMHN. Recovery academy. Greater Manchester Mental Health NHS FT. https://www.gmmh.nhs.uk/recovery
51. Verseone VerseOneUser. Recovery is a personal journey towards a meaningful and satisfying life, living as well as possible whatever symptoms or difficulties are present. http://Slam.nhs.uk. 2022. https://slam.nhs.uk/recovery-college
52. Collaborative Learning College. Centre for Addiction and Mental Health (CAMH) [Internet]. Toronto: CAMH; 2019 [cited 2025 Nov 21]. Available from: https://clc.camh.ca
53. WA Recovery College Alliance (WARCA) [Internet]. Perth (WA): HelpingMinds; 2025 [cited 2025 Nov 21]. Available from: http://www.warecoverycollege.org.au
54. A recovery approach within the Irish mental health services: a framework for development [Internet]. Dublin: Health Service Executive; 2025 [cited 2025 Nov 21]. Available from: https://www.lenus.ie/bitstream/handle/10147/75113/Framework%20for%20%20mental%20health%20services.pdf?sequence=1&isAllowed=y
55. Hayes, D., Henderson, C., Bakolis, I. et al. (2022). Recovery colleges characterisation and testing in England (RECOLLECT): rationale and protocol. *BMC Psychiatry* 22 (1): 627. https://doi.org/10.1186/s12888-022-04253-y.
56. Storm, M. and Edwards, A. (2012). Models of user involvement in the mental health context: intentions and implementation challenges. *Psychiatric Quarterly* 84 (3): 313–327. https://link.springer.com/article/10.1007/s11126-012-9247-x.
57. Health Education England (2021). Framework for involving people with lived experience in education and training. NHS HEE. https://www.hee.nhs.uk
58. Carr, S. (2019). 'I am not your nutter': a personal reflection on commodification and comradeship in service user and survivor research. *Disability & Society* 34 (7–8): 1–14. https://doi.org/10.1080/09687599.2019.1608424.
59. Faulkner, A. and Kalathil, J. (2012). *The Freedom to Be, the Chance to Dream: Preserving User-Led Peer Support*. London: Together for Mental Wellbeing.

60. Kivistö, M., Martin, M., Hautala, S., and Soronen, K. (2023). Facilitators and challenges of integrating experts by experience activity in mental health services: experiences from Finland. *Community Mental Health Journal.* https://doi.org/10.1007/s10597-022-01039-0.

61. Burridge, S. Experts by Experience Involvement Handbook: Healthcare for Homeless People [Internet]. London: Pathway; n.d. [cited 2025 Nov 21]. Available from: https://www.pathway.org.uk/wp-content/uploads/2013/05/EbE-Involvement-Handbook.pdf

62. Mavis, B., Holmes Rovner, M., Jorgenson, S. et al. (2015). Patient participation in clinical encounters: a systematic review to identify self-report measures. *Health Expectations* 18 (6): 1827–1843.

PART 3

ADVANCED PRACTICE IN MENTAL HEALTH AND SPECIFIC POPULATIONS

PART 2

CHAPTER 13

Perinatal Mental Health

Claire Hargrave
Central and North West London Foundation Trust, London, UK

Aim

The aim of this chapter is to review the unique mental health needs for women and birthing people during the perinatal period (pregnancy and up to 2 years postnatal). We will explore the responsibility of the advanced practitioner in mental health to confidently identify, assess and co-ordinate perinatal care across multiple agencies and settings.

LEARNING OUTCOMES

After reading this chapter, the reader will be able to:

1. Understand factors that increase the risk of perinatal mental illness.
2. Provide trauma-informed care for women/birthing persons in the perinatal period.
3. Be confident in co-ordinating multi-agency care which supports a woman/birthing person's mental and physical health needs.
4. Be confident in completing a thorough perinatal assessment encompassing perinatal risk.
5. Understand the stark differences in maternity outcomes based on ethnicity.
6. Have an awareness of the provision of mother and baby units and the purpose of a dual admission for mother and baby.
7. Be able to identify the perinatal red flags and respond appropriately.
8. Be able to identify child safeguarding risks during the perinatal period and support the professional network to understand how mental illness can impact on parenting ability.
9. Understand the importance of assertive treatment of mother/birthing person in the perinatal period.

The Advanced Practitioner in Mental Health, First Edition. Edited by Clare Allabyrne.
© 2026 John Wiley & Sons Ltd. All rights reserved, including rights for text and data mining and training of artificial intelligence technologies or similar technologies. Published 2026 by John Wiley & Sons Ltd.

TABLE 13.1 Four pillar capabilites.

Clinical practice

4   Utilise clinical reasoning and decision-making skills to make a differential diagnosis and provide rationales for person-management plans, through critically reflecting on and evaluating their own role in relation to challenging traditional practices, new ways of working and the impact upon the multidisciplinary team.

Leadership and management

3   Demonstrate teamworking, leadership, resilience and determination, managing situations that are unfamiliar, complex or unpredictable.

Education

3   Effectively utilise a range of evidence-based educational strategies/interventions to support person-centred care with individuals, their families and carers and other healthcare colleagues.

Research

1   Critically appraise and apply the evidence base in influencing engagement, recovery, shared decision-making, transference and safeguarding.

Source: Adapted from [1].

These are in line with Health Education England's Mental Health Advanced Practice area specific curriculum and capabilities framework [1]. This chapter will meet capabilities from across the four pillars, and examples are detailed in Table 13.1.

We will also consider perinatal mental healthcare from the capabilities across the six domains [1] later in the chapter.

INTRODUCTION

This chapter will highlight the needs of this specialist population of women and birthing people during the perinatal period. The perinatal period covers pregnancy and childbirth up until 2 years postnatal. (Please note that the terms 'mother', 'woman' and 'birthing person' will be used interchangeably in this chapter). This chapter is focused on the United Kingdom NHS provision, but many of the principles can be applied internationally. The following have useful global information. The International Marcé Society for Perinatal Mental Health [2] is a multidisciplinary organisation that promotes research and high quality perinatal mental healthcare across the world. The Maternal Mental Health Alliance (MMHA) [3] is based in the United Kingdom, but this has prompted the launch of the Global Alliance for Maternal Mental Health (GAMMH) [4] and the African Alliance for Maternal Mental Health (AAMMH) [5].

Links for more information are as follows:

The International Marce Society for Perinatal Mental Health|Perinatal Mental Health Home|Maternal Mental Health Alliance. https://marcesociety.com/

Global Alliance for Maternal Mental Health (GAMMH)|Maternal Mental Health. https://www.gammh.org/

Though perinatal provision has changed substantially over the last 10 years due to increased investment; generic mental health services will always provide care for women of childbearing age and some of these women will become pregnant, so services need to be able to 'think family' and deliver care within a life course lens [6]. As an advanced practitioner, you may be asked to lead care for women in the perinatal period due to the additional knowledge and skills possessed by advanced practitioners in mental health (AMPHs) which are required in order to ensure that all aspects of care are met. Therefore, it is important that APMHs are confident to assess women in the perinatal period, identify their needs and compile a risk assessment which includes risk to their unborn child. Working with women in the perinatal period can be highly emotive for practitioners. Some women may not be able to parent their child due to their mental health difficulties. What is in the best interests of the mother may not be in the best interests of the child, and this can result in a conflict where practitioners are split. Although as an APMH you may be predominately responsible for the mother's mental health, you still have a duty of care to report any child safeguarding concerns [7].

In some situations, you may be required to support a mother and baby being separated. This is an extremely difficult, challenging situation for all involved. For practitioners, it can evoke thoughts of their own childhood or traumatic experiences. It is important to ensure that there are opportunities for individual and group supervision to be able to have a space to share difficult feelings [8].

Working in the perinatal period can be both challenging and emotive [8]; however, it can also be extremely rewarding to be part of a woman and family's life at such a life changing point.

FUNDAMENTALS FOR ADVANCED PRACTICE IN PERINATAL MENTAL HEALTH

Policy Context

Key Points

- One in five women in the United Kingdom will experience perinatal mental health problems.
- Cost of £8.1 billion per year to UK society – 28% costs to the mother and 72% costs to the child.
- 40% of women in the United Kingdom had no access to a specialist community perinatal service.
- Cost of perinatal mental health problems to society is five times the cost of improving services.

Source: The Cost of Perinatal Mental Health Problems [9].

The MMHA commissioned a report in conjunction with the London School of Economics in 2014 which outlined the costs of perinatal mental health problems in the United Kingdom [9]. The report explained the risk to the child for untreated mental health problems in the mother and estimated that the current cost to society was five times the cost of improving services. This seminal report brought increased focus to perinatal mental health services, and this was reflected in the NHS Long Term Plan [10].

The NHS Long Term Plan [10] outlined the aspiration to increase access to perinatal specialist care for an additional 24,000 women per year by 2023/24, in addition to 30,000 getting specialist help by 2020/21. It outlined that perinatal provision should be widened to be available from preconception to 24 months after birth to support the cross-government commitment to women and children in the first 1001 critical days of a child's life [11].

Perinatal mental health services received significant investment of £365 million from 2016 to 2021 [12]. This improved access to specialist community perinatal services in the United Kingdom. In 2023, in England, Wales and mainland Scotland, every woman irrespective of where they live had access to a specialist community perinatal service [13]; however, within Northern Ireland and the Scottish Islands, some areas still do not have access to a community specialist perinatal team. A freedom of information request outlined that spending had increased for specialist perinatal services but there has been an underspend due to difficulty in recruiting specialist perinatal staff [13]. Four new psychiatric mother and baby units (MBUs) had opened in England by 2018/19 which has meant more women have been able to receive inpatient mental health treatment whilst remaining with their child nearer to their home.

In 2017, the incumbent government at the time set a national target to reduce maternal deaths (during pregnancy and 1 year post-birth) by 50% between 2010 and 2030 [14]. Paradoxically, during this time maternal mortality has increased by 8% [15]. In 2018–2020, the leading cause of death from 6 weeks post-delivery to 1 year post-delivery was mental health related, either suicide or other mental health causes. In the 2024 report [16], mental health-related causes (suicide and substance misuse) continued to be a predominant cause of death, accounting for 34% of all deaths occurring from 6 weeks to 1 year post-birth. Thrombosis and thromboembolism were the leading direct cause of maternal death across all ethnicities [16]. The All-Party Parliamentary group (ARPPG) published the first birth trauma inquiry report in 2024 [17] which drew on over 1300 women who have experienced traumatic births and highlighted the need for a national strategy for maternity care, continuity of care and addressing inequalities.

Perinatal Professional Network

One of the challenges in working in perinatal mental health services is that there are a lot of different professionals involved across mental health, maternity, health visiting and social services requiring leadership and co-ordination of care across multiple clinicians and services (see Figure 13.1). There can often be differences of opinion and priorities for treatment which can result in difficulties in agreeing a collaborative care plan.

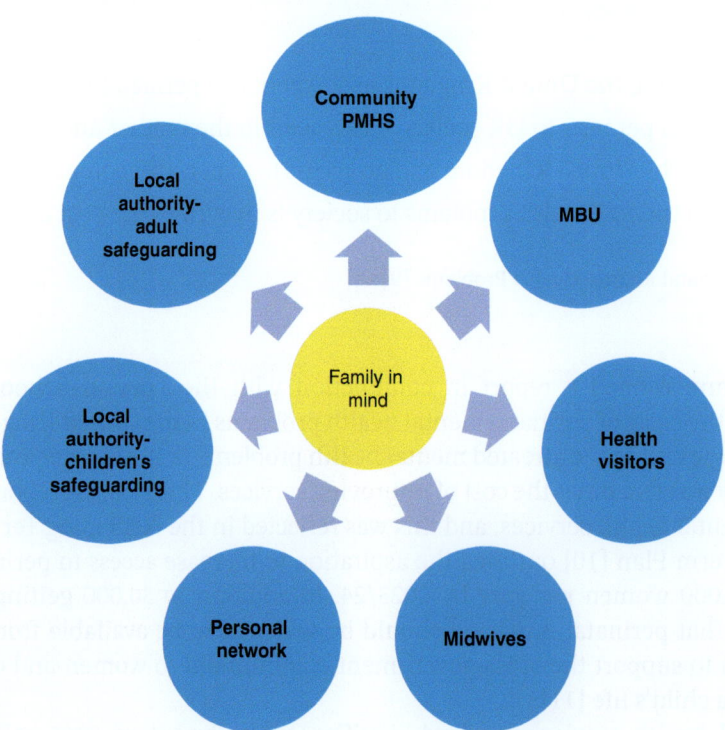

FIGURE 13.1 Professional network during the perinatal period.

Prevalence

During pregnancy approximately 12% of women experience depression and 13% experience anxiety and many will experience both [18]. In the postnatal year, depression and anxiety affect between 15 and 20% of women. Postpartum psychosis affects between 1 and 2 in 1000 women who have given birth. Women with a diagnosis of bipolar or schizoaffective disorder have a much higher risk of developing postpartum psychosis of 25%, so 1 in 4 women and this rises to 50%, 1 in 2 women if their mother or sister has had postpartum psychosis [19]. However, women can experience postpartum psychosis with no previous mental health history. Women can also experience anxiety disorders including panic disorder, obsessive compulsive disorder, post-traumatic stress disorder and tokophobia (extreme fear of childbirth). 15% of women had an eating disorder at some point in their lifetime but around 5% have an eating disorder during pregnancy [20] and 12% of mothers show significant post-traumatic stress symptoms in relation to a childbirth event [21].

The main perinatal red flags are:

- Recent significant change in mental state or emergence of new symptoms.
- New thoughts or acts of violent self-harm.
- New and persistent expressions of incompetency as a mother or estrangement from their infant [15].

When a woman becomes mentally unwell during pregnancy, there is a strict timeline from identification of symptoms to intervene and treat mother in order for her to be in the best possible mental state at the birth of her child. If a mother is mentally unwell at the point of delivery of her child, a capacity assessment will be required as outlined in the Mental Capacity Act [22]. This is usually done in collaboration with a consultant obstetrician. If a mother does not have capacity to consent to the mode of delivery of her child, an application to the court of protection may be required in order to decide the safest way for the child to be delivered [23] (see Table 13.2).

TABLE 13.2 Factors associated with increased risk of perinatal mental illness.

Factors associated with increased risk of perinatal mental illness:
- History of mental illness [18]
- Family history of mental illness [18]
- Low levels of social support
- Adverse childhood experiences (ACEs) [24]
- Domestic abuse [25]
- Single parent
- Unplanned pregnancy [26]
- Socioeconomic disadvantage, history or current substance misuse, lower education level [27]
- Recent stressful events
- Previous children being removed from care [28]
- Traumatic birth [17]

Suicidality and Suicide in the Perinatal Period

In the United Kingdom, an annual report is conducted which compiles the care of women who died during pregnancy or in their first year postnatal and the causes of those deaths. In the period 2018–2020, maternal suicide was the leading cause of direct death [15]. Deaths from mental health related causes as a whole (suicide and substance misuse) account for nearly 40% of deaths in the first postnatal year. This is a very concerning statistic particularly given that this includes death for all causes including physical health reasons. In 2024, a summary report outlined that mental health related causes were still a leading cause of death (34%) in the postnatal year [16]. The recommendations are listed from the 2022 report which included more detail about the demographics of women that died [15].

Demographics of Women That Died from Mental Health Related Causes (Suicide and Substance Misuse) [15]

- Majority not known to specialist perinatal services
- 86% were from white ethnic backgrounds
- Median age 30
- Increase in number of women under the age of 20 that died
- Very few had formal mental health diagnosis
- Majority known to children's social services
- High documented levels of domestic abuse
- A number of women had a history of childhood and/or adult trauma
- Most used a violent method to end their life.

Key Recommendations from Report [15]

- Women with persistent and severe insomnia should be assessed for underlying mental illness.
- Services should work in a trauma-informed way.
- Be alert to cultural stigma, fear of child removal, feelings of maternal incompetence – these may prevent a woman disclosing symptoms of mental illness, thoughts of self-harm or substance use

Other Existing Recommendations

- Women are at higher risk of suicide if there is a loss of a child (either by miscarriage, stillbirth or a child being removed by children's services).
- Perinatal services are only able to work with the mother or birthing person if she is the main carer of her child. If she no longer has care of her child, then perinatal services are no longer able to continue working with a parent, and she will need to be referred to a community mental health team for ongoing support. This transition of care can increase risk to the mother at a time of acute stress following the loss of her child. If a woman has stopped psychiatric medication during pregnancy, a prompt postnatal review should consider whether medication should be recommenced.

Health Inequalities

In 2023 about 40% of babies born in England and in Wales were from an ethnic minority group [29] and one-third of live births were born to non-UK born mothers [30]. There are considerable ethnic inequalities during the maternity period and although they have improved, black women are still twice as likely to die compared to white women during pregnancy in the United Kingdom from 2021 to 2023 [31]. Asian women had a slightly increased risk compared to white women, though white women are the most likely to die from suicide. Unfortunately, the report does not break down causes of death by ethnicity in the report. Women in the most deprived areas have a maternal mortality rate twice as high as those women living in the least deprived areas. In the Mothers and Babies: Reducing Risk Through Audits and Confidential Enquiries Across the UK (MBRRACE) report [28], differences between ethnic groups in the risk factors have not been adjusted for. Women who died during pregnancy had multiple social, personal and physical health problems often before conception. When adjustment has been made for some risk factors there is still excess maternal mortality in women from black and Asian ethnicities. In 2023, babies of Asian and black ethnicities have much higher mortality rates than babies of white ethnicity. Infant mortality rates in babies of Pakistani, Bangladeshi and black ethnicity are double the rate in babies for white British ethnicity [32].

Maternity services have been identified as a clinical area of focus for accelerated improvement in the CORE 20 plus 5 approaches to reduce healthcare inequalities [33]. The aim for maternity is to ensure 75% of women from black and Asian communities and most deprived groups have continuity of care. There are local policies to implement this based on the local population.

FivexMore is an organisation which is focused on black maternal health [34]. The name of the organisation was derived from the original statistic that in 2018, black women were five times more likely to die than white women during their pregnancy. FivexMore conducted a national survey of black women and made a number of key recommendations, including that staff should be aware of the disparities in maternity outcomes. Professionals should have increased knowledge in identifying and diagnosing conditions that disproportionally affect black women such as sickle cell anaemia and uterine fibroids [35].

It is important as an AMPH to understand the stark ethnic inequalities in the United Kingdom for black and Asian women during pregnancy. As an AMPH it is part of your role to act as an advocate to ensure that a woman's maternity needs are met whilst she is under your care.

Access to Perinatal Services

Access to specialist perinatal services is outlined in the perinatal mental healthcare pathways in Figure 13.2 [36].

These pathways outline the routes into perinatal services and when the pathway stops.

1. Preconception – women with a serious mental illness who are planning a pregnancy can be referred for specialist consultation for review of medication and care by a perinatal consultant psychiatrist.
2. Specialist assessment – conducted by perinatal service.
3. Emergency assessment – this may be conducted by secondary mental health services such as psychiatric liaison or home treatment team.

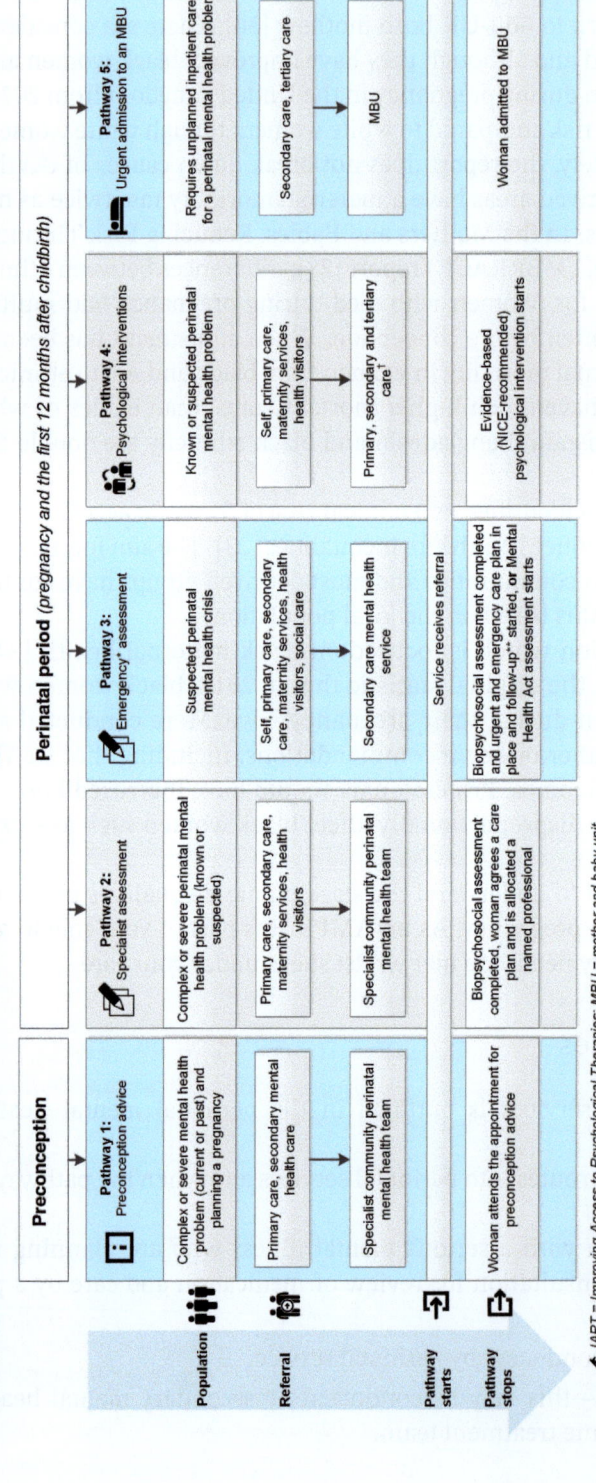

FIGURE 13.2 Perinatal mental healthcare pathways. Source: Adapted from [36].

As an APMH you may be asked to complete this assessment, which is detailed later in the chapter. This may result in a referral to home treatment team, perinatal services, informal inpatient admission or referral for a Mental Health Act assessment.

4. Psychological interventions – these can be provided by primary services such as talking therapies or secondary MH perinatal services
5. Urgent admission to an MBU – admission can be provided from 32 weeks gestation to 1 year postnatal. During early pregnancy and post 1 year mother would need to be admitted to an acute inpatient unit. There are other inclusion and exclusion criteria (please refer to inpatient section).

Alignment to the Mental Health Advanced Practice Area-Specific Capability and Curriculum Framework [1]

This chapter will now consider perinatal mental healthcare in relation to the domains as follows: [1]

A. Person-centred therapeutic alliance
B. Assessment and investigations
C. Formulation
D. Collaborative planning
E. Intervention and evaluation
F. Leadership and management and education and research

A. Person-centred alliance:

At the core of providing healthcare to an individual, a trusting relationship between practitioner and service user is imperative, so that the service user is able to share their concerns and needs. As an APMH, you will be familiar with how to build therapeutic relationships, though it can sometimes be difficult with a mother in the perinatal period to establish a relationship during a period of uncertainty and complexity. Women can be reluctant to engage with mental health services for a variety of reasonings such as mental health stigma, fear of removal of their child, substance misuse, previous experiences of poor care and trauma history.

A listening project with women who have experienced child removal due to substance misuse stated that they were not able to access appropriate mental health support and felt 'invisible' [37, 38]. They shared feeling judged and their feelings were dismissed. It is important to be able to build trust and be non-judgemental and non-discriminatory, utilising advanced communication skills.

B. Assessment and investigations:

Conducting an assessment in the perinatal period

As an APMH you will already be an expert in conducting thorough, holistic mental health assessments. The purpose of this section is to explore some of the additional aspects which should be explored when assessing a woman or birthing person during the perinatal period. Table 13.3 outlines some helpful acronyms which you may come across in documentation.

National Institute of Clinical Excellence (NICE) antenatal and postnatal mental health provides a good oversight on considerations for care planning [38]. It is important to remember that perinatal community services are not equipped to respond in an emergency and most services operate on the timeline of an assessment within a month.

TABLE 13.3 Commonly used acronyms.

Acronyms

CIN – child in need plan

CP – child protection plan

EDD – estimated date of delivery

Gravida – number of times they have been pregnant (regardless of whether they have resulted in live births)

LA – local authority

LMP – last menstrual period – used to calculate gestation

Parity – number of times that they have been pregnant beyond 24 wks

TFMR – termination of pregnancy for medical reasons

TOP – termination of pregnancy (abortion)

VBAC – vaginal birth after caesarean section

Specific assessment information

Contact details of any professionals currently involved in care:

- Midwife/obstetrician
- Health visitor
- Social worker
- Charity support

Current children
- Names, dates of birth, have they been known to children's social services?
- Are they currently in the mother's care?
- Are they in a relationship with the father/s?

Obstetric history
- **Current pregnancy:** number of weeks pregnant, estimated date of delivery (EDD). Booked maternity hospital and contact details, dates of upcoming maternity appointments, any current issues or concerns with the pregnancy such as gestational diabetes, pre-eclampsia for example. Is this a planned or unplanned pregnancy?
- **Previous pregnancies:** number of times pregnant, exploration of loss (either miscarriage, termination or removal).
- **Previous deliveries:** vaginal or C-section.
- **Perinatal trauma:** experience of delivery, was this traumatic and does it have lasting impact?
- **Method of feeding:** breastfeeding, formula feeding or mixed feeding. How do they feel feeding is going?

Mental Health and Physical Health History
- **Mental health history:** including whether a first-degree female relative has had a serious perinatal serious illness. This increases the risk of perinatal mental illness [18].
- **Physical health history:** any significant physical health history or illnesses.

Risk and red flags
- **Thoughts of harm to self: new feelings of self-harm or suicidal ideation is a significant perinatal red flag** [15]
- **Unborn baby/child:** how do they feel about the unborn/baby? Do they feel affectionate or bonded to their unborn/child? Do they have any thoughts of harming their baby?
- **Delusional beliefs:** do they have any unusual beliefs about their child – for example, believing their child has special powers or is the devil.
- **Harm from others:** domestic abuse from partner or other family members. History of domestic abuse in previous relationships. Include coercive control. Consideration of honour-based violence.
- **Child safeguarding:** is this woman known to children's services? Do the concerns warrant a child safeguarding referral and has this been discussed with the woman and her family [7]?
- **Perinatal Information:** baby care – who is doing the baby care? Has there been changes? for example has mother been preventing others from caring for the child or has she been withdrawing from care?
- **Parenting:** how is the mother feeling about the pregnancy/being a mother? Does she feel able to cope? **Feelings of incompetence as a mother is a significant perinatal red flag.**
- **Sleep:** pregnancy often affects sleep. Postnatally, where is the baby sleeping? Are they co-sleeping? How often is baby feeding and waking through the night? Is anyone able to support at night?

Case Example
- Sally is a Romanian woman who is 13 days postnatal with her first child. She has no previous history in mental health services and was brought in via ambulance to the Urgent Care Department due to concerns about postpartum psychosis. She delivered via emergency C section 13 days ago and her family report that she has been having hallucinations, delusional behaviour and mania. She was assessed by psychiatric liaison services and has been discharged home on a Saturday morning with Home Treatment Team (HTT) support and referral to community perinatal services.

What actions would you take as an APMH within the HTT?

C. Formulation

Based on your assessment as a result of compiling information from different sources, you will need to make an appropriate formulation and decide on a care plan going forward. This should include mental health, physical health and maternity considerations.

In contrast to working in adult mental health, the formulation needs to consider the risk to the baby and this should influence your decision-making when compiling a care plan. It is advised to be more conservative when considering care plan options following assessment.

For example, MBU admission may be the most appropriate recommendation for a new parent with severe depression as the risk to the child may be too high to be contained in the community. In contrast an adult without caring responsibilities may be able to be appropriately contained with HTT support. Other aspects to consider is whether the woman has support at home or whether she is the sole carer for her child. If a woman presents with symptoms of postpartum psychosis, this should be considered as a medical emergency which requires treatment in hospital. It is not appropriate for postpartum psychosis to be treated in the community. Consideration of method of feeding has an impact on prescribing and mental state. For example, if a mother is exclusively breastfeeding a newborn baby, she is unlikely to be able to get more than 2 hours of consecutive sleep.

D. Collaborative planning

Women in the perinatal period will always have as a minimum their GP and either maternity or health visiting involved. In many cases the family will also have children's social care involvement. All services will have different priorities and there will have to be a shared agreement on the care plan. It is imperative as an APMH to be able to co-ordinate care across agencies and ensure that the responsibilities of each service are understood. These cases are highly complex with high risk from both a mental health and obstetric perspective. It is important to try and contain emotions and facilitate open communication, keeping the mother and baby at the centre of the care.

As an APMH, you should be able to demonstrate that you can lead effective intervention, demonstrate good knowledge of the systems involved and manage any expectations of the intervention and service [1]. All decisions should be promoting safety and mitigating risk. You will be required to make decisions on the best setting for a pregnant person (for example, in maternity or an acute mental health ward) and balance the mental health and physical health needs. See the following for case example and considerations.

Case example

Sally is 35 weeks pregnant and is currently admitted to an acute Mental Health ward under Section 2 of the Mental Health Act [39]. She has a diagnosis of bipolar affective disorder and is currently manic, over-intrusive and sexually disinhibited. There have been concerns that she is displaying symptoms of pre-eclampsia at her recent maternity appointment which pose a risk to her and her baby. The midwives have requested that she should have physical health monitoring using the National Early Warning Score (NEWS) at least three times a day and ask for readings to be shared with them. The mental health ward has mentioned that she has been declining observations but are concerned about the risk to her and her baby. They would like her to be transferred to a maternity ward as they think that maternity will be more able to safely manage the physical health of both Sally and her baby. Maternity do not feel that she needs admission to obstetric ward and do not feel they would be able to safely manage her mental health on a busy ward.

How would you support the professional network to meet Sally's needs?

E. Intervention and evaluation

As an APMH, you may be required to lead care, prescribe the intervention and critically evaluate the plan. The care plan will need to be dynamic and changing as a woman's perinatal journey through pregnancy, birth and postnatal period progresses.

Inpatient care

Women may need inpatient treatment during pregnancy and the postnatal period. During this period, there should be a lower threshold for admission due to the risks to unborn/young child. MBUs are NHS run specialist psychiatric inpatient units which are able to admit mothers with mental health difficulties with their babies for assessment and treatment of their illness until the child is 1 year old [40]. These are specialist units that are funded nationally but many are moving to be part of an NHS provider collaborative [41].

MBUs are able to facilitate admission for women in their final trimester of pregnancy from 32 weeks gestation. It is important to seek advice on where the nearest MBU is as this may be not within your trust, and bed allocation is managed by the MBU themselves and not a central bed management system.

There is a website which states current bed availability and all the contact details for the MBUs in the United Kingdom.

perinatal.cpms.necsu.nhs.uk.

Exclusion criteria for MBUs:

- For sole purpose of a parenting assessment.
- Women with severe personality disorder, learning disability or substance misuse unless they are also suffering from, or there is suspected, serious mental illness.
- If there is evidence that the mother will not be capable of independent functioning in caring for her infant in the community with reasonable support.
- If there is evidence of serious violence/aggressive behaviour that might pose a risk of harm or injury to her own or other babies on MBU.

Admission is subject to risk assessment that they will not pose a risk to other mothers or babies.

There is a national referral form: www.nhswebbeds.co.uk/PerinatalFiles/cpms-referral-form.pdf

Figure 13.3 outlines where a pregnant woman/birthing person can be admitted across the perinatal period.

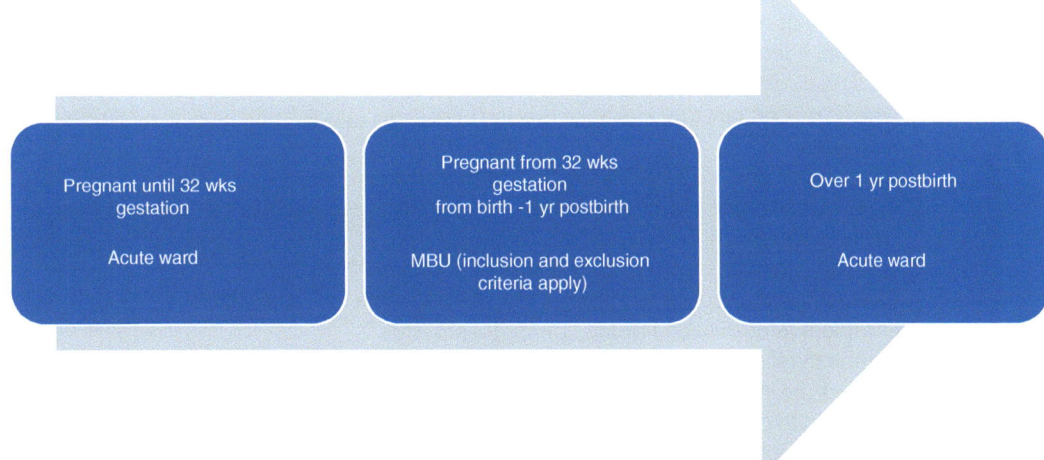

FIGURE 13.3 Admission during the perinatal period.

During pregnancy and until 32 weeks gestation, the woman would need to be admitted to an acute ward. From 32 weeks pregnant until 1 year postnatal a woman can be admitted to an MBU. Post baby's first birthday, the mother would have to be admitted to an acute ward and the baby would need to be cared for by family or social services if there is no family available.

There is a gap of provision for women who are inpatients during their early pregnancy. They are unable to be admitted to the MBU but often do not receive specialist community perinatal input whilst an inpatient. There is local variance on whether the community perinatal service remains involved whilst a mother is admitted to an acute ward. The care needs to be led by the Responsible Clinician and treating ward team, but they may seek specialist advice on care provision and treatment from perinatal services.

Considerations for Care Planning for Pregnant Woman/Birthing Person on an Adult Acute Ward

An acute mental health ward is not an ideal environment for a pregnant person to be admitted as there is not specialist perinatal trained staff and the pregnant person could be at risk from other unwell patients. Health professionals have understandable concerns about safely managing a pregnant woman and ensuring their physical health needs are met. Staff can feel ill equipped to manage the risk and close observations can be difficult due to staffing levels and they can feel intrusive to the pregnant service user. There are also concerns about prescribing and administering medication including under restraint if required. There can be difficulties in facilitating travel to antenatal visits on a different site due to staffing and managing an acutely unwell woman in a maternity setting. There is a national shortage of acute beds, and there can be considerable pressure to discharge pregnant women as soon as possible.

Actions to consider on admission
All women of childbearing age that are admitted should have a routine pregnancy test.

Maternity booking	• It is important that the woman/birthing person is booked for maternity care. Discuss with the woman whether they have booked and what maternity care they have, if any. Most hospitals accept online referrals but it would be advisable to call maternity and provide a verbal handover and ask whether they need urgent maternity care based on their gestation or current physical health. Some hospitals have a specialist perinatal midwife which you can ask to speak to. If this isn't possible, speak to the specialist safeguarding midwives. • Women can choose where to book their pregnancy. • If the woman does not have capacity to make this decision, it is advisable to book at their local maternity unit.
Perinatal services	• Consideration of referral to community perinatal and/or MBU. • Clinicians within perinatal services may be available for consultation. • Complete referral to community perinatal services. • Complete referral to MBU if they are approaching 32 wks. gestation
Child safeguarding	• Contact the local authority's emergency duty desk to see whether the woman is known and open to children's services. Make them aware of the admission • If they are not known to children SG services complete referral. • Discuss case with trust safeguarding lead for children. • Invite children's services to ward round meetings.

Care Planning

Care planning should incorporate mental health, physical health and maternity aspects, and this should be collaborative with the mother and other professionals.

Mental health	- Medication: are the medicines safe to be taken in pregnancy? - Observation levels: consider risk from others. - Restraint
Physical health	- Blood tests: are there any additional blood tests required (e.g. to test for anaemia or HbA1c)? - Frequency of NEWS - Plan for labour
Maternity care	- Upcoming antenatal appointments - Include guidance from midwives about any additional monitoring, for example, due to pre-eclampsia or gestational diabetes

Planning for Birth

If a mother is still an inpatient around the time of delivery, it is important to have an explicit care plan about the birth specifically. Please refer to the best practice toolkit for pre-birth planning [42]. A formal meeting should be set up between 28 and 32 weeks gestation with all clinicians involved to discuss antenatal, birth and postnatal plans.

Capacity should be assessed about delivery options in conjunction with maternity services. This should be independent of consent to treatment for mental health treatment and should be in line with the Mental Capacity Act [22].

Postnatal Period

If a mother is admitted to an acute ward instead of an MBU postnatally, this can be due to bed availability, current risk or safeguarding concerns. The mother may be too unwell to be safely managed on an MBU and may pose a risk to other mothers and babies. In this situation it is important to assertively treat the mother so she can get better and potentially be transferred to an MBU at a later date. A mother and her family may choose to be admitted to an acute ward due to distance to the nearest MBU or bed availability. In some circumstances, there are child safeguarding concerns which may mean that mother is viewed as not able to care for baby at present. In this situation, it isn't appropriate for a mother to be admitted with her baby if she isn't going to be the main carer.

If there is a plan for mother to be the main carer for baby when she improves, then re-referral to an MBU can be considered once mum has improved and she consents. After risk assessment has been completed, try to facilitate visits so that the mother can see her child, and liaise with community perinatal team and wider professional network.

PHARMACOLOGY

Prescribing should be carefully considered during pregnancy and the postnatal period. Due to ethical considerations, there have been limited studies on the effects of medication on the foetus and transference across breastmilk. Antenatal and postnatal mental health [18] outlines considerations for prescribing during pregnancy and the postnatal period. Another excellent resource is the United Kingdom Teratology Information Service (UKTIS) website which has evidence-based safety information about medication in pregnancy:

UKTIS – Evidence-based safety information about medication, vaccine, chemical and radiological exposures in pregnancy. https://uktis.org/

There is a partnered website for patients Best Use of Medicines in Pregnancy (BUMPs) website:

Bumps – Best use of medicines in pregnancy. https://www.medicinesinpregnancy.org/

This covers information about all medications including physical health medications.

In addition, the Maudsley Prescribing Guidelines have a comprehensive chapter on Pregnancy and Breastfeeding [43]. Women are often ill advised to stop medications at the start of pregnancy. However, most medications should not be abruptly stopped and may be able to be cross titrated across to medicines which have better profiles during pregnancy. Women may choose to stop taking medication during pregnancy due to concerns about the impact on their unborn child. This should be continually reviewed and explored. It is important to assertively treat women who are acutely unwell as they may not be able to exercise their parental responsibility when unwell, which can result in decisions being made about their child that they may not agree with.

> ### Principles for Prescribing During Pregnancy [43]
>
> - Medication should be at the lowest effective dose.
> - Monotherapy – prescribe as few drugs as possible.
> - Consider that doses may need increasing during the final trimester as blood volume increases by 30%.
> - Depots – ideally depots should not be initiated during pregnancy, but it may be important to continue if compliance is an issue and increasing risk.
>
> Source: Taylor et al. [43].

> ### Important Note on Valproate
>
> 1. If valproate is taken during pregnancy, up to 4 in 10 babies are at risk of developmental disorders and approximately 1 in 9 are at risk of birth defects [44].
> 2. Women of childbearing age should not be prescribed valproate unless two prescribers agree that there is no other option and a pregnancy prevention programme should be in place.
> 3. If you become aware of a woman who is pregnant and is prescribed valproate, please seek specialist advice from pharmacy and/or specialist perinatal services.

Management of Acute Agitation in Pregnant Women

Observation levels should be considered and documented in the care plan with consideration given to the risk posed from other service users on the unit. As with all service users, restraint should be the last option when other interventions have not been successful [45]. During pregnancy it is important to restrain in a safe way that does not pose a risk to the unborn. A pregnant person should not be restrained in the prone position as this can lead to airway obstruction. The mother should not be restrained in the supine position as she may develop supine hypotensive syndrome [46.] This is when the weight of the baby and uterus press on internal organs which can compress the aorta and interior vena cava. This can affect circulation and cause blood pressure to fall. If restraint is required, the mother should be restrained on their left side on the ground, with the right side up. This is to ensure that the uterus does not compress the vena cava.

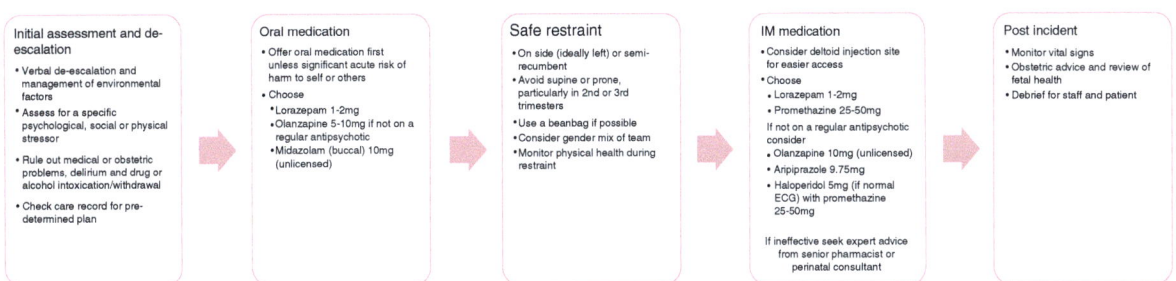

Source: Algorithm for management of acute agitation in pregnant women [45] / With Permission of Cambridge University Press.

SAFEGUARDING

Child

It is important to work in collaboration with children's services during the perinatal period. They will require information from mental health services to support the Children and Families assessment. However, if you are not sure what level of information should be shared, please discuss with Trust Safeguarding Lead for Children or Trust legal advice. Information sharing must be proportionate, and it may be appropriate to consider whether the court should order information to be shared.

It is imperative that mental health services should lead on mental healthcare and treatment. Children's services' primary responsibility is safeguarding the child. In some of these cases, the situation can become very complex and blurred responsibilities can happen. Open communication, trust and transparency are key to good quality care and working relationships with families [46].

In supporting women with serious mental illness or significant substance misuse, the unborn child may be placed on a Child Protection Plan. It is important that you are present at the initial child protection conference (ICPC) and ongoing core group meetings [7]. Children's services are unable to apply for a court order until the child is born, but they can prepare the paperwork to submit to court once baby is born. In serious cases, they may apply for a court hearing as soon as the baby is born and a possible outcome is that an Interim Care Order (ICO) is granted. This grants the local authority shared parental rights over the child. An ICO can stipulate that the child remains with the parent or that the child is based either with a family member who has passed a viability assessment or a foster carer. This is an interim arrangement until the next court hearing.

If the local authority are planning for separation at birth, an MBU admission is not appropriate. In some situations where the local authority may have concerns, they may commission a parenting assessment which takes place in a residential setting.

Adult (Mother) and Child

Domestic Abuse

60–70% of women accessing mental health services will have experienced domestic abuse. It is estimated that 30% of domestic abuse starts in pregnancy [47]. The recent Domestic Abuse bill [48] recognises that children affected by domestic abuse as victims themselves. The briefing conducted by the MMHA [47] highlighted the importance of consistent inquiry and professional curiosity. This may indicate a training need within the service.

F. Leadership and Management, Education and Research

Whilst providing care for women in the perinatal period the APMH may identify opportunities to improve pathways and care for women across services. This may be in the form of authoring a policy based on good practice examples. APMHs are also in a position to ensure that staff receive regular supervision given the emotive nature of this work. You should consider whether there are additional training needs for staff to ensure they are providing evidence-based care. It is important to keep up-to-date with the latest evidence for women and birthing people.

CONCLUSION

This chapter provided an outline of the role of the APMH caring for women in the perinatal period. The work is challenging and complex, and it requires excellent co-ordination skills to ensure that the mother, any family and all agencies are included in order to collate all information and then work out a collaborative care plan. This care plan needs to encompass mental health, physical health and maternity care aspects. Risk assessment needs to incorporate risk to baby, and safeguarding procedures must be followed.

It is important to remember that the APMH is in a unique position to challenge bias and act as an advocate. Well organised, joined up care can make a substantial difference to a mother's mental health, and this can have lasting effects on her ability and opportunity to parent her child and lasting effects on the child's mental and physical health.

HELPFUL RESOURCES

5xmore – Organisation supporting black maternal mental health https://fivexmore.org

PANDAs – Charity support to parents affected by perinatal mental illness https://pandasfoundation.org.uk

Action on Postpartum Psychosis (APP) – Charity for mums and families affected by postpartum psychosis https://www.app-network.org

Maternal OCD – Charity supporting women with maternal OCD https://maternalocd.org

Birth Trauma Association – https://www.birthtraumaassociation.org

Maternal Mental Health Alliance – Network of 130 charities and organisations working to ensure that women with perinatal mental health difficulties have access to good quality care https://maternalmentalhealthalliance.org

REFERENCES

1. Health Education England (2020). Advanced practice mental health curriculum and capabilities framework. https://www.hee.nhs.uk/sites/default/files/documents/AP-MH%20Curriculum%20and%20Capabilities%20Framework%201.2.pdf
2. Marcé (2025) Perinatal mental health. https://marcesociety.com
3. Maternal Mental Health Alliance (2023) https://maternalmentalhealthalliance.org
4. Global Alliance for Maternal Mental Health (2023) https://www.gammh.org
5. African Alliance for Maternal Mental Health (2025) https://aammh.org
6. Howard, L.M. and Khalifeh, H. (2020). Perinatal mental health: a review of progress and challenges. *World Psychiatry* 19 (3): 313–327. https://doi.org/10.1002/wps.20769.
7. Children's Act (2004). Available at: www.legislation.gov.uk/ukpga/2004/31/contents
8. De Backer, K., Rayment-Jones, H., Lever Taylor, B. et al. (2024). Healthcare experiences of pregnant and postnatal women and healthcare professionals when facing child protection in the perinatal period: a systematic review and critical interpretative synthesis. *PLoS One*. https://doi.org/10.1371/journal.pone.0305738.
9. Bauer A, Parsonage M, Knapp M, Iemmi V, Adelaja B, Hogg S. (2014). The costs of perinatal mental health problems. www.centreformentalhealth.org.uk/wp-content/uploads/2018/09/costsofperinatal.pdf
10. NHS England (2019) The NHS long term plan. https://www.england.nhs.uk/wp-content/uploads/2022/07/nhs-long-term-plan-version-1.2.pdf (August 2019).
11. Department of Health and Social Care. (2021). The best start for life: a vision for the 1,001 critical days. https://assets.publishing.service.gov.uk/media/605c5e61d3bf7f2f0d94183a/The_best_start_for_life_a_vision_for_the_1_001_critical_days.pdf
12. House of Commons Library (2021). Debate pack: maternal mental health. https://researchbriefings.files.parliament.uk/documents/CDP-2021-0025/CDP-2021-0025.pdf
13. Maternal Mental Health Alliance (2023). Specialist perinatal mental health care in the UK 2023. https://maternalmentalhealthalliance.org/media/filer_public/9a/51/9a513115-1d26-408a-9c85-f3442cc3cb2b/mmha-specialist-perinatal-mental-health-services-uk-maps-2023.pdf
14. Department of Health (2017). Safer maternity Care – progress and next steps. https://assets.publishing.service.gov.uk/media/5a74eacbe5274a3cb286839b/Safer_maternity_care_-_progress_and_next_steps.pdf
15. Knight M, Bunch K, Felker A, Patel R, Kotnis R, Kenyon S, Kurinczuk JJ (Eds.) (2022). On behalf of MBRRACE-UK. Saving lives, improving mothers' care core report – lessons learned to inform maternity care from the UK and Ireland confidential enquiries into maternal deaths and morbidity 2018–20. https://www.npeu.ox.ac.uk/assets/downloads/mbrrace-uk/reports/maternal-report-2022/MBRRACE-UK_Maternal_CORE_Report_2022_v10.pdf
16. Felker, A Patel, R, Kotnis, R, Kenyon, S, Knight, M (Eds.) on behalf of MBRRACE-UK. Saving Lives, Improving Mothers' Care Compiled Report – Lessons learned to inform maternity care from the UK and Ireland Confidential Enquiries into Maternal Deaths and Morbidity 2020–22. (2024). https://www.npeu.ox.ac.uk/assets/downloads/mbrrace-uk/reports/maternal-report-2024/MBRRACE-UK%20Maternal%20MAIN%20Report%202024%20V2.0%20ONLINE.pdf
17. All party parliamentary group of birth trauma (2024). Listen to Mums: Ending the postcode lottery on perinatal care. https://www.theo-clarke.org.uk/files/2024-05/Birth%20Trauma%20Inquiry%20Report%20for%20Publication_May13_2024.pdf

18. National Institute for Health and Care Excellence (NICE) (2016). Antenatal and postnatal mental health: clinical management and service guidance. www.nice.org.uk/guidance/qs115/resources/antenatal-and-postnatal-mental-health-pdf-75545299789765
19. Action for Postpartum Psychosis (2014). Insider guide: planning pregnancy: a guide for women at high risk of postpartum psychosis. https://www.app-network.org/wp-content/uploads/2011/10/2018-Insider-guide_PlanningPregnancy.pdf
20. Bye, A., Martini, M.G., and Micali, N. (2021). Eating disorders, pregnancy and the postnatal period: a review of the recent literature. *Current Opinion in Psychiatry* 34 (6): 563–568. https://doi.org/10.1097/YCO.0000000000000748.
21. Heyne, C.S., Kazmierczak, M., Souday, R. et al. (2022). Prevalence and risk factors of birth-related post-traumatic stress among parents: a comparative systematic review and meta-analysis. *Clinical Psychology Review* 94: 102157. https://doi.org/10.1016/j.cpr.2022.102157.
22. Mental Capacity Act (2005) www.legislation.gov.uk/ukpga/2005/9/contents
23. Court of Protection Handbook (2014). Court sanctioned interventions during childbirth guidance. https://courtofprotectionhandbook.com/2014/08/29/court-sanctioned-interventions-during-childbirth-guidance
24. Foti, T.R., Watson, C., Adams, S.R. et al. (2023). Associations between adverse childhood experiences (ACEs) and prenatal mental health and substance use. *International Journal of Environmental Research and Public Health* 20: https://doi.org/10.3390/ijerph20136289.
25. Maternal Mental Health Alliance (2023). Briefing perinatal mental health and domestic abuse. https://maternalmentalhealthalliance.org/media/filer_public/79/63/79635e45-1797-4729-a18b-2ab4c46f4cde/mmha-briefing-perinatal-mental-health-and-domestic-abuse-jan-23.pdf
26. Qiu, X., Zhang, S., Sun, X. et al. (2020). (2020) unintended pregnancy and postpartum depression: a meta-analysis of cohort and case-control studies. *Journal of Psychosomatic Research* 138: 110259. https://doi.org/10.1016/j.jpsychores.2020.110259.
27. Yang, K., Wu, J., and Chen, X. (2022). Risk factors of perinatal depression in women: a systematic review and meta-analysis. *BMC Psychiatry* 22: 63. https://doi.org/10.1186/s12888-021-03684-3.
28. MBRRACE-UK (2023). Saving lives, improving mothers' care. Lessons learned to inform maternity care from the UK and Ireland Confidential Enquiries into Maternal Deaths and Morbidity 2019–21. https://www.npeu.ox.ac.uk/assets/downloads/mbrrace-uk/reports/maternal-report-2023/MBRRACE-UK_Maternal_Compiled_Report_2023.pdf
29. Office for National Statistics (ONS) (2024). Births in England and Wales: 2023 www.ons.gov.uk/peoplepopulationandcommunity/birthsdeathsandmarriages/livebirths/bulletins/birthsummarytablesenglandandwales/2023
30. Office for National Statistics (ONS) (2024). Births by parents' country of birth, England and Wales: 2023 www.ons.gov.uk/peoplepopulationandcommunity/birthsdeathsandmarriages/livebirths/bulletins/parentscountryofbirthenglandandwales/latest
31. National Perinatal Epidemiology Unit, MBRRACE – UK Mothers and Babies: Reducing Risk through Audits and Confidential Enquiries across the UK (2025) Maternal mortality 2021-2023. https://www.npeu.ox.ac.uk/mbrrace-uk/data-brief/maternal-mortality-2021-2023#maternal-mortality-amongst-different-population-groups-in-2021-2023
32. King's Fund (2025). The health of women from ethnic minority groups in England. www.kingsfund.org.uk/insight-and-analysis/long-reads/the-health-of-women-from-ethnic-minority-groups-england
33. Vousden, N., Bunch, K., Kenyon, S. et al. (2024a). Impact of maternal risk factors on ethnic disparities in maternal mortality: a national population-based cohort study. *The lancet regional health – Europe* 40: https://www.thelancet.com/journals/lanepe/article/PIIS2666-7762(24)00059-0/fulltext.

34. NHS England (2021). Core 20 PLUS 5 An approach to reducing health inequalities. https://www.england.nhs.uk/wp-content/uploads/2021/11/core20plus5-online-engage-survey-supporting-document-v1.pdf
35. 5xMore (2022). The black maternity experiences report. https://fivexmore.org/blackmereport
36. NHS (2018) The Perinatal Mental Health Care Pathways. https://www.england.nhs.uk/wp-content/uploads/2018/05/perinatal-mental-health-care-pathway.pdf (england.nhs.uk)
37. Maternal Mental Health Alliance (2024). Listening to the stories of women who have experienced child removal due to drug and alcohol use. https://maternalmentalhealthalliance.org/media/filer_public/35/9a/359a2b64-8d0f-4136-bd91-8f2926937ab3/mmha-womens-reform-addiction-child-removal-maternal-mental-health-august-2024.pdf
38. NICE (2020). Antenatal and postnatal mental health: clinical management and service guidance. www.nice.org.uk/guidance/cg192/resources/antenatal-and-postnatal-mental-health-clinical-management-and-service-guidance-pdf-35109869806789
39. Mental Health Act (1983) Section 2. www.legislation.gov.uk/ukpga/1983/20/section/2
40. Royal College of Psychiatrists (2018) Mother and Baby Units (MBUs). www.rcpsych.ac.uk/mental-health/treatments-and-wellbeing/mother-and-baby-units-(mbus)
41. NHS England (2020). NHS-led provider collaboratives: specialised mental health, learning disability and autism services. https://www.england.nhs.uk/mental-health/nhs-led-provider-collaboratives
42. Healthy London Partnership and NHS London Clinical Networks (2019). Pan-London perinatal mental health networks pre-birth planning: Best practice toolkit for oerinatal mental health services. https://www.transformationpartners.nhs.uk/wp-content/uploads/2019/01/Pre-birth-planning-guidance-for-Perinatal-Mental-Health-Networks.pdf (Accessed on 13/12/24).
43. Taylor, D.M., Barnes, T.R.E., and Young, A.H. (2024). Pregnancy and breastfeeding. In: *The Maudsley Prescribing Guidelines in Psychiatry* (ed. D.M. Taylor, T.R.E. Barnes, and A.H. Young). https://doi.org/10.1002/9781119870203.mpg007.
44. UK Government (2024). Guidance valproate use by women and girls. https://www.gov.uk/guidance/valproate-use-by-women-and-girls#information-about-the-risks-if-valproate-is-taken-during-pregnancy-
45. Powell, J., Taylor, D., and Manoharan, M. (2024). The pharmacological management of acute behavioural disturbance in pregnancy. *BJPsych Advances* 30 (1): 67–70. https://doi.org/10.1192/bja.2023.7.
46. De Backer, K., Rayment-Jones, H., Lever Taylor, B. et al. (2024). Healthcare experiences of pregnant and postnatal women and healthcare professionals when facing child protection in the perinatal period: a systematic review and critical interpretative synthesis. *PLoS One*. https://doi.org/10.1371/journal.pone.0305738.
47. Maternal Mental Health Alliance (2023). Briefing perinatal mental health and domestic abuse. https://maternalmentalhealthalliance.org/media/filer_public/79/63/79635e45-1797-4729-a18b-2ab4c46f4cde/mmha-briefing-perinatal-mental-health-and-domestic-abuse-jan-23.pdf
48. Domestic Abuse Act (2021). www.legislation.gov.uka/ukpga/2021/17/pdfs/ukpga_20210017_en.pdf

CHAPTER 14

Child and Adolescent Mental Health Services (CAMHS)

Ann Cox[1] and Narenza Dhanasar[2]

[1] *Derbyshire Healthcare NHS Foundation Trust, Derby, UK*
[2] *East London NHS Foundation Trust, London, UK*

Aim

The aim of this chapter is to provide an overview of working in Child and Adolescent Mental Health Services (CAMHS) as an advanced practitioner in mental health (APMH), including exploring some of the knowledge and skill set that is required to work in this specialist field of practice. This chapter will introduce the reader to some of the operational, cultural and societal challenges that the advanced practitioner faces when working in CAMHS. Consideration is given to the level of complexity contributed by child development, neurodivergence, working systemically and the need for the advanced practitioner who has a prescribing function to have confidence in prescribing off label and off licence. This chapter will provide a comprehensive overview of the opportunities and challenges in working in CAMHS as an advanced practitioner. For the purposes of this chapter, we will use the term child or child and young person (CYP) interchangeably to refer to any person who is under the age of 18 years.

LEARNING OUTCOMES

After reading this chapter, the reader will be able to:

1. Have knowledge of the contextual history of CAMHS and its implications for the APMH working in CAMHS currently.
2. Have an introduction to the theoretical underpinnings and legal frameworks that orientate and inform the clinical decision-making by the APMH in CAMHS.
3. Understand the breadth and depth of clinical assessment for a child with a mental health difficulty.

The Advanced Practitioner in Mental Health, First Edition. Edited by Clare Allabyrne.
© 2026 John Wiley & Sons Ltd. All rights reserved, including rights for text and data mining and training of artificial intelligence technologies or similar technologies. Published 2026 by John Wiley & Sons Ltd.

4. To have an awareness of the breadth of investigations and clinical decision-making that a CAMHS advanced practitioner would undertake.
5. To have an understanding how the systemically driven nature of working with children is paramount to a successful outcome of care delivery.

This chapter will embody the following competencies within the Advanced Practice Mental Health Curriculum and Capabilities Framework [1] (see Table 14.1).

TABLE 14.1 How this chapter meets the APMH curriculum and capabilities framework.

Clinical practice
1. Work autonomously within professional, ethical codes and legal frameworks, being responsible and accountable for their decisions, actions and omissions at this level of practice.
2. Demonstrate the underpinning psychological, biological and social knowledge required for advanced practice in mental health.
3. Demonstrate comprehensive knowledge of, and skills in, systematic history taking and clinical examination of patients who are culturally diverse and/or have complex needs in challenging circumstances, to develop a co-produced management plan.
4. Utilise clinical reasoning and decision-making skills to make a differential diagnosis and provide rationales for person-management plans, through critically reflecting on and evaluation of their own role in relation to challenging traditional practices, new ways of working and the impact on the multidisciplinary team.
5. Initiate, evaluate and modify a range of interventions, which may include therapies, medicines, lifestyle advice and care.

Leadership and management
1. Identify, critically evaluate and reformulate understanding of professional boundaries to support new ways of working within the context of organisational and service need.
2. Exercise professional judgement and leadership to effectively promote safety in the presence of complexity and unpredictability.
3. Demonstrate team working, leadership, resilience and determination, managing situations that are unfamiliar, complex or unpredictable.

Education
1. Facilitate collaboration of the wider team to support individual or interprofessional learning and development.
3. Effectively utilise a range or evidence-based educational strategies/interventions to support person-centred care with individuals, their families and carers and other healthcare colleagues.

Research
1. Critically appraise and apply the evidence base in influencing engagement, recovery, shared decision-making, transference and safeguarding.
3. Demonstrate the application of quality improvement methodologies in improving service.

INTRODUCTION

The Contextual History of CAMHS

It is important to understand the historical context of Child and Adolescent Mental Health Services (CAMHS) as a specialist service in England, how its strategy and service provision have developed over the years and its subsequent impact on advanced practice roles. Historically, CAMHS were understood to be specialist mental health services that supported children with severe and enduring mental health difficulties [2, 3]. Originally operating as child guidance clinics, CAMHS was established as a four tier model following the Together We Stand Health Advisory Service Report in 1995 [4]. Tier one was identified as universal services, Tier 2 services were established as low-level mental health intervention services, Tier 3 CAMHS was positioned as being the service that provided bespoke specialist assessment and intervention for children with severe and enduring mental health difficulties [5] and Tier 4 were specialist CAMHS inpatient services (see Figure 14.1).

However, in more recent years, CAMHS has been redefined to include all services and agencies across the community, ascending from primary care to specialist psychiatric inpatient services that provide assessment and treatment for children's mental health difficulties and therefore, CAMHS as it is now includes children's mental health distress in all its forms of severity. The change in the context of CAMHS also involved moving to the position of children's mental health being everyone's business [6] and should be considered across the full scope of what we now call CAMHS. However fundamentally, the services that support children with severe and enduring mental health difficulties are mostly unchanged and sit within specialist CAMHS services within NHS Trusts [7]. It is currently within these services where the most advanced practice roles for CAMHS are situated [8].

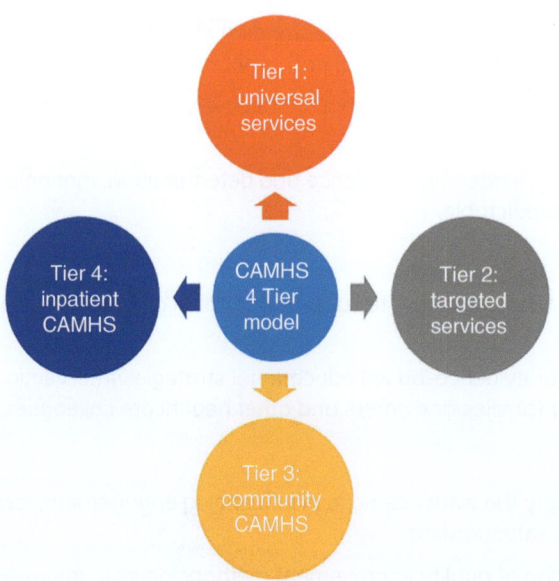

FIGURE 14.1 CAMHS tiers.

Following the CAMHS review in 2008 [9], the Children's and Young Peoples' improving access to psychological therapies (CYP-IAPT) was launched. This was a whole service transformation model, incorporating training which is still in place today and it focuses on five main principles:

- Evidence-based practice
- Participation
- Outcome measurement
- Leadership
- Accessibility [10]

What the CYP-IAPT strategy doesn't do is support the development of specific core professionals in advanced practice which is a significant omission from the strategy [10]. The CYP-IAPT strategy contextualises some of the challenges for advanced practice roles in CAMHS and associated career structures. There are some professionals that have used these training offers to add additional skills and qualifications to their professional roles as a stepping stone into advanced practice roles; however, as the CYP-IAPT strategy does not contribute to the development of advanced roles specifically, CAMHS practitioners have struggled previously to access opportunities to develop. Professionals have had to gain additional qualifications outside of the training strategy and profession specific career structures have equally had to be developed outside of the strategy.

There is significant importance placed on multi-professionals in advanced practice roles within CAMHS to lead, shape and develop sustainable career pathways for future generations of practitioners. These roles are crucial not only for the delivery of expert clinical care but also for driving innovation, influencing service design and mentoring the emerging workforce. Advanced practitioners are often at the intersection of clinical expertise and leadership, expected to balance complex caseloads while contributing to policy, training and interagency collaboration. However, working in an advanced practice capacity within CAMHS can present considerable challenges—particularly when national or local service strategies lack a clear, structured approach to the development and support of these roles. The absence of consistent frameworks, defined competencies and protected leadership time can result in role ambiguity, underutilisation of skills and difficulties in retention and succession planning. Additionally, limited strategic investment in advanced roles may lead to disparities across regions, with some practitioners working in well-established, supportive environments while others face systemic barriers to progression.

To ensure the future viability of CAMHS, it is essential that service strategies begin to prioritise the formal recognition and development of advanced practice roles. This includes embedding clear career structures, offering ongoing professional development and fostering environments where experienced clinicians can lead, change and inspire the next generation of mental health professionals.

Advanced practice roles in CAMHS can incorporate a variety of roles, and these roles include professionals that have dual qualified in an evidence-based therapy, independent prescribers, advanced practitioners in mental health (APMHs), which are the group we are specifically focusing on for the purposes of this chapter, and consultant practitioners who have developed their expertise through completing clinical master's degrees and in some case professional doctorates or PhDs. Some of these practitioners have become Approved and Responsible Clinicians [11] that have been approved by the secretary of state to undertake specific responsibilities in assessing and treating children who are detained under the Mental Health Act,1983, amended 2007 [12]. Advanced practice in CAMHS is a challenging role, in that there are multiple theoretical underpinnings and legal frameworks that need to be understood and applied by the practitioner to properly assess and treat the child's mental health difficulty that a practitioner may not necessarily require in other service areas. Such theoretical underpinnings and legal frameworks will include:

- critically understanding child development in relation to physical and cognitive developmental stages.
- the ability to define and assess the social and emotional competence of a child.
- understanding the nuances of neurodivergence in the developing brain [13].
- having an understanding of the accountability and impact of frequently prescribing off label and off licence medications [14].
- understanding contextual aspects of societal cultural shifts [15].
- having significant and applied knowledge of legal frameworks such as Gillick Competency [16], the Mental Capacity Act [17], the Mental Health Act [12], the Children Act [18] United Nations Conventions on the Rights of the Child (UNCRC) [19] and the Human Rights Act [20].
- having a significant understanding of physical health and how this is potentially impacted by the key developmental stages of a child.
- understanding the critical need for systemic and multi-agency working [21].

Whilst this list of frameworks and theories is not exhaustive, it provides an understanding of the multi-layered theoretical perspective that needs to be understood and applied when working in advanced practice roles in CAMHS. The ability for the advanced practitioner to understand, process and apply these frameworks to inform their clinical decision-making is critical to working in CAMHS. We will now consider these different theoretical underpinnings and legal frameworks to better understand how they are used in clinical practice.

SYSTEMIC AND MULTI-AGENCY WORKING

When working with children, the consideration of the system around the child is imperative as all the systems around the child will impact the child in some way. Bronfenbrenner's ecological systems theory is helpful to consider when working in CAMHS as it explores different impacts from different aspects of the system, starting with the child's system at home, then moving outwards to include wider family, school, community, culture, laws, media and societal norms and how this is impacted over time [22]. Time is an important factor; as systems that impact a 6 year old to those that impact a 14 year old will be very different. Whilst we need to consider the systems that impact the child, we also need to consider the systemic and multi-agency working that is required from a professional perspective. Mirroring Bronfenbrenner's [22] systems, the APMH will also need to work with the relevant family members and professionals in the system. This may include siblings, parents and wider family members, general practitioners (GPs), paediatricians, education, social care or other professionals that are required to support the child or the family in some way. The systemically driven approach in CAMHS can be far reaching at times [23].

Whilst the systemically driven approach is paramount for working in CAMHS, there is an importance that the child's voice remains central and heard. Children and parents can have very different perspectives of the child's difficulties. At times the impact of the child's difficulties on the parent can be significant but the child may not find their difficulties too impactful. Therefore, managing these differences in perceptions and ensuring the appropriate support is provided for both the child and the parent may mean supporting the parent to access support for themselves outside of CAMHS or considering a family therapy approach. When these situations do occur, it is the APMH's role to work with the parents to see the perspective of the child and care plan and develop goals accordingly. Of course, if the child's difficulties do not impact the child much at all, then the likelihood of the child making any changes will be limited as they would not see the need. In situations such as these, there would need to be support for the parent to accept the situation and if required support the parent to manage their feelings about the child's difficulty differently [24].

CHILD DEVELOPMENT THEORIES

There are many theories around child development and many theories around the different aspects of the development of the child, and there is no scope in this chapter to go into these theories in detail.

Most theories 'stage' the different aspects of development, demonstrating that the child's development is multi-layered and multi-faceted. It may be helpful to explore these in depth. Some of the most prominent theorists in this field are mentioned in Table 14.2.

Many early theories of child development have been criticised for being too linear and the research now explores children's development both chronologically as in physical maturation and also in breadth, which would include experiential learning. This is termed as dual processing theory [32]. Therefore, not only will children develop because they are evolutionary programmed to do so but they will also develop through experiential learning. Klaczynski [32] refers to this as developing heuristics which are memories of stored events that children can draw on to inform future behaviour. For example, if a child is involved in making a decision in CAMHS about treatment, then the child will store this memory and use it at a time in the future to inform future decision-making or behaviours; therein the more we involve children in decision-making, the more heuristics the child will store and have available to them for future reference and so will be a better decision-maker moving forward through developing their decision-making experience [33]. In understanding this, the APMH has a legal, moral and ethical obligation to involve children in their healthcare decisions as much as possible to help understand the needs from the child's perspective and inform the care plan [18–20, 34]. The ISupportRights standards are a helpful tool to aid the APMH in ensuring children's rights are being upheld in practice [35].

TABLE 14.2 Child development theoretical approaches and theorists.

Theoretical approach	Theorist
Maturation	Arnold Gessell [25]
Psychodynamic	Sigmund Freud [26]
Psychosocial	Erik Erikson [27]
Cognitive	Jean Piaget [28]
	Lev Vygotsky [29]
Behaviourist	John Watson [30]
	B.F. Skinner [31]
Dual process	Paul Klaczynski [32]
Ecological	Bronfenbrenner [22]

Understanding the different child development stages and expected maturation stages will underpin the clinical decision-making for an advanced practitioner in children's mental health, and they will need to understand how the development of the child may influence the mental health difficulty.

The presentation of children's mental health difficulties can be very different to that of adults; and younger children or those that are chronologically and/or socially and emotionally developmentally younger can present differently to those who present more maturely [36]. Therefore, having this understanding will help inform the assessment and intervention offered by the advanced practitioner. Developmentally younger children are more likely to present with more somatic symptoms, stomach aches, headaches and generally feeling physically unwell, alongside anger issues; older children can present with psychosocial and emotional difficulties and regularly present with emotional dysregulation. It is important to differentiate between what dysregulation is as a normal part of adolescence, to that which is driven by mental health and emotional difficulties.

NEURODIVERGENCE

Neurodevelopmental difficulties are lifelong difficulties that include diagnoses of autism spectrum disorder (ASD), attention deficit hyperactivity disorder (ADHD) and Tourette's syndrome which is a tic disorder. There are many other neurodevelopmental disorders, however, these are the ones that are most regularly seen in CAMHS [37]. Ambitious about autism [38] reported that a study they had undertaken had shown that four out of five young people with autism has experienced a mental health difficulty; so many of the children that are supported in CAMHS do have comorbid neurodiversity. Being able to adapt engagement, language and make reasonable adjustments [39] to ensure that interventions are accessible for all children dependent on their developmental stage and their emotional literacy is a key skill that is nurtured in advanced practice. This may be using creative methods of engagement, rather than just talking, it could include using art materials, using flashcards, worksheets and toys and puppets [24]. One example of a creative activity from practice is when trying to elicit negative automatic thoughts from a child: with the child we bounced a ball against a wall and got them to share the first thought that came into their head, demonstrating to the child what a negative automatic thought is and how quickly they are produced. Using a ball in this way helps connect the theory to practice in a session with a child and shows how our brain works through a physical activity, rather than just explaining it in words. Helping the child understand theory in this way, is far more engaging and helpful for some children that discussing it purely through conversation [40].

Learning Difficulties vs. Learning Disabilities

Advanced practitioners in CAMHS hold pivotal clinical and leadership roles in addressing the complex needs of CYP with learning difficulties and learning disabilities. While the terms are sometimes used interchangeably in clinical and educational contexts, they refer to distinct conditions, each with unique implications for assessment, diagnosis and intervention. Recognising and responding appropriately to these differences is essential for delivering accurate, effective and person-centred care within CAMHS (see Table 14.3) [41].

Learning difficulties – a broad term used to describe problems in acquiring knowledge and skills to the expected level for a child's age. These difficulties may affect literacy, numeracy, memory, concentration or social skills [42]. Some examples include dyslexia, dyspraxia, ADHD or mild language processing

TABLE 14.3 Key differences between learning difficulties vs. learning disability [42, 43].

Feature	Learning difficulty	Learning disability
Impact on IQ	No impact	Significantly low IQ
Scope	Often domain specific	Global impact on learning and daily living
Permanence	May improve with support	Lifelong
Examples	Dyslexia, ADHD	Intellectual disability, Down's syndrome

difficulties. CYP with learning difficulties may experience associated mental health challenges such as low self-esteem, anxiety or behavioural difficulties due to frustration and academic failure.

Learning Disabilities – A significantly reduced ability to understand new or complex information, learn new skills and cope independently, which started before adulthood and has a lasting effect on development [43]. Some examples include moderate to severe intellectual disability, Down's Syndrome and Global Developmental Delay. CYP with learning disabilities are at significantly higher risk of mental health conditions and often require adapted assessments, accessible communication and coordinated multi-agency care.

PRESCRIBING IN CAMHS AND PSYCHOPHARMACOLOGY

Independent prescribing in CAMHS is a highly autonomous and accountable skillset that is a qualification open to some professionals who work in advanced practice roles, particularly nurses and pharmacists that work in CAMHS [44]. Understandably, there are limited research studies on effects of medication on children, as generally randomised control trials (RCTs) of medication are not authorised to be undertaken on children. What this means in CAMHS is that there are few licenced medications available for prescribing for children's mental health, including ADHD and tic disorders. This in turn means that prescribing in CAMHS can be challenging and requires significant understanding of the effects of medication on the developing child, with at times, limited evidence to support prescribing decision-making [45].

There are **five main types of medications** that are prescribed in CAMHS:

- Antidepressants that also target anxiety disorders.
- ADHD medications, stimulant and non-stimulant medications.
- Antipsychotic medications, which are at times used outside of the prescribed licence for psychosis and are used for symptoms of dysregulation and trauma presentations.
- Hypnotics and medications to induce sleep/sedation, for example, melatonin and promethazine.
- Benzodiazepines that are used in mainly crisis situations to help reduce severe agitation and distress [46].

There are a number of medications that are licenced for prescribing in ADHD (methylphenidate, amphetamines, atomoxetine, guanfacine), and there is one antidepressant (fluoxetine) that is licenced for 8 years old and over. All other medications in CAMHS are generally prescribed either off licence or off label, making it a very challenging and skilled area to work in [46]. The majority of prescribing off licence or off label is undertaken through experience and CAMHS culture. It is imperative to ensure that when prescribing in CAMHS, that all prescribing guidance, supervision and regular continuing professional development in this area of practice is up to date to ensure best practice at all times [47]. The APMH really has to understand the implications of prescribing off licence and off label, interactions, sensitivities of children with neurodevelopmental difficulties and how to explain the associated risks and benefits to children and their parents.

SOCIETAL CULTURAL SHIFTS AND THEIR IMPACT ON CHILDREN'S MENTAL HEALTH

Childhood in today's society in the United Kingdom is very different to what a childhood was like 40 years ago. The evolution of the games console and the introduction of social media have changed the way children interact and view the world. Forty years ago, children were only comparing themselves to their classmates, whereas now children compare themselves to people everywhere and to filtered and artificial intelligence (AI) developed images. Children are spending more time indoors playing on games consoles than going out and socialising with friends [48]. The introduction of games consoles and the use of the internet and social media have significantly changed the experience of the developing child [48]. With children spending more time indoors that outside, there is evidence of a negative impact on child development. In one particular study, The Natural Childhood report by Stephen Moss [49], Moss makes reference to nature deficit disorder and how this has impacted on delays in motor and cognitive development; including children having lost skills in tree climbing, den building, the team work approach that this required and the dexterity in some motor skills development that playing outside helped children develop. Moss also refers to an underdeveloped ability for decision-making and mentalising, for example being able to plan ways to get home from the park, as children these days are reliant on being driven in cars and spend less time in the outdoors [49].

One also has to consider the impact of using games consoles, social media and the internet and its' fast pace, overloaded with information and the associated reduction in physical activity and the increase in referrals for ADHD [50]. With screen use identified as impacting on children's health such as sleep, mood dysregulation and over stimulation of the developing brain, these can mirror many of the symptoms of ADHD and so it is possible some of the increase in referrals could be pathologising what is being created from significant screen use and associated sensory needs, as opposed to it being a neurodevelopmental disorder [48].

We cannot look at recent cultural shifts without examining those experienced during and after the COVID 19 pandemic which have been and continue to be hugely significant. These include increased anxiety due to the change in routines and demands to not socialise; disruption for children in their social lives and education; more forced interaction on the internet, games consoles or social media; and is a hangover for children communicating in this way [51]. These cultural shifts have contributed to increases in severity and complexity in children's mental health presentations. It is important for the APMH to have an awareness of these cultural shifts and the associated impact that these will have on children's mental health [52].

PHYSICAL HEALTH AND ISSUES SPECIFIC TO CHILDREN

When assessing children, it is important to undertake a holistic assessment that involves understanding both the physical and mental health of the child. This is of course good practice across all fields of mental health. In particular for children there can be a variety of causes for a presentation that could be due to either mental health or physical health cause.

A comprehensive, holistic assessment is a cornerstone of effective practice within CAMHS. Completing a robust initial holistic assessment is imperative to ensure the right intervention is offered. This type of assessment involves gathering detailed information across multiple domains including emotional well-being, cognitive functioning, physical health, developmental history, family dynamics, education and social circumstances to gain a full understanding of the young person's needs, strengths and vulnerabilities [53, 54].

One of the most critical, yet sometimes underemphasised, components of a holistic assessment is physical health. CYP presenting with emotional or behavioural difficulties may also be living with chronic health conditions such as asthma, diabetes, epilepsy or undiagnosed neurodevelopmental conditions. These physical health issues can influence mood, energy levels, concentration, behaviour and sleep factors which may be misinterpreted if considered only through a psychological lens [55]. Furthermore, side effects from medication, nutritional deficiencies and pain or discomfort may also manifest in ways that mimic or exacerbate mental health symptoms. For this reason, assessing physical health and liaising with primary and secondary healthcare professionals is vital to creating a safe and accurate formulation [56].

Developmental and Age-Specific Considerations

Children and adolescents must be assessed within a developmentally appropriate framework. Their psychological presentation is closely tied to their stage of cognitive, emotional and social development. For example, identity formation, dependency on caregivers, emerging autonomy and susceptibility to peer influences are all features of adolescence that must inform how risks and resilience are understood [57]. Additionally, certain behaviours may be developmentally normal at one age but clinically concerning at another. APMHs must be sensitive to these distinctions to avoid pathologising normal developmental variations or, conversely, missing early signs of significant difficulties. For example, during adolescence, there are significant changes in hormones and at times this can impact on thyroid function [58]. Thyroid dysfunction can present with psychiatric difficulties such as hyperactivity, anxiety and depression and in rare cases psychosis, so it is important to ensure you rule out such physical health causes for these difficulties [59]. Other physical health considerations include vitamin deficiencies such as Vitamin D and B12 which are known to contribute to low mood and associated symptoms [60].

APMHs in CAMHS are uniquely positioned to lead and coordinate holistic assessments. Their role involves drawing together insights from families, schools, GPs, paediatrics and social care to create a nuanced and multi-layered understanding of the child's needs [61]. They are also responsible for identifying health inequalities, safeguarding concerns and gaps in service provision. A holistic perspective enables APMHs to develop trauma-informed, culturally sensitive and person-centred care plans that support both symptom reduction and wider developmental outcomes [62].

Since the COVID 19 pandemic there has been an increase in the diagnosis of paediatric acute onset neuropsychiatric syndrome/paediatric autoimmune neuropsychiatric disorders associated with streptococcal infections (PANS/PANDAS) [63]. These are post-infection presentations that have a rapid onset and present as psychiatric difficulties including obsessive compulsive disorder (OCD), irritability, urinary difficulties, mood dysregulation, disordered eating and in 25% of cases psychosis [63]. Whilst this is a physical health reaction to infection, that requires treatment with antibiotics, the symptoms can present as mental health difficulties, therefore it is important for the APMH to rule out physical causes for the symptoms the child presents with and ensure the appropriate intervention is offered. If it is suspected that a child has PANS or PANDAS then this should be treated by the GP or paediatrician depending on the service criteria in the local area. Many children with PANS/PANDAS are not diagnosed quickly enough and this results in children being accepted in CAMHS who are offered treatment interventions based on their symptoms, such as eating disorder or OCD intervention pathways [64]. Whilst these interventions may help with some of the symptoms, they will not treat the underlying infection and therefore results in children being supported by CAMHS for long periods of time and not being effectively treated for the underlying physical health cause [64].

Other physical health knowledge and investigations that the APMH would need to be able to undertake in CAMHS are:

1. Consider the possibility of physical illness and include in differential diagnosis.
2. Conduct a physical examination (blood pressure, pulse, weight, height) including a neurodevelopmental/neurological examination, but know limitations and when to refer to paediatrics (MRI, CT scan).
3. Request relevant blood tests for baselines and medication reviews and interpret blood test results. Where this is out of the APMH's scope of practice, then request appropriate investigations (blood tests, ECG, genetic testing) from GP, paediatrics in hospital or in the community.
4. Maintain up-to-date knowledge with the effects, interactions and side effects of all prescribed medication, including physical health medications, especially those that can have psychiatric symptom side effects such as those medications with steroids including asthma medications.
5. Recognise acute medical illnesses, including those needing urgent attention for example eating disorders.
6. Liaise with other experts in the fields of paediatrics, pharmacy or medicine as necessary.
7. Recognise the possibility of safeguarding concerns associated with physical symptoms or injuries and liaise with other agencies (social care, paediatrics) as appropriate.
8. Manage side effects of medication such as tachycardia with stimulant medication and increased prolactin levels in antipsychotic use.
9. Assess self-harm wounds for infection or need for a referral to the GP or an acute hospital if required and apply dressings if appropriate.
10. Assessing and providing dietary advice for children with eating difficulties or prescribed stimulant medication that may supress appetite.
11. Providing psychoeducation to inform daily structured activities and sleep hygiene intervention.

This list is not exhaustive but provides an idea of the physical health aspects of care required in CAMHS by the APMH. APMH's should also consider the developmental and emotional needs of children subject to physical examination and investigations and conduct these in a sympathetic way with appropriate chaperoning; particularly those that may have significant sensory needs and find it difficult to cope with interventions such as blood pressure cuffs tightening. Implementing a physical health clinic for children who have neurodevelopmental disorders and/or sensory needs can be a helpful resource for CAMHS services so that time can be provided for children who have these difficulties and they can be better supported to have their physical observations completed, this may be with using social stories to help orientate the child or some graded exposure to help them get used to the equipment [65]. Using the ISupportRights standards can additionally ensure children's views and wishes are considered during such interventions [35]. Children who are prescribed psychotropic and/or stimulant medications require frequent physical health monitoring including height, weight and other physical measurements;

blood tests; and ECGs as per NICE guidance [66, 67], and therefore the APMH would be expected to undertake these and ensure that they are completed within the agreed time frames. The APMH would also be expected to act upon any results that require intervention to ensure the child's physical health is maintained whilst taking medication [67].

OUTCOME AND EXPERIENCE MEASURES SCREENING TOOLS

Implementing the CYP-IAPT strategy involves the use of outcome measures and validating children's and families' experience of services [4]. Seeking valuable feedback and using this to clinically inform care is important at all stages of assessment and formulation, planning and review and discharge.

The Child Outcomes Research Consortium (CORC) [68] has developed a data set of outcome measures for children's mental health and well-being. These outcome measures can be used face to face or online in consultation with children and their families. See Table 14.4 for examples. It should be noted that CAMHS

TABLE 14.4 Examples of outcome and experience measures screening tools, listed alphabetically [68].

Name of tool	Age range	Suitability/domains
Beck Youth Inventory (BYI) (Self)	Age 7–18	The BYI is a 100-item self-report measure comprising five self-report inventories that can be used separately or in combination to assess symptoms of depression, anxiety, anger, disruptive behaviour and self-concept.
Behavioural and Emotional Rating Scale (BERS-2) (Self and parent)	Age 5–18	A strength-based approach to assessment which covers domains such as interpersonal strengths, functioning at school, affective strength, intrapersonal strength, family involvement and career strength.
Behavioural and Emotional Rating Scale (BERS-2) (Self and parent)	Age 5–18	A strength-based approach to assessment and provides an overall index of a child's strengths and competencies from three perspectives: self, parent and teacher. Items cover domains such as interpersonal strengths, functioning at school, affective strength, intrapersonal strength, family involvement and career strength.
Brief Parental Self-Efficacy Scale (BPSES) (Parent/Carer)		Five-item measure of parental self-efficacy that can be completed by parents or carers of children and young people.
Children's Global Assessment Scale (CGAS)	Age 4–16	A rating of general functioning. The clinician assesses a range of aspects if psychological and social functioning and gives the child or young person a single score between 1 and 100, based on their lowest level of functioning. The score puts them in one of 10 categories that range from 'needs constant supervision' (1–10) to 'superior functioning' (91–100).
Current View (Practitioner)		Current view is a practitioner-completed tool that captures information on four components: Provisional problem descriptions, selected complexity factors, contextual problems and EET (education, employment or training) difficulties.

(Continued)

TABLE 14.4 (Continued)

Name of tool	Age range	Suitability/domains
Experience of Service Questionnaire (ESQ)	Age 9–18	This includes 12 items and three free text sections looking at what the respondent liked about the service, what they felt needed improving and any other comments.
Revised Children's Anxiety and Depression Scale (and Subscales) (RCADS)	Age 8–18	A 47-item, youth self-report questionnaire with subscales including separation anxiety disorder, social phobia, generalised anxiety disorder, panic disorder, obsessive compulsive disorder and low mood (major depressive disorder).
Outcome Rating Scale (ORS) & Child Outcome Rating Scale (CORS)	Age 5–18	Measures used to monitor children's, young people and their families' or carers' feedback on therapeutic progress.
Strengths and Difficulties Questionnaire (SDQ)	Age 2–17	A brief emotional and behavioural screening questionnaire with 25 items in the SDQ comprise 5 scales of 5 items each.

Source: Adapted from [68].

has a specific data set that is uploaded to national level to inform clinical strategy, so it will be expected that the APMH will be using outcome measures on a regular basis. It is important that the APMH uses their skills of engagement to engage children and families of differing abilities to be able to complete the outcome measures.

In CAMHS there is an expectation that there will be an outcome measure collected over two time periods as a minimum to demonstrate progress in their mental health distress. The two periods are done typically at intake and follow-up, to track progress and assess the effectiveness of interventions. In CAMHS the RCADS and the associated symptom trackers, SDQ, ORS and CORS are some of the most utilised questionnaires to do this. On discharge, the Chi-Esq is used to ascertain experience of the service. Outcome measures should be used to clinically inform care and orientate intervention; they should not be used as a stand-alone intervention [69].

AN OVERVIEW OF SPECIFIC RISKS IN CAMHS

One in six adolescents are living at home and face multiple forms of neglect and abuse [70]. Forms of neglect and abuse include lack of warmth, love, encouragement, inadequate supervision, exposure to parents/carers using substances and physical, emotional, sexual and verbal abuse. This can result in no interest in their education. With the previous risk identified around internet use, social media, the development of AI and the pressures within education, children can find life difficult. The internet, social media and AI can be used to inform or increase risk. Examples of this include pro-ana (pro-anorexia, urging people to lose weight and not eat) and suicide inciting websites. Young people will also use group chats on social media to compete with each other in causing the most injury to themselves. There are also concerns about online exploitation from games and there is further concern about AI exploitation in online child sexual abuse, including developing deep fakes and impersonations [71]. The risks for children are extensive and any risk assessment and safety plan will need to be considerate of these issues.

The Department of Health highlights that a risk assessment and management plan is only as effective as the quality of communication used to share its findings with those involved in the child's care [72].

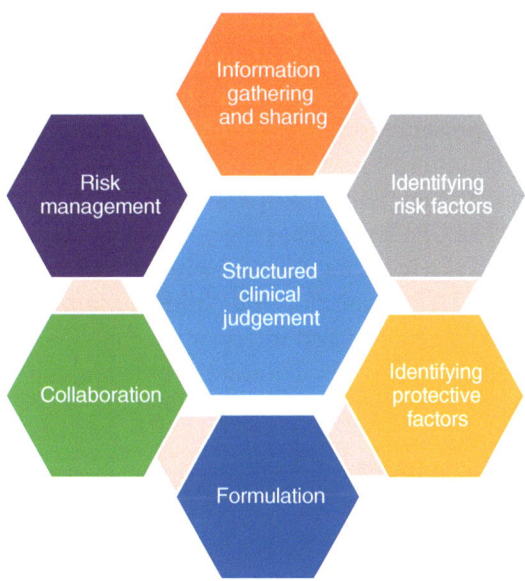

FIGURE 14.2 Structured clinical judgement.

APMHs should consider best practice using structured clinical judgement based on research risk factors, understanding of child development, social and family context and assessment of mental state. Structured clinical judgement is showcased in Figure 14.2 and used when assessing and managing risk for children.

Effective risk assessment and management is a collaborative process. The APMH should facilitate the collaborative process with the child and family and must be aware of any legal frameworks that will underpin the process. This may be the consideration of Gillick competence [16] or the Mental Capacity Act [17]; it should definitely include the Children Act [18] and the UNCRC (United Nations Convention on the Rights of a Child) [19]. The level of legal involvement is often proportionate to the degree of identified risk, for example, safeguarding concerns, suicidality or severe neglect may necessitate formal interventions, multi-agency action or legal orders. APMHs must be proficient in interpreting and applying these legal principles to ensure that their clinical decisions are ethically sound, legally defensible and prioritise the best interests of the young person [17].

The 5 'P's' model by McNeil et al. [73] is a helpful tool when collaborating on the discussion around formulating risk and safety planning.

The five P's are:

- Presenting factors – past and current risk factors
- Predisposing – vulnerabilities
- Precipitating – what triggers the behaviour
- Perpetuating – issues that maintain the risk
- Protective factors [73]

There has been a move away from stratifying risk into groups (low, medium, high) as it is felt that this way of determining risk is subjective and does not convey the context and the detail of the risk of a child [74]. It is important that the risk assessment includes the detail of the risk, how the risks have been assessed and then a safety plan provided to manage the identified risks [74].

The Dynamic Support Register (DSR) and Care (Education) and Treatment Review (CETR) have been put in place to support CYP with a diagnosis of autism and learning disability [75] who are at risk. Risk stratification is used in DSR and CETR to identify children who are risk of admission to hospital, who have a history of multiple presentations to accident and emergency and have high complex care needs. In DSR, CYP are stratified into risk levels (e.g. red, amber, green) to highlight those most likely to need inpatient care if no action is taken. This allows agencies to respond early and coordinate support to avoid unnecessary admissions. The CETR panel has the power to demand that services and organisations attend the CETR or can instruct a service to be involved with a child or family to mitigate any presenting risks. The APMH's role in the CETR is to support the child and family during the process and provide the overview of the assessment, formulation and intervention that has been provided in CAMHS and to relay the outcome back to the clinical team. Explaining the outcome to the child and family may also be required if they have not understood it fully from the panel feedback.

Red Flags [76]

- Suicidal intent, plan or ideation
- Abuse (physical, sexual, emotional, verbal)
- Difficulty in going to sleep, staying asleep or waking up, persistent nightmares
- Sudden outbursts or explosive emotional reactions
- Avoiding friends or family and wanting to be alone all of the time
- Seeing or hearing things
- Significant changes in behaviour over a short period of time
- Eating problems including eating too much or too little
- Violence towards oneself, others, animals or property
- Refusal to go to school on a regular basis
- Ongoing decline in school performance
- Deliberate disobedience or aggression
- Opposition to authority figures and little or no remorse for breaking rules
- Cutting or other self-injury
- Isolation, loneliness and a lack of friends
- Risky or dangerous behaviour including sexually acting out, recklessness, running away, setting fires and knife crime
- Feeling hopeless or worthless
- Abuse of alcohol and/or drugs or heavy tobacco use
- Frequent outbursts of anger or inability to cope with problems
- Obsession with weight, constant dieting, purging food or vomiting [76]

SAFEGUARDING

In the United Kingdom, there is an estimated 14 million children. Of these, one-third are said to be living in poverty and extremely vulnerable. These vulnerabilities include:

- Current awareness of safeguarding concerns (child protection or child in need)
- Known to local authority care and looked after child (LAC)/Child in Care (CIC)

- Disability and/or chronic long-term health conditions
- Adverse economic, family circumstances and characteristics, including parental physical and mental health
- Non-engagement in education
- Offending and/or antisocial behaviour
- Abuse and higher risk of exploitation
- Missing and absent children and minority populations [77]

Safeguarding is not a one-off event, but a continuous process of vigilance, professional curiosity and accountability. Documentation and communication are vital and safeguarding is a shared responsibility amongst the child's network. APMHs play a pivotal role in recognising these risks, making timely referrals to children's social care and contributing to multi-agency safeguarding processes. This includes involvement in strategy meetings, child protection conferences, LAC/CIC reviews and Multi-Agency Risk Assessment Conferences (MARACs) [78]. APMHs also lead on safeguarding supervision, policy development and staff training within CAMHS teams, ensuring that services are compliant with Working Together to Safeguard Children (2018) guidance and local safeguarding partnerships [78, 79].

CASE STUDIES

Case Study 14.1

Pseudonyms are used to protect the anonymity of CYP, and confidentiality has been fully maintained in line with ethical and professional standards (Adapted from [80]).

Ben is a 14-year-old male who has a diagnosis of ADHD and ODD. Ben lives in a two-bedroom flat with his single mother and five siblings; he is the eldest. Ben's mother was aged 16 when he was born. Ben has been excluded from three mainstream schools and is now in a Pupil Referral Unit (PRU). Ben is under a Child in Need Plan due to allegations of his mother physically abusing him. Ben has been exposed to violent or graphic content, including videos depicting acts of killing since the age of 10. He is aggressive towards his mother and younger siblings in the home. He hits, shouts, swears, bangs his head on the wall, punches the wall and has self-harmed by cutting his wrists in the past. He has been in fights at school and hence has exclusions, but recently there was an alleged stabbing of his school teacher, which has resulted in Ben being placed on bail and now known to multiple services including the YOT (Youth Offending Team).

He has been on ADHD medication, both stimulant (methylphenidate) and non-stimulant (atomoxetine) with no effect. Ben reported that his appetite was poor, and he described feeling numb inside. Ben also struggles with his learning and his understanding of language and concepts. He is now undergoing an ASD assessment and cognitive assessment. He has hearing difficulties in his left ear, severe food allergies including to nuts and seeds, long sightedness (corrective glasses to be worn which he refuses to wear) and has a history of fainting episodes and chest pain.

Ben presents with suicidal ideation with no plans, poor sleep, poor appetite and the emotion he feels is anger. He has limited eye contact and engagement is poor. He is now in a relationship with a female peer and has expressed that he wishes to have a baby with her.

Case Study 14.2
Millie was a 14 year old girl who lived at home with her mum. Millie was reported to have rapid onset anxiety within the last 2 months which has become progressively worse to the point of crisis. Millie's presentation included her screaming and shouting as she couldn't cope with the emotions she was experiencing. Millie would be observed kneeling on the floor rocking backwards and forwards whilst holding her hands over her ears screaming for 'it' to stop; Millie is struggling to eat and sleep. Millie would constantly say that she wanted to die. Millie had difficulties in urinating, and she was repeatedly going to the toilet multiple times a day; she had a fear that if she urinated, she would die. Millie was also presenting with ritualistic-type behaviours, pacing in one room; she felt she couldn't go to other rooms as something bad would happen. Millie couldn't explain what was going on for her, but she felt very frightened and felt that bad things were happening to her. At times Millie was so distressed that her mum could not calm her down. On meeting with Millie, she had not been to sleep for the past 48 hours and was in a very distressed state. Millie had COVID within the last month which included a sore throat and fever. There is no evidence of any neurodevelopmental difficulties for Millie.

REFLECTIVE QUESTIONS FOR APMHS IN CAMHS

1. Clinical Formulation and Assessment
   - What factors (biological, psychological, social) are contributing to this young person's current presentation?
   - What further assessments might be required (e.g. neurodevelopmental, trauma-informed, physical health)?
   - How do I ensure the child's voice and lived experience are central to formulation and planning?
2. Risk Assessment and Management
   - How am I identifying and responding to risks of harm to self, others and from others (e.g. safeguarding)?
   - How do I maintain a balance between therapeutic engagement and necessary information sharing under safeguarding responsibilities?
3. Multi-Agency Working
   - Are all relevant services (e.g. education, YOT, social care, paediatrics) actively involved in this case? If not, what is missing?
   - How am I contributing to effective communication and collaboration across systems?
4. Professional Role and Leadership
   - What leadership behaviours am I demonstrating in this case, and how do they align with the expectations of advanced practice?
   - Am I modelling trauma-informed, anti-discriminatory and child-centred care?
5. Ethics and Legal Considerations
   - How do I apply relevant legal frameworks (e.g. Children Act, MHA and MCA) to this case?

6. Supervision and Self-Care
   - How might these cases be affecting me emotionally and professionally?
   - What support or supervision do I need to manage the complexity and risk involved?
   - How do I maintain resilience, boundaries and reflective capacity in high-pressure situations?

CONCLUSION

Working in CAMHS as an APMH requires a dynamic combination of clinical expertise, leadership and adaptability within a complex and evolving service landscape. This chapter has outlined the multi-faceted nature of the role, highlighting the interplay between developmental, systemic and pharmacological considerations, as well as the operational and societal factors that influence practice. A systemically informed, evidence-based and legally sound approach ensures that APMHs can make meaningful clinical decisions that lead to better outcomes for children and young people.

REFERENCES

1. Health Education England (2020). Advanced practice mental health curriculum and capabilities. https://www.hee.nhs.uk/sites/default/files/documents/AP-MH%20Curriculum%20and%20Capabilities%20Framework%201.2.pdf
2. Williams, R. and Kerfoot, M. (2005). *Child and Adolescent Mental Health Services: strategy, Planning, Delivery, and Evaluation*. Oxford; New York: Oxford University Press.
3. Department of Health (2004). *CAMHS Standard, National Service Framework for Children, Young People and Maternity Services*. London: DH.
4. Williams, R. and Richardson, G. (1995). *Together we Stand: the Commissioning, Role and Management of Child and Adolescent Mental Health Services: An NHS Health Advisory Service (HAS) Thematic Review*. London: HMSO.
5. House of Commons Health Committee. Children's and adolescents' mental health and CAMHS: CAMHS as a whole system [Internet]. London: UK Parliament; 2014 [cited 2025 Feb 15]. Available from: https://publications.parliament.uk/pa/cm201415/cmselect/cmhealth/342/34206.htm
6. Department of Health (2004). *National Service Framework for Children, Young People and Maternity Services*. London: HMSO.
7. Wolpert M, Harris R, Jones M, et al. (2014). The AFC–Tavistock model for CAMHS. Tavistockandportman.ac.uk. Available from: https://repository.tavistockandportman.ac.uk/941/1/Thrive%20model%20for%20CAMHS.pdf
8. Health Education England (2022). Advanced practice in mental health implementation guide. Available from: https://advanced-practice.hee.nhs.uk/advanced-practice-in-mental-health-implementation-guide
9. UK Parliament. *CAMHS Review* [Internet]. Hansard – House of Commons; 2008 Nov 18 [cited 2025 May 4]. Available from: https://hansard.parliament.uk/commons/2008-11-18/debates/08111871000014/CAMHSReview
10. Department of Health & NHS England. *Future in Mind: Promoting, protecting and improving our children and young people's mental health and wellbeing* [Internet]. London: H.M. Government; 2015 [cited 2025 Feb 15]. Available from: https://assets.publishing.service.gov.uk/government/uploads/system/uploads/attachment_data/file/414024/Childrens_Mental_Health.pdf

11. Health Education England. *Approved Clinicians and Responsible Clinicians (AC/RC)* [Internet]. London: NHS England workforce, training & education; 2022 [cited 2025 Feb 16]. Available from: https://www.hee.nhs.uk/our-work/mental-health/new-ways-working-mental-health/approved-clinicians-responsible-clinicians-acrc
12. Mental Health Act 1983 [Internet]. London: UK Government; 1983 [cited 2025 Feb 8]. Available from: https://www.legislation.gov.uk/ukpga/1983/20/contents
13. Levin, E. (2011). Child development. In: *Encyclopaedia of Child Behaviour and Development*, 337–339. Boston, MA: Springer US.
14. Medicines and Healthcare products Regulatory Agency (MHRA). *Off-label or unlicensed use of medicines: prescribers' responsibilities* [Internet]. London: Gov.uk; 2014 [cited 2025 Feb 15]. Available from: https://www.gov.uk/drug-safety-update/off-label-or-unlicensed-use-of-medicines-prescribers-responsibilities
15. Bornstein, M.H. (2013). Parenting and child mental health: a cross-cultural perspective. *World Psychiatry* 12 (3): 258–265. https://doi.org/10.1002/wps.20071.
16. Scarman, Lord, Harwich LBOF, Oakbrook LBOF, Templeman, Lord (1985). Gillick v West Norfolk and Wisbech Area Health Authority and another. http://Globalhealthrights.org. [cited 2025 Feb 8]. https://www.globalhealthrights.org/wp-content/uploads/2013/01/HL-1985-Gillick-v.-West-Norfolk-and-Wisbech-Area-Health-Authority-and-Anr.pdf
17. Mental Capacity Act 2005 [Internet]. London: UK Government; 2005 [cited 2025 Feb 8]. Available from: https://www.legislation.gov.uk/ukpga/2005/9/contents
18. Children Act 1989 [Internet]. London: UK Government; 1989 [cited 2025 Feb 8]. Available from: https://www.legislation.gov.uk/ukpga/1989/41/contents
19. UNICEF UK. (2010). UN convention on rights of a child (UNCRC). www.unicef.org.uk/what-we-do/un-convention-child-rights
20. Brammer A. (1998). Human Rights Act 1998. The Negligence Liability of Public Authorities, Second Edition. www.legislation.gov.uk/ukpga/1998/42/contents
21. Hoyos, C., El-Masry, A., Harrison, D. et al. (2020). Systems thinking: from child and adolescent mental health to medicine. *Journal of the American Academy of Child and Adolescent Psychiatry* 59 (8): 911–913. https://doi.org/10.1016/j.jaac.2020.02.006.
22. Bronfenbrenner, U. (2009). *The Ecology of Human Development: Experiments by Nature and Design*. London: Harvard University Press. https://doi.org/10.2307/j.ctv26071r6.
23. Department for Education. *The multi-agency response to children and families who need help* [Internet]. London: Gov.uk; [cited 2025 Feb 22]. Available from: https://www.gov.uk/government/publications/the-multi-agency-response-to-children-and-families-who-need-help/the-multi-agency-response-to-children-and-families-who-need-help
24. Cox A. (2021). How can children aged 8-12 years be involved in decision-making and consent processes in outpatient Child and Adolescent Mental Health Services (CAMHS). Derby University.
25. Gesell, A. (2021). *Child Development*. Prabhat Prakashan.
26. Freud, S. (1917). *A General Introduction to Psychoanalysis*. United States: S. Freud, North Charleston, South Carolina.
27. Erikson, E.H. (1959). *Identity and the Life Cycle*. New York: Norton.
28. Piaget, J. (1926). *The Language and Thought of the Child*. London: Routledge.
29. Vygotsky, L. (1978). *Mind in Society: the Development of Higher Psychological Processes*. Cambridge: Harvard University Press.

30. Watson, J.B. (1957). *Behaviourism*. Chicago, IL: University of Chicago Press.
31. Skinner, B.F. (1976). *About Behaviourism*. Pimlico.
32. Klaczynski, P.A. (2004). A dual process of adolescent development. Implications for decision-making, reasoning and identity. In: *Advances in Child Development and Behaviour* (ed. R.V. Kail), 73–123. Oxford: Academic Press.
33. Larcher, V. and Hutchinson, A. (2010). How should paediatricians assess Gillick competence? *Archives of Disease in Childhood* 95 (4): 307–311. https://doi.org/10.1136/adc.2008.148676.
34. Rushforth, H. (1999). Practitioner review: communicating with hospitalised children: review and application of research pertaining to children's understanding of health and illness. *Journal of Child Psychology and Psychiatry* 40 (5): 683–691. https://doi.org/10.1111/1469-7610.00485.
35. ISUPPORT. www.isupportchildrensrights.com
36. Singh, S.P., Evans, N., Sireling, L., and Stuart, H. (2005). Mind the gap: the interface between child and adult mental health services. *Psychiatric Bulletin* 29 (8): 292–294. https://doi.org/10.1192/pb.29.8.292.
37. Waiting times for children and young people's mental health services, 2022-23. NHS England Digital. https://digital.nhs.uk/supplementary-information/2024/waiting-times-for-children-and-young-peoples-mental-health-services-2022-23
38. Ambitious about Autism (2017). Four out of five young people with autism experience mental health issues. https://www.ambitiousaboutautism.org.uk/about-us/media-centre/news/four-out-five-young-people-autism-experience-mental-health-issues#:~:text=According%20to%20a%20new%20report%20commissioned%20by%20Ambitious,people%20with%20autism%20have%20experienced%20mental%20health%20issues
39. UK Government. *Equality Act 2010: Guidance* [Internet]. London: Gov.uk; 2010 [cited 2025 Feb 16]. Available from: https://www.gov.uk/guidance/equality-act-2010-guidance
40. PositivePsychology.com. *Cognitive Therapy Techniques* [Internet]. [cited 2025 Feb 16]. https://positivepsychology.com/cognitive-therapy-techniques
41. British Psychological Society (2015). *Children and Young People with Learning Disabilities and Severe Complex Needs: Integrated Working and Workforce Development*. Leicester: BPS.
42. Mencap (2024). *Learning difficulties [Internet]*. London: Mencap [cited 2025 Nov 22]. https://www.mencap.org.uk/learning-disability-explained/learning-disability-and-conditions/learning-difficulties.
43. Mencap (2024). What is a learning disability?. Mencap. www.mencap.org.uk/learning-disability-explained/what-learning-disability
44. NICE (2025). Non-medical prescribing Org.uk. https://bnf.nice.org.uk/medicines-guidance/non-medical-prescribing
45. Sharma, A.N., Arango, C., Coghill, D. et al. (2016). BAP position statement: off-label prescribing of psychotropic medication to children and adolescents. *Journal of Psychopharmacology* 30 (5): 416–421. https://doi.org/10.1177/0269881116636107.
46. BNFC content published by NICE. Org.uk. https://bnfc.nice.org.uk
47. Rpharms.com (2021). A competency framework for all prescribers. https://www.rpharms.com/Portals/0/RPS%20document%20library/Open%20access/Prescribing%20Competency%20Framework/RPS%20English%20Competency%20Framework%203.pdf?ver=mctnrKo4YaJDh2nA8N5G3A%3d%3d
48. Acpeds.org (2020). https://acpeds.org/position-statements/media-use-and-screen-time-its-impact-on-children-adolescents-and-families

49. Moss, S. (2012). http://friendsofhaileypark.org.uk/uploads/1/9/5/1/1951271/naturalchildhood_stephen moss_nationaltrust.pdf
50. NIHR (2023). Significant rise in ADHD diagnoses in the UK. http://Nihr.ac.uk.2023 www.nihr.ac.uk/news/significant-rise-adhd-diagnoses-uk
51. Mesce, M., Ragona, A., Cimino, S., and Cerniglia, L. (2022). The impact of media on children during the COVID-19 pandemic: a narrative review. *Heliyon* 8 (12): e12489. https://doi.org/10.1016/j.heliyon.2022e12489.
52. The role of paediatricians in children and young people's mental health – position statement 2024. RCPCH. www.rcpch.ac.uk/resources/role-of-paediatricians-child-mental-health-position
53. Department of Health (2015). *Future in Mind: promoting, Protecting and Improving our Children and Young People's Mental Health and Wellbeing*. London: Department of Health.
54. National Institute for Health and Care Excellence (NICE) (2008). Social and emotional wellbeing in children and young people [PH12]. London: NICE.
55. Royal College of Paediatrics and Child Health (2018). *Facing the Future: Standards for Children with Ongoing Health Needs*. London: RCPCH.
56. British Medical Association (2017). *Recognising the Importance of Physical Health in Mental Health Care*. London: BMA.
57. Viner, R.M., Ozer, E.M., Denny, S. et al. (2012). Adolescence and the social determinants of health. *Lancet* 379 (9826): 1641–1652.
58. Campbell, P.J., Brown, S.J., Kendrew, P. et al. (2020). Changes in thyroid function across adolescence: a longitudinal study. *The Journal of Clinical Endocrinology & Metabolism* 105 (4): e1162–e1170. https://doi.org/10.1210/clinem/dgz331.
59. Samuels, M.H. (2014). Psychiatric and cognitive manifestations of hypothyroidism. *Current Opinion in Endocrinology, Diabetes and Obesity* 21 (5): 377–383. https://doi.org/10.1097/MED.0000000000000089.
60. Zielińska, M., Łuszczki, E., and Dereń, K. (2023). Dietary nutrient deficiencies and risk of depression (review article 2018–2023). *Nutrients* 15 (11): 2433. https://doi.org/10.3390/nu15112433.
61. NHS England (2017). *The Role of the Advanced Clinical Practitioner in Multi-Professional Teams*. London: NHS England.
62. Munro, E. (2011). *The Munro Review of Child Protection: Final Report – A Child-Centred System*. London: Department for Education.
63. Kids LC. (2022). Are we facing a surge of Long Covid with Paediatric Acute-Onset Neuropsychiatric Syndrome (PANS)?. Long Covid Kids. https://www.longcovidkids.org/post/what-is-paediatric-acute-onset-neuropsychiatric-syndrome-pans-and-how-is-it-treated
64. Bruce, H., Mansoor, S., and Evans, S. (2021). Implementing a physical healthcare clinic in a CAMHS neurodevelopmental population. *BJPsych Open* 7 (S1): S312–S313. Available from: https://doi.org/10.1192/bjo.2021.825.
65. Bestbier, L. and Williams, T.I. (2017). The immediate effects of deep pressure on young people with autism and severe intellectual difficulties: demonstrating individual differences. *Occupational Therapy International* 2017: 1–7. https://www.ncbi.nlm.nih.gov/pmc/articles/PMC5612681.
66. Quality statement 6: monitoring for side effects of antipsychotic medication | Bipolar disorder, psychosis and schizophrenia in children and young people | Quality standards | NICE. www.nice.org.uk/guidance/qs102/chapter/quality-statement-6-monitoring-for-side-effects-of-antipsychotic-medication
67. Recommendations | Attention deficit hyperactivity disorder: diagnosis and management | Guidance | NICE. www.nice.org.uk/guidance/ng87/chapter/Recommendations

68. Anna Freud Centre (2025). http://Corc.uk.net. www.corc.uk.net
69. Rossiter, R. and Tait, N. (2021). *Gathering feedback and measuring outcomes and change with Children and Young People with Learning Disabilities (CYP-LD), their families and networks: revised guidance*. London: British Psychological Society Division of Clinical Psychology/Child Outcomes Research Consortium.
70. Simpson F. NSPCC (2020). Adolescents four times more at risk of physical abuse than younger children. CYP Now. www.cypnow.co.uk/content/news/nspcc-adolescents-four-times-more-at-risk-of-physical-abuse-than-younger-children
71. Child Rescue Coalition (2024). The dark side of AI: risks to children]. https://childrescuecoalition.org/educations/the-dark-side-of-ai-risks-to-children
72. National Mental Health Risk Management Programme (2009). Best Practice in Managing Risk Gov.uk. https://assets.publishing.service.gov.uk/government/uploads/system/uploads/attachment_data/file/478595/best-practice-managing-risk-cover-webtagged.pdf
73. Macneil, C.A., Hasty, M.K., Conus, P., and Berk, M. (2012). Is diagnosis enough to guide interventions in mental health? Using case formulation in clinical practice. *BMC Medicine* 10 (1): 111. https://doi.org/10.1186/1741-7015-10.111.
74. England NHS (2024). NHS England Principles for assessing and managing risks across integrated care systems. Nhs.uk. https://www.england.nhs.uk/long-read/principles-for-assessing-and-managing-risks-across-integrated-care-systems
75. Nhs.uk. https://www.england.nhs.uk/wp-content/uploads/2023/01/Dynamic-support-register-and-Care-Education-and-Treatment-Review-policy-and-guide.pdf
76. ACMH. Possible Red Flags | Children's Mental Health. https://www.acmh-mi.org/get-information/childrens-mental-health-101/possible-red-flags
77. Lalljee J. (2023). Red flags in child safeguarding. Pulse Today. www.pulsetoday.co.uk/clinical-feature/clinical-areas/paediatrics/red-flags-in-child-safeguarding
78. HM Government (2018). *Working Together to Safeguard Children: a Guide to Inter-Agency Working to Safeguard and Promote the Welfare of Children*. London: Department for Education.
79. Royal College of Psychiatrists (2019). *Child Protection and the Role of Child and Adolescent Mental Health Services*. London: RCPsych.
80. Nursing & Midwifery Council (2018). The code: Professional standards of practice and behaviour for nurses, midwives and nursing associates.

CHAPTER 15

Mental Health in Older People and the Advanced Practitioner

Kirstie Tomlinson
Nottinghamshire Healthcare NHS Trust, Nottingham, UK

> **Aim**
>
> This chapter explores the role of the advanced practitioner in mental health (APMH) working in the field of older people's mental healthcare. Illustrated by case examples, the chapter describes the clinical role of the APMH in older people's mental health services, placing this within the wider context of the Advanced Practice Mental Health Curriculum and Capabilities Framework [1]. The chapter also aims to reflect on some of the complexities of working in the field of older people's mental health and some of the specific challenges an APMH might be asked to address.
>
> By exploring the social, physical and psychological factors relevant to older age and applying this in the context of assessing, formulating and intervening to address an older person's mental health issue, the chapter hopes to demonstrate how the APMH might structure and develop their knowledge base in this area of practice, emphasising how the skills of the APMH are ideally placed to contribute to high-quality mental healthcare.

LEARNING OUTCOMES

After reading this chapter, the reader will be able to:

- Be reminded of the normal processes of ageing, of issues of loss and other social and emotional factors that impact a person and their mental health in later life and be able to apply them in the context of advanced practice in older people's mental health.
- Know the importance of a person-centred approach and be able to appreciate the complexity of the life stories of older people in the context of their current presentation.

The Advanced Practitioner in Mental Health, First Edition. Edited by Clare Allabyrne.
© 2026 John Wiley & Sons Ltd. All rights reserved, including rights for text and data mining and training of artificial intelligence technologies or similar technologies. Published 2026 by John Wiley & Sons Ltd.

- Understand that mental health presentations in later life can present differently to those in a younger adult and adapt practice in relation to need.
- Be able to comprehensively assess cognition, work sensitively with a person experiencing cognitive impairment and be able to identify and respond to delirium when it impacts an older adult's mental health.
- Have an understanding of the physical health changes that can impact a person in later life, the relationship between long-term health conditions and mental health and be able to develop collaborative treatment plans that take account of both physical and mental health.
- Understand the concept of frailty and be able to take this into account when working with an older adult with mental health problems.
- Understand and be able to apply legal frameworks in the context of working in the field of older peoples' mental health.

Health Education England (HEE) Advanced Practice Mental Health Curriculum and Capabilities Framework [1]:
This chapter supports the following Domains:

Domain A: This chapter illustrates the role of the advanced practitioner in advocating for potentially vulnerable people or groups, highlighting the importance of understanding social, psychological and biological issues that may impact older people with mental health problems, supporting the person to maximise well-being and recovery (1.9, 1.10, 1.11, 1.15, 1.16, 1.17, 1.18).

Domain B: It emphasises the importance of comprehensive assessment and history-taking in the older adult, highlighting the interplay between physical and mental health and considering the importance of cognition and of considering capacity and consent (2.1, 2.2, 2.3, 2.4, 2.7, 2.8, 2.9, 2.10, 2.11, 2.12, 2.13, 2.14).

Domain C: Formulation is considered across both physical and mental health presentations, illustrated through a case where the APMH needs to revisit formulation as patient need changes (3.1, 3.2, 3.3, 3.4).

Domain E: The impact of pharmacological treatment and associated adverse effects, with specific reference to an older person, is illustrated through the interventions in the same case (5.1, 5.2, 5.3, 5.4, 5.7, 5.8).

INTRODUCTION

In the United Kingdom, 65 years of age is accepted to be the marker for the start of older age, perhaps because it was once the official retirement age for men and the age at which they could draw their state pension [2]. However, there is no longer an official retirement age and people are also living longer, healthier lives. In 2018, a man aged 65 could expect to live for another 18.6 years, while a woman could expect to live for 21 more years [3].

In 2020, 1 billion people in the world were aged 60 years or over. According to the World Health Organisation, by 2050 that figure will have doubled to reach 2.1 billion, while the number of people aged 80 years or older is expected to triple between 2020 and 2050 to reach 426 million [4]. In the United Kingdom, the proportion of those aged 65 and older is increasing, and the proportion of those aged 85 is also increasing in similar trajectories to those globally. Understandably, these increasing numbers are associated with an increasing associated demand for health and social care to meet need [5].

Not only are the number of older people in our populations increasing, but the prevalence of mental health conditions is higher among specific groups of older people than in the general population. For example, some research suggests that 40% of older people who are living in care homes have depression, while 30% of older carers experience depression at some point during their caring experience [6]. Similarly, older people experiencing bereavement are up to four times more likely to experience depression than older people who haven't been bereaved [7].

The NHS Long Term Plan recognises the importance of improving mental health in the older population and articulates an intention to ensure consistent access to mental healthcare for older adults with mental health problems, embedding it as a 'silver thread' across all of the adult mental health Long Term Plan ambitions [8].

The APMH working within older people's mental health services has a complex task; not only do they need to understand and work with complex mental health problems, understanding how these might present differently in an older person, but they must also be able to evaluate this in the context of the normal processes of ageing and understand some of the social and emotional factors that impact people in later life [9].

They need to be able to comprehensively assess cognition, cognitive impairment and delirium and their implications for mental health. They must also be able to treat mental health problems whilst understanding physical health changes in the older person – adapting practice to take account of multiple physical health comorbidities and polypharmacy. They need a detailed grasp of the concept of frailty and its social implications, and they should be able to work with all these issues within supportive legal frameworks.

Finally, but first and foremost, working in a person-centred and family-centred way requires an ability to appreciate the complexities of an older person's life story, ensuring they are seen as an individual with experiences, aspirations and opinions.

PERSON-CENTRED CARE AND THE OLDER PERSON: NORMAL AGEING, LIFE STORIES AND SOCIAL AND EMOTIONAL FACTORS IMPORTANT IN LATER LIFE

As we age, biological, psychological, social, environmental and financial changes can all potentially impact on mental well-being. While individual experiences of ageing vary, as do responses to them, certain events are more likely to occur with increasing age, including bereavement, retirement, changes in mobility, increasing caring responsibilities, development of long-term physical health conditions and loss of autonomy (for example, moving into care). Mental health problems, however, are not an inevitable part of ageing, and an APMH needs to be able to identify aspects of normal individual ageing in the context of an older person's overall health and well-being to be able to identify mental health problems when they do occur. They need to be ready to actively challenge age-related stigma and the impact this stigma has on older people, their families, carers and other professionals. Most importantly, they need to be able to instill hope to overcome the barriers older people experience when accessing support for their mental health, promoting a message of well-being by helping an older person work towards developing life satisfaction, optimism, purpose and a sense of belonging and support [9].

Health Education England Older Adults Mental Health (HEE OAMH) Competency Framework [10] highlights the importance of practitioners being able to differentiate between an older person with existing or emerging mental health needs, who is ageing and an individual whose mental health is affected by the process of ageing.

For both presentations, an older person's baseline needs to be identified by the APMH. Healthcare professionals who work in mental health services for older people need to be skilled at understanding the importance of eliciting a person's life story, weaving this into collaborative assessment processes to make what can be a difficult process more individually meaningful [11]. The skilled APMH also needs to recognise the importance of triangulation of data sources to navigate such detailed complexity [12]. To accurately identify increased need and effectively care plan, the APMH needs to work collaboratively with families, carers and healthcare professionals to increase their awareness of out-of-the-ordinary changes brought about or exacerbated by the ageing process, and the subsequent coping and defence mechanisms that might be used by older people.

Clinical situations in the context of working with older people and their families often provide an opportunity for the APMH to apply their leadership and teaching pillars [13] that truly emphasise the building of a person-centred therapeutic alliance. They must be able to offer expert advice to families and non-specialist staff in contact with older people, providing thought leadership and best practice examples on the topic of ageing, whilst advocating for age awareness in the context of sometimes challenging individual and societal determinants of health and social care [14].

Learning Event – Applying Advanced Level Communication Skills

Take, for example, a family who have lived a very private life where they have avoided healthcare services for many years, holding a degree of suspicion and cynicism about the usefulness of doctors. Thus far, they have enjoyed good health, with a mother and wife who is a strong and opinionated matriarch of the family, and a quieter husband, daughter and son. Mum has strong and, perhaps, inflexible values and opinions that have shaped the family around her.

How then, do they respond when mum's behaviour changes following the death of her own mother and she starts displaying strange behaviour, such as chopping down a garden tree in the middle of the night, taking risks she wouldn't normally take, such as walking outside at night without shoes and in her nightwear, and being aggressive to those around her?

We might reasonably assume that this acute change in behaviour would cause the family so much concern that they would be worried about mum's health and would contact a doctor, but what if their family narrative means they decide to manage this within the family, keeping mum in her room with the door locked to keep her safe until her behaviour settles? What if this was how mum used to respond to her children when they were unsettled growing up, and if this is considered normal for the family?

A concerned neighbour rings the GP when she sees mum climbing a tree at nighttime.

How should the APMH, who has been asked to engage mum and her family in healthcare by the concerned GP, navigate safeguarding concerns whilst respecting that professional values and perspectives may differ from long-held family beliefs and practices?

Through the application of advanced-level communication skills, the APMH is able to take a history from the husband and daughter by using a skilled but non-judgemental approach, whilst at the same time ensuring that mum is not at risk of immediate harm. The daughter and husband describe mum's behaviour having changed over the last year, initially in small but strange ways, such as her wearing strange clothing or having new likes and dislikes that were unusual for her. These changes would increase in frequency over time and became more bizarre, such as her buying a chainsaw to chop down all the trees in the garden. The family became concerned when mum started putting herself at risk, and would lock her in her bedroom to keep her safe. They also noticed that she seemed to be having difficulty talking, with her words no longer appearing to form full sentences.

The APMH spends time discussing the risks of mum staying at home with the family, and suggests that a period in hospital would allow for a full assessment of the reasons for mum's change in behaviour, which could have several different causes. The family are very reluctant for mum to be admitted to hospital, and the APMH attempts to reassure them, whilst also explaining to them that their mum's current behaviour is of a nature and degree that might need hospital admission to keep her safe.

Here, the APMH has demonstrated sensitivity in a complex and uncertain situation, has managed distress and potential conflict, whilst being accountable and responsible for their decisions [13]. All this, while continuously building therapeutic partnerships, understanding what is normal for the family, what is now different and the factors that have impacted on this change. The APMH needs to know when to seek help, be able to critically reflect on their own actions, whilst keeping the older person's needs and the needs of their family, front and central.

Questions for Reflection

Do you think mum is presenting with a mental health problem and associated risks that might need admission to hospital, or might there be a less restrictive option available to support mum and her family with their current difficulties?

Could mum be reacting to the recent death of her mother, and might this reaction be understandable in the face of loss and grief?

Might there be concerns about her cognition in relation to her altered behaviour?

How might the APMH assess this further, help the family make sense of this change and help them access the help that might be needed, despite their preference for privacy?

The APMH needs to be able to recognise and challenge more widely held barriers that can occur when working within older people's mental health services. One in three people in the United Kingdom report experiencing age prejudice or age discrimination [15]. Exposure to negative age stereotypes has been associated with worse health outcomes [16], including a reduction in longevity [17]. Ageism directed towards the self may discourage older people from embracing the behaviours and opportunities that would enable them to fully participate in society, including accessing healthcare [18].

Ageism might lead older people and their families to think that mental health problems are an inevitable part of ageing 'my husband has died, of course I'm going to feel sad', or an older person might hold a more traditional attitude to a healthcare professional 'I don't want to bother the doctor'. They may misattribute their symptoms to a physical cause 'I'm tired and aching because my arthritis is playing up, I just need to accept I can't get about the way I used to'. They may be ashamed that they are experiencing frightening symptoms 'I can't tell anyone I'm going crazy, what would they think? I need to pull myself together'. All these beliefs could place the recognition of serious mental health problems at risk [19, 20].

The APMH should take time to sensitively identify any barriers to engagement for each older person, taking time to understand a lifetime of experiences and values formed. They should not only aim to build a person-centred therapeutic alliance with the older person in a way that empowers and engages them, but do this in conjunction with a detailed and critical appraisal of individual and societal approaches to ageing, which can be negative; for example, associating ageing with decline and ill-health, frailty, vulnerability and dependency on others [21].

ASSESSMENT OF MENTAL HEALTH PROBLEMS IN THE OLDER PERSON

As well as being able to demonstrate clinical expertise in the assessment, diagnosis and treatment of complex mental health problems [1], the APMH engaged in the assessment of older people's mental health problems needs to be able to apply specific skills and knowledge that are not always routinely practiced in general adult psychiatric services. This next section takes us through some of the complexities of assessing an older person who has been referred to mental health services by her GP, by exploring a case study and its intricacies as it unfolds. The case is adapted from examples drawn from clinical practice but does not identify any individual person or their family, in line with Nursing and Midwifery Council guidelines regarding confidentiality [22].

> ### Case Study: Mary, an Initial Referral
>
> Mary is a 78-year-old lady who lost her husband, Graham 2 years ago to lung cancer. They had been married for 48 years and Mary reports they had a happy marriage. They were not able to have children but enjoyed their time together, travelling abroad frequently and enjoying time with groups of friends. Since Graham's death, Mary has lived alone in their marital home. She has close and supportive neighbours, and she also volunteers twice a week at a local charity shop.
>
> Two months ago, Mary tripped over a rug in the charity shop and fell, banging the back of her head on the counter. She was reviewed in the emergency department where physical causes for her fall were excluded, and she was diagnosed with a mild concussion. Mary has no other past medical history, other than a diagnosis of hypertension in 2017, which is well-controlled by medication. Mary has stayed at home since the fall, worrying that if she goes out again, she will fall and hurt herself. Her friend delivers her shopping and spends time at home with her to keep her company.
>
> For the past 2 weeks, Mary has been waking in the morning in a confused and anxious state. She does not know where she is for some minutes and is becoming increasingly distressed about this. She is worried that the bang on her head has caused some permanent damage. Mary telephones her GP and tells her she is worried that she has dementia. She can't concentrate and is frightened.
>
> The GP refers Mary to the community mental health team for assessment.

Mental health conditions affecting older people include anxiety and stress-related disorders, bipolar affective disorder, depression, dementia, delirium, personality disorders, psychosis, schizophrenia and substance misuse disorders [23].

The APMH who is assessing and managing mental health conditions in older people must consider complex interlinking biological, psychological and social factors that can be both qualitatively and quantitatively different to those presenting in a younger person.

Case Study: Mary, Assessment

Mary is assessed by an APMH in a community mental health clinic.

She comes alone and is agitated and restless, insisting to the APMH that she has dementia. She tells the APMH that her mother died in her 80s of dementia, and that she can tell she is 'going exactly the same way'. She has downloaded a list of dementia-related symptoms from the internet and has ticked each one to show the APMH. Mary remains preoccupied with her symptoms throughout the assessment and is hard to deflect from this focus.

The APMH takes a short history as Mary's level of distress makes it challenging to elucidate any detail and conducts a mental state examination [24].

Mental State Examination

Mary presents as agitated and preoccupied in the clinic, rubbing her hands together and appearing to find it hard to sit still. She makes good eye contact and responds to questions appropriately but appears facially unreactive. She appears underweight and her mucous membranes appear dry. Mary's speech is rushed and repetitive, but not pressured, and the content remains focused on reporting dementia-related symptoms. It appears fluent and is normal in volume. Her affect is agitated and anxious but she self-reports that her mood is 'fine'. Mary's thoughts appear preoccupied with a fixed idea she has dementia, and she is not open to discussion or reassurance about this. She is convinced that she will decline rapidly and asks the APMH to help her find a care home. She denies any suicidal ideation and denies any perceptual abnormality. The APMH was unable to formally assess her cognition as Mary declined to complete an ACE-III [25] saying she would be unable to complete it as she is 'too far gone'. Mary's judgement and insight appears partial – she accepts she has a mental health problem, but remains fixed on a singular explanation for this, believing nothing can help her.

Mary consents to a blood sample being taken and the APMH takes FBCs, U&Es, CRP, LFTs, TFTs, HbA1c, Vit B12 and folate and bone profile. All results are within normal parameters. Mary has a history of hypertension for which she is prescribed ramipril but does not take any other medication.

The APMH formulates psychiatric differentials with reference to the ICD-11 [26] for Mary's presentation, considering a possible dementia, mild cognitive impairment, generalised anxiety disorder, adjustment disorder and a depressive episode. As Mary attends the appointment alone, the APMH is unable to gain a collateral history at this stage but asks Mary if she can speak to her friend after the appointment, to which Mary agrees.

CLINICAL HISTORY TAKING AND ASSESSMENT TOOLS IN MENTAL HEALTH

The APMH could use several assessment tools available to help them when assessing an older person, but emphasis, as with any other assessment in mental health, should first be on clinical history-taking. The diagnostic interview will help the APMH review specific symptoms, durations and rule out other causes that might better account for a clinical presentation [27].

When assessing older people, the APMH needs to be aware of not just psychiatric differentials for mental illness but also be aware of any physical health and iatrogenic causes that can lead to psychiatric symptoms. They must be able to conduct appropriate examinations and interpret appropriate investigations to rule these out. Changes in mental state associated with infection are very common in older people and should be ruled out with any new-onset presentation. Even constipation may present as confusion or low mood [28].

PSYCHIATRIC PRESENTATIONS RESULTING FROM PHYSICAL ILLNESSES AND MEDICATIONS

Condition	Physical conditions	Medications
Depression	Brain lesion, CVA, Cushing's disease, Huntington's disease, multiple sclerosis, hypothyroidism, vitamin (B, D) deficiency, Parkinson's disease, angina and myocardial infarction, anaemia, diabetes mellitus, pain, malignancy (esp. pancreas, lung), electrolyte disturbance	Steroids, anticholinergics, alcohol
Mania	Brain lesion, CVA, Cushing's disease, Huntington's disease, hyperthyroidism, multiple sclerosis, temporal lobe epilepsy, vitamin (B,D) deficiency, Parkinson's disease	Antiparkinsonian medication, steroids, antidepressants, alcohol, caffeine
Anxiety	Brain lesion, CVA, phaeochromocytoma, Huntington's disease, hyperthyroidism, Parkinson's disease, heart disease (angina, myocardial infarction, heart failure, arrhythmias), hypoglycaemia, lung disease (COPD, pneumonia, pulmonary embolism)	Steroids, antidepressants, thyroxine, anticholinergics, sympathomimetics, alcohol, caffeine
Psychosis	Brain lesion, CVA, Cushing's disease, Huntington's disease, temporal lobe epilepsy, Parkinson's disease, angina and myocardial infarction	Antiparkinsonian medication (dopamine agonists)

Source: [29] / With Permission of NHS.

When collateral history and assessment tools can be used to support a clinical diagnosis. The same psychiatric symptom can present in several different mental health conditions, and eliciting and understanding a detailed narrative history is of prime importance [30], as the APMH needs detail to be able to formulate in the context of what can often be a degree of diagnostic ambiguity [31]. The RIME (reporter, interpreter, manager, educator) framework [32] can offer the APMH a systematic approach in the context of this uncertainty, which proposes consistent gathering of accurate information and interpreting this information against a knowledge base to interpret the clinical meaning and significance of the symptoms that present. A systematic phenomenological approach to understanding symptoms in mental health has been documented by authors such as Oyabede [33].

Red flag presentations also need to be carefully considered in the context of older people's mental health. Risks that are a consequence of the degree of severe mental illness, such as suicide, violence to others or responding to command hallucinations, may present more acutely in an elderly, frail or confused person, while risks that are inherent to the nature of specific conditions such as eating disorders, alcohol misuse and delirium have particular risk emphasis in an older person [34–38].

Assessment tools can then be used to support a working diagnosis, including widely used tools such as the Beck Depression Inventory (BDI-II) [39], the Hamilton Depression Rating Scale (HAM-D) [40], the Young Mania Rating Scale (YMRS) [41] and the Positive and Negative Syndrome Scale (PANSS) [42], or those adapted specifically for use in an older person such as the Geriatric Depression Scale (GDS) [43], the Geriatric Anxiety Inventory (GAI) [44] and the Confusion Assessment Method (CAM) [45].

DEPRESSION IN LATER LIFE

Depression in later life is common and can be associated with a variety of losses and age-related changes [46]. For example, moving into a care home is a major life event, often associated with other multiple losses (bereavement, physical health decline, reduced mobility), all of which can increase the risk of a depressive episode occurring. The APMH needs to be able to recognise and respond to this complexity. In an older person, depression may not present with classic diagnostic symptoms. A depressed older person can present with anxiety and agitation rather than low mood, depression can be hidden behind physical health symptoms and the impact it has on concentration and motivation means it can often be confused with the onset of dementia. How then, does the APMH identify depression in the older person who has experienced loss? They must be alert to the possibility, listening in detail to the person and their presenting complaint. Depression is quite different from grief or sadness – it is more intense, pervasive, less variable and lasts longer. Typically, a depressive episode develops over weeks to a few months, and importantly, it can be associated with a significant and new level of impairment for the older person. Signs of depression in an older person can include unexplained day-to-day functional decline such as reduced self-care and a neglected appearance, reduced mobility or new problems with continence. At home, there may be evidence of empty fridges and cupboards, or a person may show little joy in seeing people they love, such as their grandchildren [47].

Anxiety is often the most prominent symptom of depression in an older adult and importantly, can be an indicator of severity. Agitation is common and can present with a person pacing up and down or wringing their hands. Increasing irritability, withdrawal and alcohol use can also be present [48].

A preoccupation with physical complaints often presents in the depressed older person. Delusions or over-valued ideas can focus on beliefs they have a serious illness. Memory problems can also occur but often have a more acute onset than they would in dementia and the depressed older person is often very worried about them [48].

Case Study: Mary, Treatment and Monitoring

After gaining a collateral history from Mary's friend, and supporting this with application of the Beck Depression Inventory, the APMH diagnoses Mary with a moderate depressive episode, and spends time talking to her about treatment, recommending, in line with NICE Guidance [49], cognitive behavioural therapy (CBT) and a prescription of an antidepressant, sertraline. Mary does not want to engage in therapy, as she is not fond of talking to people she doesn't know, and is still preoccupied with the belief she has dementia, but she agrees to start a prescription of sertraline. After 3 months of treatment Mary's mood improves and her worries about dementia are no longer evident. The APMH discharges her to the care of her GP.

Six months later Mary's GP re-refers her to the Community Mental Health Team (CMHT). Mary has reported to the GP that her memory is worsening again, and the GP has recently increased her sertraline. Mary does not attend her CMHT appointment, and the APMH arranges a home visit. When she arrives, she finds Mary acutely distressed. Her house is in disarray, her speech is confused and she appears to be trying to wind invisible string around her arms and hands without anything being outwardly observable to the APMH.

The APMH is concerned that Mary is acutely confused and visually hallucinated and arranges for her to be transferred to the Emergency Department (ED) for review. Bloods taken in the ED show:

- SODIUM 125 mmol/L [133–146]
- POTASSIUM 5.0 mmol/L [3.5–5.3]
- UREA 8.5 mmol/L [2.5–7.8]
- CREATININE 93 umol/L [64–104]
- C-REACTIVE PROTEIN 2 mg/L [0–5]
- HAEMOGLOBIN 127 g/L [130–175]
- WBC 9.68 10 E9/L [4.00–11.00]
- PLATELETS 235 10 E9/L [150–450]
- RBC 3.87 10 E12/L [4.20–6.50]
- EGFR BY CKD-EPI/1.73M2 59 mL/min 1.73 m [60–200]

A working diagnosis of delirium secondary to hyponatraemia is proposed, following the recent increase in sertraline, and her dose is reduced. Mary is admitted to an inpatient healthcare of the elderly ward, where her presentation settles, and she is discharged home 2 weeks later.

FORMULATION AND COLLABORATIVE TREATMENT AND CARE PLANNING

As with all treatment and care planning in mental health, the most important step is supporting the person and their care givers to understand their mental health problem, educating them where needed, so they have full involvement in treatment decisions. The APMHs teaching pillar [13] can be applied in more formal situations, such as delivering sessions to placement care givers, but the skills can also be applied to patients and their families on a case-by-case basis. This means exploring the individual's understanding of their mental health problem, including its causes, and working through any beliefs that may create barriers to accessing treatment. It may also mean that the APMH has to accept the expertise of the older person, without losing the critical listening faculties [1] that might alert them to worsening hopelessness or self-destructive thinking.

PHYSICAL HEALTH COMPLEXITY AND FRAILTY IN LATER LIFE

Frailty and multimorbidity are not an inevitable part of ageing, but the APMH working with older people needs to have an awareness of the complex relationship between physical and mental health in later life, and of the interplay of age-related changes in older people.

The prevalence of long-term physical health conditions increases as a person ages. These conditions also increase the risk of an older adult developing a common mental health problem. The reverse is also a concern: People with a diagnosis of serious mental illness are at increased risk of developing a chronic physical health condition. For example, a diagnosis of schizophrenia is associated with an increased risk of physical comorbidity, such as cardiovascular disease [50], while people with diagnoses of chronic physical health conditions such as COPD or cardiovascular disease have a high risk of developing depression [51]. Musculoskeletal conditions, such as arthritis, are common in older people and the associated pain impacts both physical and mental health and can predispose individuals to depression and substance misuse [52]. Acute illnesses, such as urinary tract infections, may present with psychiatric and behavioural symptoms in an older person including visual hallucinations and extreme agitation. The APMH needs to be able to recognise and respond to concerns about multimorbidity, identify urgent physical health concerns and adapt their mental health treatment to best impact on both physical and mental health.

Similarly, frailty is a multidimensional clinical syndrome characterised by a progressive decline in physiological function across multiple body systems, leading to a state of reduced resilience and an impaired capacity to maintain or regain health following physiological or psychological challenges. A person identified as frail is at high risk of adverse outcomes such as falls, immobility, delirium incontinence and the side effects of medication, with an increased risk of admission to hospital or a need for long-term care [53]. The APMH must be adept at recognising frailty-related concerns, able to use appropriate assessment tools [54] and able to access the appropriate intervention across multiple services when they identify concerns.

PRESCRIBING IN OLDER PEOPLE'S MENTAL HEALTH

The Maudsley Prescribing Guidelines [55] provide guidance and detailed information regarding the prescription of psychiatric medication in the older person. The APMH must take into account that the pharmacokinetics and pharmacodynamics of most drugs are altered in older people as kidney function and other age-related physical changes develop [56]. Physical health multimorbidity in the older person also increases the chances of polypharmacy and the APMH must be mindful of drug interactions, taking the recommended approach of start low, go slow [28]. When an APMH prescribes medication as part of an intervention for a mental health problem in an older person, they must be vigilant for potential adverse effects [57]. In Mary's case, The Maudsley Practice Guidelines for Physical Health Conditions suggests any degree of hyponatraemia should prompt a medication review and recommends a rationalisation of treatments where one or more medications may be involved [58]. There is more information on prescribing for older adults in Chapter 8.

SSRIs and Hyponatraemia

Sertraline is a selective serotonin reuptake inhibitor (SSRI). The underlying mechanism for SSRI-induced hyponatremia is thought to be the syndrome of inappropriate antidiuretic hormone secretion (SIADH), where the body retains water excessively due to abnormal antidiuretic hormone secretion, leading to dilutional hyponatremia [59].

DELIRIUM

Delirium is characterised by a presentation of increased confusion which fluctuates and is often worse in the evening. Hyperactive delirium presents with multiple psychiatric symptoms, which may include restlessness, agitation, rapid mood changes, paranoid delusions, hallucinations or refusal to cooperate with care. Hypoactive delirium may present with inactivity or reduced motor activity, abnormal drowsiness or a refusal to eat and drink. It can be missed as it can mimic the symptoms of depression. [60] The APMH working with older people should consider delirium in any new or deteriorating physical illness, a recent change in medication, a recent admission to hospital or recent surgery. They should also consider it when a person's mental state acutely changes when they have dementia, a sensory impairment, have had a previous stroke, are dehydrated, in pain or have had a recent change in environment.

> ### Case Study: Mary, Review and Changing Concerns
>
> Three months later, Mary's friend takes her back to the GP. She is concerned that Mary has never recovered from her hospital admission, she sits in her chair for much of the day, she no longer does any household activities and she seems to struggle with day-to-day things. She says she can't remember how to use the TV remote control, and she made her friend a cup of coffee but made it with cold water. Last night, her friend stayed at her house, and she reports Mary put her coat on and tried to leave the house at 2 a.m. as she said she 'had to go catch a train'.
>
> The GP is concerned that Mary may be cognitively impaired. She completes a Mini-ACE assessment and Mary scores 8/30 [24]. The GP contacts the community mental health team and asks them to assess.

COGNITIVE IMPAIRMENT, DEPRESSION AND THE IMPORTANCE OF HISTORY TAKING

For any older person who shows a significant decline in mood, cognition and function, the APMH should be mindful that a differential diagnosis may be depression or dementia. There is a complex relationship between depression and dementia which the APMH needs to have awareness of when assessing an older person [61]. Depression can be a reaction to cognitive decline, but it can also be a prodrome of an emerging dementia itself. The occurrence of a first major depressive episode in an older adult is also a risk factor for developing dementia.

The APMH must use cognitive assessment tools with caution in the older person and they should not replace clinical history taking. Common tests used to screen for depression are less efficient in people with dementia, while the depressed older person may score very poorly in a cognitive screening test. Cognition may be impacted detrimentally due to the depression alone, while some signs of dementia may mimic depression such as social withdrawal, apathy, lack of interest in self or others and poor motivation. In addition, dementia may develop insidiously over months or years and be slow in progression [62].

Depression can also occur as dementia advances, and family or carers may notice a change in behaviour [63]. When this occurs, early recognition and assessment of any contributing physical and social factors is crucial.

> ### Case Study: Mary, Dementia and Safety Concerns
>
> The APMH takes a further collateral history from Mary's friend, asking specific questions related to cognition and functioning. This details a history of progressive memory impairment and associated functional decline over the last year.
>
> The APMH completes an ACE-III [25] with Mary, which scores 54/100 and a subsequent head CT reports bilateral hippocampal atrophy and a Medial Temporal Atrophy score of 3.
>
> The APMH formulates a differential diagnosis [26] for Mary of probable dementia in Alzheimer's disease and suggests prescription of a medication, donepezil. Mary becomes very distressed when the APMH discusses this diagnosis with her, as she no longer thinks there is a problem with her memory, and wishes to be left at home, alone, in peace. Her friend is becoming increasingly concerned as she reports that Mary was spotted by a neighbour last night walking down the street in her night clothes and she had to bring her back to the house. She is worried she is not safe to stay at home alone.
>
> Mary declines any further intervention and asks the APMH to leave.

While diagnostic separation of depression and emerging dementia can be challenging, the APMH has all the tools available to them to provide a comprehensive, person-centred assessment. Clinical history-taking is key, from both the patient and carers, cognitive and functional assessment can support a clinical diagnosis, and imaging, if indicated, can further help firm up diagnosis. A multidisciplinary team approach is key to dementia assessment and a subsequent, holistic care plan, and the APMH should be able to lead on treatment approaches, using evidence-based guidelines to ensure the delivery of comprehensive and individualised care to the older person under their care.

COGNITIVE SCREENING TESTS IN THE OLDER ADULT

Cognitive screening tests play a crucial role in the assessment of older adults, particularly for the detection of mild cognitive impairment (MCI) and neurodegenerative disorders such as Alzheimer's dementia. Tools such as the Addenbrookes Cognitive Examination (ACE-III) help identify individuals who may require further diagnostic evaluation, intervention or support. Screening is not diagnostic, but helps guide whether further comprehensive neuropsychiatric testing or diagnostic imaging is warranted [64].

INTERVENTION, EVALUATION AND SAFETY PLANNING

The APMH needs to remain informed about current treatment strategies and associated research to be able to provide the best service to the people in their care and their families. Interventions to manage and treat mental health conditions should consider current evidence-based guidance [65] and where possible, be incorporated as part of a holistic care plan. Interventions may be pharmacological, psychological or social and should be delivered in a safe and appropriate manner.

Mary's presentation has changed and there are now significant risks to her safety in the context of a progressive cognitive impairment. When balancing a person's safety with their need for independence, all care should be underpinned by an understanding, and appropriate use, of relevant legislation and guidelines. The APMH now needs to consider Mary's rights and needs under the context of the appropriate legal frameworks: the Mental Capacity Act (MCA) [66] and where necessary, the Mental Health Act 1983, amended 2007 [67]. Here, the APMH must not only be skilled in assessing capacity related to a specific presenting issue but also be able to identify when risks increase and a different approach to management is needed.

CAPACITY ASSESSMENT IN THE OLDER ADULT WITH COGNITIVE IMPAIRMENT

Assessment of capacity is important in older adults with cognitive impairment because it ensures their autonomy is respected whilst also protecting them from harm. Many individuals with cognitive impairment may retain the ability to make certain decisions. A capacity assessment provides the basis for invoking substitute decision-making, when the person needs it, in their best interests. Assessing capacity helps identify when protective interventions are needed, while avoiding unnecessary restrictions on liberty. The Mental Health Act 1983, amended 2007 [67], is also sometimes used in the care of a person with dementia, but it should only be applied when frameworks such as the MCA are not sufficient. In Mary's case, she is refusing treatment and intervention and is behaving in a way that is risky (wandering outside at night), so detainment in hospital for further assessment under the Mental Health Act may be deemed appropriate following a Mental Health Act Assessment.

SUMMARY AND CONCLUSION

Mary's case is a changing but simplified example of the complexities that can arise when working with an older person with mental health problems. Although an APMH is trained to assess undifferentiated presentations, this complexity can prove challenging, both in assessment and subsequent treatment and care planning.

Older people can present with both functional and organic mental disorders, and an overlap between symptoms can complicate diagnosis further. Older people with a lengthy history of serious mental illness can present with a sudden deterioration in mental state due to delirium or a more protracted decline when they develop a cognitive impairment. Comorbid physical health conditions and the medications prescribed to treat them have also to be considered when an older person presents with a concerning change in mental state, while reported concerns with physical health can, conversely, have their basis in a mental health condition.

The APMH must always be prepared to listen, question and constantly reassess their treatment plan in collaboration with the patient, their family and the many members of the multidisciplinary team that work with them. They must keep in mind, at all times, an awareness of wider determinants of older people's mental health but also the detail and context of the older person's life story, in order to provide the best possible levels of person-centred care. They must be able to synthesise and apply evidence to provide effective interventions and be ready to use their leadership and teaching skills to promote best practice for patients, their families and their colleagues.

In many ways, the complexities inherent in working with older people with mental health problems lends itself to advanced practice in mental health. It offers us the opportunity to think critically across different schools of thought and areas of practice and asks us to strive to improve and build on our knowledge and skills in a variety of areas. The multifactorial nature of the problems that an older adult presents with, across mental, physical and social domains, asks us to continually reflect on all six domains of the Advanced Practice Mental Health Framework, but most importantly, it offers the practitioner the chance to share in the challenges, but also the joys, of lives well-lived.

FURTHER RESOURCES

Information

Home | British Geriatrics Society – Useful source of information for all aspects of health in older people. Training courses also available.

Alzheimer's Society – Excellent source of information related to dementia. Alzheimer's Society.

BMJ Best Practice – online app available for download. Useful resource on up to date information about most aspects of physical healthcare. Homepage| BMJ Best Practice.

Training and teaching Resources

E-Learning for health website – Home – elearning for healthcare Useful resource for training. Search: 'older people mental health' to access targeted resources.

NHS e-learning hub – another website that gives access to training resources. Search: 'Older Adults' Mental Health' https://learninghub.nhs.uk/catalogue/olderadultsmentalhealth Make a difference: Think Depression in Older People. Online training resource, useful for teaching/ training and family work. Available on Spotify at: Make a difference: Think depression in older people | Podcast on Spotify and You tube at: 1.2 Depression in Older People.

Royal College of Psychiatry – Old age psychiatry training packs Old age psychiatry training packs Resources align with the Older People's Mental Health Competency Framework.

Journals

International Journal of Geriatric Psychiatry. Access online at International Journal of Geriatric Psychiatry | Wiley Online Library.

Age and Aging (Journal of the British Geriatrics Society): Access many articles for free online at Age and Ageing | Oxford Academic.

The Journal of Dementia Care. Access online at Current Issue – Dementia Community.

Aging and Mental Health. A journal that investigates the relationship between the aging process and mental health, and explores mental changes associated with ageing. Available online at Aging & Mental Health | Taylor & Francis Online.

REFERENCES

1. HEE (2022). Advanced practice mental health curriculum and capabilities framework. https://www.hee.nhs.uk/sites/default/files/documents/AP-MH%20Curriculum%20and%20Capabilities%20Framework%201.2.pdf
2. Office for National Statistics (2019) Living longer: is age 70 the new age 65? https://www.ons.gov.uk/peoplepopulationandcommunity/birthsdeathsandmarriages/ageing/articles/livinglongerisage70thenewage65/2019-11-19
3. Office for National Statistics (2019). National Life Tables, UK 2016 to 2018, data and analysis from census 2021. https://www.ons.gov.uk/peoplepopulationandcommunity/birthsdeathsandmarriages/lifeexpectancies/bulletins/nationallifetablesunitedkingdom/2016to2018
4. DESA Population (Population Division of the United Nations Department of Economic and Social Affairs) (2022). World Population Prospect 2022: release note about major differences in total population estimates for mid-2021 between 2019 and 2022 revisions. New York: United Nations Department of Economic and Social Affairs, Population Division. https://population.un.org/wpp/Publications/Files/WPP2022_Release-Note-rev1.pdf (accessed 30 September 2024).
5. Age Concern (2019). Later Life in the United Kingdom 2019. Factsheet. https://www.ageuk.org.uk/globalassets/age-uk/documents/reports-and-publications/later_life_uk_factsheet.pdf (accessed 30 September 2024).
6. Joint Commissioning Panel for Mental Health (2013), 'Guidance for commissioners of older people's mental health'. https://www.jcpmh.info/wp-content/uploads/jcpmh-olderpeople-guide.pdf
7. Independent Age (2018). Good grief: older people's experiences of bereavement, London: Independent Age. https://independent-age-assets.s3.euwest1.amazonaws.com/s3fs-public/2018–04/Good%20Grief%20report.pdf
8. NHS England (2019). NHS mental health implementation plan 2019/20–2023/24. p. 36. https://www.england.nhs.uk/wp-content/uploads/2022/07/nhs-mental-health-implementation-plan-2019-20-2023-24.pdf
9. National Institute for Clinical Excellence (NICE) (2018). Promoting positive mental wellbeing for older people. https://www.nice.org.uk/Media/Default/About/NICE-Communities/Social-care/quick-guides/Mental-wellbeing-in-care-homes.pdf
10. Health Education England (HEE) (2020). Older people's mental health competency framework. https://www.e-lfh.org.uk/wp-content/uploads/2020/04/OlderPeoplesMentalHealthCompetencyFramework-V1.8.pdf
11. Alzheimer's Society (2021). This is me: a support tool to enable person centred care. https://www.alzheimers.org.uk/get-support/publications-factsheets/this-is-me
12. Budson, A.E. and Solomon, P.R. (2015). Evaluating the patient with memory loss or dementia. In: *Memory Loss, Alzheimer's Disease, and Dementia*, 4–36. Elsevier Health Sciences.

13. HEE (2017). Multi-professional framework for advanced clinical practice in England. https://www.hee.nhs.uk/sites/default/files/documents/multi-professionalframeworkforadvancedclinicalpracticeinengland.pdf
14. Age UK (2024). Age UK's blueprint for improving the lives of older people. https://www.ageuk.org.uk/globalassets/age-uk/documents/campaigns/ge-202425/general_election_manifesto_2425.pdf
15. Centre for Ageing Better (2020). Doddery but dear? Examining age-related stereotypes. https://www.ageing-better.org.uk/sites/default/files/2020-03/Doddery-but-dear.pdf
16. Levy, B. (2009). Stereotype embodiment: A psychosocial approach to aging. *Current Directions in Psychological Science* 18 (6): 332–336.
17. Levy, B.R., Slade, M.D., Kunkel, S.R., and Kasl, S.V. (2002). Longevity increased by positive self-perceptions of aging. *Journal of Personality and Social Psychology* 83 (2): 261–267.
18. Swift, H.J., Abrams, D., Lamont, R.A., and Drury, L. (2017). The risks of ageism model: How ageism and negative attitudes toward age can be a barrier to active aging. *Social Issues and Policy Review* 11 (1): 195–231.
19. World Health Organisation (2021). *Global Report on Ageism*. Geneva: World Health Organization. https://iris.who.int/bitstream/handle/10665/340208/9789240016866-eng.p.
20. Lyons, A., Alba, B., Heywood, W. et al. (2017). Experiences of ageism and the mental health of older adults. *Well-Being and Mental Health* 1456–1464.
21. Centre for Ageing Better (2020). An old age problem? How society shapes and reinforces negative attitudes to ageing. https://www.ageing-better.org.uk/publications/old-age-problem-how-society-shapes-and-reinforces-negative-attitudes-ageing
22. Nursing and Midwifery Council (NMC) (2023). The code: professional standards of practice and behaviour for nurses, midwives and nursing associates. https://www.nmc.org.uk/standards/code/
23. Reynolds, C.F., Jeste, D.V., Sachdev, P.S., and Blazer, D. (2022). Mental health care for older adults: recent advances and new directions in clinical practice and research. *World Psychiatry* 21 (3): 336–363.
24. Soltan, M. and Girguis, J. (2017). How to approach the mental state examination. *British Medical Journal* 357. https://doi.org/10.1136/sbmj.j1821.
25. Beishon, L.C., Batterham, A.P., Quinn, T.J. et al. (2019). Addenbrooke's Cognitive Examination III (ACE-III) and mini-ACE for the detection of dementia and mild cognitive impairment. *Cochrane Database of Systematic Reviews* 12: CD013282.
26. World Health Organisation (WHO) (2022). ICD-11 INTERNATIONAL CLASSIFICATION OF DISEASES – mortality and morbidity statistics. https://icd.who.int/en
27. Goldberg, J. and Stahl, S. (2024). Chapter 1: Making sense of the senseless: how to gather and organize pertinent information. In: *Clinical Reasoning in Psychiatry*, 1–25. Cambridge University Press. https://www.cambridge.org/core/books/clinical-reasoning-and-decisionmaking-in-psychiatry/making-sense-of-the-senseless-how-to-gather-and-organize-pertinent-information/BC35EDE101079A04B8B960E427EC2893
28. NHS England and NHS Improvement (2017). Mental health in older people a practice primer. https://www.england.nhs.uk/wp-content/uploads/2017/09/practice-primer.pdf
29. NHS England and NHS Improvement (2017). Mental health in older people a practice primer. p. 32. https://www.england.nhs.uk/wp-content/uploads/2017/09/practice-primer.pdf
30. Launer, J. (1999). A narrative approach to mental health in general practice. *British Journal of Medicine* 318 (7176): 117–119. https://doi.org/10.1136/bmj.318.7176.117.
31. Goldberg, J. and Stahl, S. (2024). Chapter 2: The approach to diagnostic ambiguity. In: *Clinical Reasoning in Psychiatry*, 26–51. Cambridge University Press. https://www.cambridge.org/core/books/clinical-reasoning-and-decisionmaking-in-psychiatry/approach-to-diagnostic-ambiguity/DE1B7BB4F7B2AB1D4FF9B60C28AB68F8

32. Johnson, H.L., Beatty, J.R., Archer, H.R. et al. (2023). Applying the RIME Framework to Level Nurse Practitioner Curriculum Competencies. *Nurse Education* 48 (1): 43–48. https://pubmed.ncbi.nlm.nih.gov/35977345/
33. Oyabede, F. (2015). *Sims' Symptoms of the Mind: Textbook of Descriptive Psychopathology*, 5th ed. Elsevier: Saunders.
34. Correia, R. and Jackson, D. (2021). Risk to self: identifying and managing risk of suicide and self-harm. *BJPsych Advances* 27 (2): 126–136. https://www.cambridge.org/core/journals/bjpsych-advances/article/risk-to-self-identifying-and-managing-risk-of-suicide-and-selfharm/7FE846E28CBEC14534E0B391F950445C
35. O'Callaghan, C., Richman, A., and Majumdar, B. (2010). Violence in older people with mental illness. *Advances in Psychiatric Treatment* 16 (5): 339–348. https://www.cambridge.org/core/journals/advances-in-psychiatric-treatment/article/violence-in-older-people-with-mental-illness/EC61BF3AB50410204AD445137DABE99F
36. Aziz, V., Rafferty, D., and Jurewicz, I. (2017). Disordered eating in older people: Some causes and treatments. *BJPsych Advances* 23 (5): 331–337. https://www.cambridge.org/core/journals/bjpsych-advances/article/disordered-eating-in-older-people-some-causes-and-treatments/0F154FFC05FD133ACAC04A19ECF3258F
37. Rao, R. and Crome, I. (2016). Alcohol misuse in older people. *BJPsych Advances* 22 (2): 118–126. https://www.cambridge.org/core/journals/bjpsych-advances/article/alcohol-misuse-in-older-people/FA7BD9C2C3CF8E393BB25E1CD39DE8D8
38. Wilson, J., Mart, M., Cunningham, C. et al. (2020). Delirium. *National Review, Disease Primers.* 6 (1): 90. https://doi.org/10.1038/s41572-020-00223-4.
39. Beck, A.T., Steer, R.A., and Brown, G.K. (1996). *Manual for the Beck Depression Inventory-II San Antonio.* TX: Psychological Corporation.
40. Hamilton, M. (1960). A rating scale for depression. *Journal of Neurology, Neurosurgery and Psychiatry* 23 (1): 56–62. https://doi.org/10.1136/jnnp.23.1.56.
41. Young, R.C., Biggs, J.T., Ziegler, V.E., and Meyer, D.A. (1978). A rating scale for mania: Reliability, validity and sensitivity. *The British Journal of Psychiatry* 133 (5): 429–435.
42. Kay, S.R., Fizbein, A., and Opler, L. (1987). The Positive and Negative Symptom Scale (PANSS) for schizophrenia. *Schizophrenia Bulletin* 13 (2): 261–276.
43. Yesavage, J., Brink, T., Rose, T. et al. (1983). Development and validation of a geratric depression screening scale: a preliminary Report. *Journal of Psychiatric Research* 17 (1): 37–49.
44. Panchana, N., Byre, G., Siddle, H. et al. (2007). Development and validation of the geriatric anxiety inventory. *Internationla Psychogeriatrics* 19 (1): 103–114.
45. Inouye, S., Van Dyck, C., Alessi, C. et al. (1990). Clarifying confusion: the confusion assessment method. *Annals of Internal Medicine* 113 (12): 941–948.
46. Manthorpe, J. and Iliffe, S. (2005). *Depression in Later Life*. London: Jessica Kingsley.
47. National Institute on Aging (2023). Depression and older adults. https://www.nia.nih.gov/health/mental-and-emotional-health/depression-and-older-adults
48. Devita, M., De Salvo, R., Ravelli, A. et al. (2022). Recognizing depression in the elderly: practical guidance and challenges for clinical management. *Neuropsychiatric Disease and Treatment* 18: 2867–2880.
49. National Institute for Health and Care Excellence (NICE) (2009). Depression in Adults: Recognition and Management (NICE Clinical Guideline CG90). https://www.nice.org.uk/guideance/cg90.

50. Correll, C.U., Solmi, M., Veronese, N. et al. (2017). Prevalence, incidence and mortality from cardiovascular disease in patients with pooled and specific severe mental illness: a large-scale meta-analysis of 3,211,768 patients and 113,383,368 controls. *World Psychiatry* 16 (2): 163–180. https://onlinelibrary.wiley.com/doi/full/10.1002/wps.20420.
51. Dhar, A.K. and Barton, D.A. (2016). Depression and the link with cardiovascular disease. *Frontiers in Psychiatry* 7: 33.
52. Brennan, P., Schutte, K.K., and Moos, R.H. (2005). Pain and use of alcohol to manage pain: prevalence and 3-year outcomes among older problem and non-problem drinkers. *Addiction* 100 (6): 777–786. https://pubmed.ncbi.nlm.nih.gov/15918808/.
53. NHS England (2024). Frail Strategy: A strategy for the development and/or improvement of acute frailty same day emergency care services. https://www.england.nhs.uk/long-read/frail-strategy/
54. Rockwood, K., Song, X., MacKnight, C. et al. (2005). A global clinical measure of fitness and frailty in elderly people. *Canadian Medical Association Journal* 173 (5): 489–495.
55. Taylor, D., Barnes, T., and Young, A. (2025). Prescribing in older people. In: *The Maudsley Prescribing Guidelines in Psychiatry*, 15th ed. Blackwell: Wiley.
56. Taylor, D., Barnes, T., and Young, A. (2025). Prescribing in older people. In: *The Maudsley Prescribing Guidelines in Psychiatry*, 15th ed, 601. Blackwell: Wiley.
57. King's Fund (2013). Polypharmacy and medicines optimisation: making it safe and sound. https://www.kingsfund.org.uk/insight-and-analysis/reports/polypharmacy-and-medicines-optimisation
58. Taylor, D.M., Gaughran, F., and Pillinger, T. (2021). Sodium Derangement. In: *The Maudsley Practice Guidelines for Physical Health Conditions in Psychiatry*, 273–227. Blackwell: Wiley.
59. Peters, N. and Thompson, C. (2020). Syndrome of inappropriate antidiuretic hormone (SIADH) induced by antidepressants: a case report and review. *Cureus* 12 (9).
60. BMJ (2015). Assessment of delirium. BMJ. http://bestpractice.com.bmj.com
61. Muliyala, K.P. and Varghese, M. (2010). The complex relationship between depression and dementia. *Annals of Indian Academy of Neurology* 13 (Suppl2): S69–S73. https://pmc.ncbi.nlm.nih.gov/articles/PMC3039168/.
62. Park, S.H. and Cho, Y.S. (2022). Predictive validity of the Cornell scale for depression in dementia among older adults with and without dementia: a systematic review and meta-analysis. *Psychiatry Research* 310. https://doi.org/10.1016/j.psychres.2022.114445.
63. Kitching, D. (2015). Depression in dementia. *Australian Prescriber* 209–2011. https://10.18773/austprescr.2015.071.
64. Jin, J. (2020). Screening for cognitive impairment in older adults. *JAMA* 323 (8): 800. https://jamanetwork.com/journals/jama/fullarticle/2761646
65. NICE (2018). Dementia: assessment, management and support for people living with dementia and their carers. NICE guideline (NG97). https://www.nice.org.uk/guidance/ng97
66. Mental Capacity Act (2005). https://www.legislation.gov.uk/ukpga/2005/9/contents
67. Mental Health Act (1983). https://www.legislation.gov.uk/ukpga/1983/20/contents

CHAPTER 16

Supporting People with Learning Disabilities and Autistic People

Jo Delrée[1] and Sue Bridges[2]

[1] Delree Training and Consultancy, London, UK
[2] Norfolk and Suffolk NHS Foundation Trust, Norwich, UK

> **Aim**
>
> This chapter will support advanced practitioners in mental health (APMH) towards an increased understanding and improved skills in working with learning disabled (LD) and/or autistic populations in order to promote safe and accurate assessment of these groups at an advanced level. It also encourages the advanced practitioner to reflect on the appropriate or inappropriate prescribing of medications for this group and the interplay between mental illness, physical illness and behaviour.

LEARNING OUTCOMES

After reading this chapter, the reader will be able to:

- Understand advanced practice in mental health in the context of people with LD and autistic people.
- Understand atypical presentations of mental illness in this population.
- Understand behaviour as communication.
- Recognise and support good practice in physical and mental health, avoiding diagnostic overshadowing and over-medication.

The Advanced Practitioner in Mental Health, First Edition. Edited by Clare Allabyrne.
© 2026 John Wiley & Sons Ltd. All rights reserved, including rights for text and data mining and training of artificial intelligence technologies or similar technologies. Published 2026 by John Wiley & Sons Ltd.

NHS England Mental Health advanced practice area specific capability and curriculum framework [1] 2022:

This chapter supports the following domains:

Domain A:
1.13 Demonstrate a critical understanding of their broadened level of critical decision-making, accountability, responsibility and autonomy, and the limits of their own competence and professional scope of practice, including when working with conflict, complexity, risk, uncertainty and incomplete information.
1.17 Promote and demonstrate action in support of marginalised, under-represented and disadvantaged people and groups.
Domain B1:
2.2 Demonstrate advanced knowledge and understanding of mental health-related presentations.
Domain B2:
2.7 Critically apply advanced knowledge of mental health and illness.
Domain C:
3.1 Use expertise and decision-making skills to inform clinical reasoning approaches when dealing with differentiated and undifferentiated individual presentations and complex situations, synthesising information from multiple sources to make appropriate, evidence-based judgements and/or diagnoses.
3.2 Develop differential judgements, recognising key biases and common errors, including diagnostic overshadowing and the issues relating to diagnosis in the face of ambiguity and incomplete data.
Domain D2:
4.4 In the presence of uncertainty/emergency/emergent risk, analyse and modify intervention to mitigate risk.

INTRODUCTION

Working with people who are mentally unwell, have a learning disability and/or are autistic requires an understanding of those conditions, an understanding of mental illness and an understanding of how those things impact the individual. This chapter cannot possibly cover the depth or breadth of knowledge that is required to fully appreciate the needs and complexities of these populations; however, it will provide some information about how mental illness impacts autistic people and people with learning disabilities, as well as some suggestions for how they can be better supported in advanced practice. It will review some underpinning principles, such as parity of esteem and diagnostic overshadowing, the need for professional curiosity and the use of reasonable adjustments.

It will also provide some statistics and information on the more common mental illnesses and give some information on good practice at an advanced level.

Oftentimes supporting a person who is mentally unwell and has a learning disability and/or is autistic requires a multidisciplinary approach, and there are of course experts in the fields of autism and learning disability who can and should be consulted alongside family, carers or whoever knows the person best.

Fundamental to the chapter is the fact that people with learning disabilities and autistic people deserve a good standard of care as equal and valued citizens.

AUTISM AND MENTAL ILLNESS

Autism is a lifelong condition believed to be caused by a diverse range of neurological differences. Autism is often described as a 'spectrum', or more recently among autistic communities a 'wheel', [2] meaning that there are wide-ranging expressions of the condition. Diagnostically, autism is characterised by social communication differences and restricted, repetitive and inflexible patterns of behaviour, interests or activities, alongside sensory processing issues; however, how the individual experiences and expresses this varies greatly. If we understand autism as a spectrum, with so-called 'low functioning' individuals at one end and 'high functioning' at the other, we risk simplifying what is in fact a complex and nuanced condition. There is a risk that people who are thought of as being 'low functioning' are not given access to opportunities that would expand or develop their skills and abilities, while those labelled 'high functioning' may be denied access to the support that they need. If we use a wheel to help us visualise the autism, it can help us to understand all of the individual variation that we see amongst autistic individuals and respond to their needs more appropriately.

As our understanding of autism and the autistic experience has grown, so has our awareness of the breadth of the spectrum. This is particularly the case when we consider how autism can present in women and girls.

Historically, it was thought that cisgender males were more commonly affected than females, with the given ratio of 4:1. Now that ratio is thought to be closer to 3:4 [3, 4], although autism is widely believed to be underdiagnosed in females, with only around 20% receiving a diagnosis before the age of 18 [4]. This is in part due to historical concepts of autism, which were based on mainly male subjects, but is also linked to the different way in which autism is expressed in women and girls [5]. This is a complex and developing field, and cannot be covered in any depth here, but it is important for the advanced practitioner in mental health to have at least a basic understanding of these differences and the potential impact that they have on mental health. One key factor in this regard is the tendency for autistic females to internalise problems, unlike their male counterparts, who tend to externalise; so, we see more behavioural outbursts or destructive/disruptive behaviour in males, which is often the prompt to pursue diagnosis. The tendency for females to internalise means that those behaviours are not present, so their autism isn't recognised and/or diagnosis is not sought. It should be noted that not all autistic males display aggressive or disruptive behaviour, however.

Internalising can also lead to mental ill health [6] as can camouflaging, or masking, which is also believed to affect females more than males [6, 7], although males do report this behaviour too. Essentially, this is when the individual learns to imitate neurotypical behaviour, particularly in social situations, in order to cope and not stand out as being different. Autistic individuals may also compensate for a lack of instinctive understanding using cognitive strategies [8]. For instance, where a neurotypical person may recognise a facial expression instinctively, an autistic person may compensate for this cognitively by learning what different expressions mean and how they should respond to them. These strategies can be very effective in masking an individual's autism, and again contribute to under-diagnosis, but are exhausting and can contribute to long-term mental illness [6, 7].

It should also be borne in mind that some, though not all, autistic people also have a learning disability, which will also affect their understanding and communication.

This knowledge should support the advanced practitioner to contextualise the following information about mental health and autism.

Autistic people experience the same range of mental illnesses as the general population and there is evidence that there is a greater prevalence of mental illness in this group [9, 10]. However, the way that autism affects an individual and their behaviour can make identifying symptoms of mental illness more complicated [11] and can potentially lead to mis- or under-diagnosis, and as a result autistic people are not getting the help that they need in a timely fashion.

Depression rates are thought to be up to four times higher in the autistic population and anxiety disorders affect 20% compared with 4% in the general population. There are also increased rates of disruptive/impulse-control/conduct disorders, obsessive-compulsive disorder (OCD) and bipolar disorders. Schizophrenia rates are increased too, at around 3.6 times the general population prevalence [9, 10, 12, 13].

Personality disorder (PD) is also more common with some studies suggesting that 50% of autistic people fulfil the diagnostic criteria for PD. It should be noted that the relationship between autism and PD is complex and requires further research [14]; however, there are some clear commonalities – for instance, atypical social approaches, altered empathy, difficulty maintaining relationships, unattainably high expectations of others' behaviour etc.; though the motivations/cognitive processes that underpin the characteristics may be different. For instance, the intense, unstable personal relationships seen in PD could be understood as an autistic special interest and the 'unreasonable and demanding' behaviour ascribed to PD could in fact be the rigid, perseverant thinking/rule adherence associated with autism [15].

One crucial point for the advanced practitioner to note is the increased trauma and suicide risk common to both groups [14].

Another example of these complex relationships and diagnostic overlaps can be seen when considering eating disorders. Autism is more common in individuals with anorexia nervosa, with some studies suggesting that 10% of females presenting to eating disorder services have an autism diagnosis, with a further 17.5% going on to receive a diagnosis of an eating disorder [16, 17]. Again, complexities and overlaps exist, and ways of discerning between disordered eating as a result of autism and eating disorders in autistic individuals continue to develop. It should be noted that in both PD and eating disorders, females are more affected than males.

AUTISM AND GENDER IDENTITY

This is a relatively new area in terms of research; however, it is generally accepted that autism is more prevalent in the transgender population, and that gender incongruence is higher in the autistic population compared with general population rates [18]. This is a complex area and though there is insufficient space in this chapter to do it justice, the advanced practitioner should be aware of issues around gender variance in autistic people, since anxiety and depression seem to be common for this specific group [19].

LEARNING DISABILITY AND MENTAL ILL HEALTH

A learning disability is defined as impaired Intelligence (IQ below 70), reduced ability to understand new or complex information and impaired ability to learn new skills, along with impaired social functioning. There is considerable overlap between autism and learning disability; exact prevalence rates are hard to establish and there is considerable variance but it is estimated that around a third of people with learning disabilities are also autistic and similarly around a third of autistic people have a learning disability [20, 21].

Overall, evidence suggests that mental illness is more common in people with learning disabilities, with studies spanning well over a decade suggesting that it is twice as prevalent compared to the general population [20, 22–27].

Increased rates of mental ill health seem to begin in childhood for this group. Buckley et al. [28] note that psychiatric symptoms in young people with learning disabilities are more than three times higher than the general population but also note that formal diagnoses are similar to the general population, suggesting that formal diagnostic processes are not capturing the full extent of mental ill health in this population. This should be a consideration for Child and Adolescent Mental Health Services (CAMHS) services, who will certainly see children and young people with learning disabilities and therefore need CAMHS practitioners to have a good understanding of the needs of young people with learning disabilities who are mentally unwell.

Depression occurs at approximately three times the general population rate in people with learning disabilities and is probably the most common mental illness in this population [22, 25, 27, 29, 30].

The prevalence of anxiety disorders in the learning disabled population is hard to establish but is generally accepted to be as prevalent as in the general population, if not more so [22, 25, 31].

Schizophrenia is three times more prevalent in people with learning disabilities [14, 22, 24, 32] but may be mis- or underdiagnosed.

THE ROLE OF THE ADVANCED PRACTITIONER IN SUPPORTING PEOPLE WITH LEARNING DISABILITIES AND AUTISTIC PEOPLE

Considering the previously presented information, the advanced practitioner is likely to come across autistic people and people with learning disabilities who are mentally unwell in the course of their work and therefore must be fully cognisant of the needs and presentations of people with learning disabilities and autistic people.

A lack of knowledge, or even more worryingly, a lack of regard for this group is dangerous, and significantly contributes to poor treatment outcomes, poor mental and physical health and the untimely deaths of people with learning disabilities and autistic people. The concept of parity of esteem, which originated in the field of learning disability nursing, has been highlighted for many years [33, 34], stating the need to place equal importance on physical and mental health and also to address the health inequalities experienced by people who are mentally ill. When advanced practitioners are working with autistic people and those with a learning disability, this takes on an additional dimension – equal weight must be given to mental and physical health, but this needs to be done in the context of the individual and how they are affected by their autism and/or learning disability, acknowledging and actively working to prevent the health inequalities experienced by people with learning disabilities and autistic people.

ATYPICAL PRESENTATIONS – AVOIDING DIAGNOSTIC OVERSHADOWING

Symptoms of mental ill health can be difficult to spot in people with learning disabilities and autistic people, especially where people do not use speech or there are communication issues. It is easy for mental illness to be overlooked or for diagnostic overshadowing to come into play.

Diagnostic overshadowing is the tendency to attribute presenting symptoms to a pre-existing condition. In autistic people and people with a learning disability, this means that psychiatric symptoms, or behaviour changes caused by underlying pain or physical ill health, may be explained away as 'autistic behaviours' or as being caused by the person having a learning disability. This is an extremely dangerous phenomenon. The LeDeR report [35] discussed in more depth later in this chapter, which looks into the deaths of people with learning disabilities, tells us that people with a learning disability are twice as likely to die an avoidable death. Much of this is due to a combination of poor treatment, a lack of reasonable adjustments, misdiagnosis and treatment delays, caused by unconscious bias and diagnostic overshadowing [36]. In psychiatric services, this same phenomenon leads to the misdiagnosis and underdiagnosis of mental illness [37].

To avoid this, it is vital that when we are working with autistic people and people with a learning disability, we engage our 'professional curiosity'. This is a term used across many disciplines, but in essence requires the practitioner to question presenting information – looking for explanations based on their knowledge of relevant evidence and good practice [38, 39]. In this instance, it requires us to ask *why?* Why would a person use that behaviour? What circumstances (internal and external) would cause a person to act that way? What symptom of a mental (or physical) illness could manifest in this way if a person does not use speech to communicate? How would a person describe that feeling if their interoception (their sense of their internal environment – how their body feels and how this interacts with emotions) is atypical? Essentially it is about understanding the commonalities of the human experience (what would make *any* person behave in that way? What would make *me* act like that?) before we look for the differences that autism and learning disability may (or may not) add. This requires an understanding of the symptoms of mental illness, an understanding of autism and/or learning disability, but most importantly, an understanding of the person at the centre of our care.

Even when we are fully aware of all of the aforementioned, it can still be difficult to differentiate the symptoms of mental illness from an exacerbation of autistic behaviours or other existing behaviours.

Diagnosing schizophrenia in a person with limited verbal 'self-report' skills can be complicated. Delusions can be mistaken for autistic idiosyncrasies and vice-versa.

Disorganised speech may be difficult to spot in a person whose speech is usually idiosyncratic, and disorganised behaviour may be interpreted as challenging behaviour due to autism and not given further thought (this would be an example of diagnostic overshadowing). Negative symptoms of schizophrenia can be particularly problematic, as they overlap with autistic responses such as social withdrawal and reduced motivation [10, 40].

OCD, post-traumatic stress disorder or mood disorders in autistic people may also be misinterpreted as psychosis, or vice versa [40–43]. Once again, the behaviours that these conditions create can look like autistic behaviour – hence the need to engage professional curiosity and make sure we know why a behaviour is occurring – particularly looking for new behaviours and behaviour change.

For the same reasons, and despite it being so common in autistic people and people with learning disabilities, depression is also easily overlooked and is thought to be mis- or under-diagnosed frequently. Again, there is overlap with some autistic behaviours, but additionally some atypical symptoms such as self- injurious behaviour, psychomotor changes or changes in autistic behaviours [44] can indicate depression in an autistic person.

For people with learning disabilities who experience communication barriers, self-report of depressive symptoms may be difficult or impossible. In such instances, changes in behaviour such as changes in appetite and weight, changes in sleep patterns, loss of interest in preferred activities, increased irritability or challenging behaviour, increased dependence on carers or skill loss should be considered as potential symptoms of depression.

Symptoms of anxiety can be similar to some characteristics of autism, which can make differentiation difficult. Preoccupations, repetitive behaviours (e.g. obsessions and compulsions), speech irregularities, deficits in emotion recognition, avoiding of social situations, being withdrawn, impairments in reciprocal social interaction and reduced eye contact and restricted, repetitive, and stereotyped behaviours are all associated with both conditions [45], so the advanced practitioner will need to be detailed in their history taking to be able to differentiate.

In people with learning disabilities who experience communication difficulties, clinicians once more need to look at behaviour and behaviour change which could indicate anxiety, such as irritability, increased challenging behaviour, sleep disturbance etc. Physical symptoms such as rapid heartbeat/palpitations, increased respiratory rate, muscle tension or weakness, digestive issues, sweating etc. should also be considered.

As previously noted, up to 50% of autistic people may fulfil the diagnostic criteria for PD. It should be noted that the relationship between autism and PD is complex and requires further research [46].

There is a particular issue with misdiagnosis of PD in autistic females who have no verbal communication issues or learning disability, since both conditions can lead to difficulties in developing and maintaining relationships, problems with identity, problems with anger and self-regulation and self-damaging behaviour [47]. This makes it important to look at the overall clinical picture and history, rather than focussing on specific/presenting symptoms before drawing any conclusions or making a diagnosis.

The identification of eating disorders presents a similar challenge in this group. Some of the cognitive features of autism are present in individuals with anorexia nervosa who are not autistic, in particular, cognitive inflexibility, weak central coherence and social cognitive impairment. It is also suggested that for some autistic people, applying strict rules to eating may have a functional role, helping the individual to cope with other stressors. This would explain why recovery from anorexia nervosa is a comparatively longer process for autistic people and highlights the importance of differentiating between disordered eating as a result of autism and eating disorders, since treatment and supports would be different [16, 17].

CLINICAL INVESTIGATIONS: TOOLS TO SUPPORT PHYSICAL HEALTH AND PAIN ASSESSMENT

Various tools have been developed to support clinicians to understand behaviour as a form of communication and reduce the risk of diagnostic overshadowing. The following are pain assessment tools that use clinician or carer reports to observe and assess behavioural manifestations of pain, such as facial expressions, vocalisations and body movements.

For children with learning disabilities/autistic children:

- the Non-communicating Children's Pain Checklist [48]
- the revised Face, Legs, Activity, Cry, Consolability Scale [49]

For adults with learning disabilities/autistic adults:

- the Non-communicating Adults Pain Checklist [50]

CLINICAL INVESTIGATIONS: MENTAL HEALTH ASSESSMENT TOOLS FOR PEOPLE WITH LEARNING DISABILITIES AND AUTISTIC PEOPLE

The are numerous mental health assessment tools but few specifically designed for people with a learning disability. Most tools can be adapted to meet the cognitive ability and communication needs of the individual.

The Moss-PAS (ID) (previously called Mini Psychiatric Assessment Schedule for Adults with a Developmental Disability [PAS-ADD]) provides a wide-spectrum mental health assessment primarily designed for people with learning disabilities who have limited language or reduced cognitive development. The tool can be used to collect symptom information directly from an individual or can be completed by staff on the basis of knowledge already possessed about the individual. The score form enables two different clinical episodes to be rated on the same form, in order to assess significant change or fluctuating mood disorder [51].

The broad areas of the checklist encompass:

- Appetite and sleep
- Tension and worry
- Phobias and panics
- Depression and hypomania
- Obsessions and compulsions
- Psychoses
- Autism

The Psychiatric Autism Checklist [52] has been found to be useful in identifying autistic adults who need psychiatric services. This uses carers and family members observations to support clinicians to build a fuller picture of the individuals mental health.

> Learning event 1: Read the RCN document on mental health assessment for people with learning disabilities. Reflect upon how you could include some of these good practice examples into your own practice.
> Conducting mental health assessments of people with learning disabilities (http://rcni.com)

PHARMACOLOGY AND STOPPING OVERMEDICATION OF PEOPLE WITH A LEARNING DISABILITY, AUTISM OR BOTH (STOMP)

The same universal principles that apply for all patients should also be followed in relation to pharmacology for both these client groups. Most psychiatric disorders use both psychosocial and pharmacological interventions. In relation specifically to mental health patients who use medication to help manage their illness, concordance may be an issue, especially for those whose symptoms are severe. Not taking a prescribed medication can lead to worsening of the illness, further interventions and admission to hospital. The input and expertise of a pharmacist is said to be good practice when prescribing and monitoring a medication for severe mental health conditions [53].

When working with people with learning disabilities, it is important to consider their ability to take oral medications, particularly in tablet form, as some may have dysphagia or other musculoskeletal or sensory issues that make swallowing tablets problematic. Liquid forms of medications can be considered or patches. Since it is known that adults with learning disabilities are more likely to be both over and underweight than the general population, this should be considered when considering dosage.

The overmedication of people with learning disabilities and/or autism has been an issue for many years [54], including the use of psychotropic drugs without a clear association with their primary indication. Prescribing such medicines as an intervention for challenging behaviour, without considering physical and environmental/contextual causes for the behaviour, is also an ongoing problem. Practitioners need to be aware of the issue of overmedication and other available interventions to ensure that questions are asked before medication is prescribed as a default, and to make sure that people receive holistic, high-quality care.

Stopping overmedication of people with a learning disability, autism or both (STOMP) is a campaign launched in 2016 by NHS England [55] to stop the excessive use of psychotropic medication with people with learning disabilities and autistic people. Psychotropic medicines affect how the brain works and include medicines for psychosis, depression, anxiety, sleep problems and epilepsy. People with a learning disability, autism or both are more likely to be given these medicines than other people often because their behaviour is seen as challenging. The campaign was launched to ensure the overuse of these medicines stops. These medicines are right for some people. They can help people stay safe and well. Sometimes there are other ways of helping people, so they need less medicine or none at all. It should be noted, however, that there is little research regarding the safety and efficacy of psychoactive medications in the learning disability population [56].

LEARNING DISABILITIES MORTALITY REVIEW (LeDeR)

Research has shown that on average, people with a learning disability and autistic people die at least 20 years earlier than the general public and do not receive the same quality of care as people without a learning disability or who are not autistic [57].

Established in 2017, and funded by NHS England, the LeDeR programme reviews all the deaths of people with a learning disability and autistic people and aims to:

- Improve care for people with a learning disability and autistic people.
- Reduce health inequalities for people with a learning disability and autistic people.
- Prevent people with a learning disability and autistic people from early deaths.

> Learning event 2: Read the information about the LeDeR programme [57].
> LeDeR – About LeDeR, consider why there are health inequalities for people with a learning disability and autistic people. What can you do to change your practice to ensure that people have a better health outcome?

GOOD PRACTICE IN MENTAL HEALTH SERVICES – THE GREEN LIGHT TOOLKIT

The Green Light Toolkit [58] provides a framework to help mental health services meet legal requirements and respond to the needs of people with learning disabilities and/or autistic people. Originally developed by the National Development Team for Inclusion (NDTI) in 2004, the Toolkit has undergone many revisions to adapt to changes in legislation and service delivery. The latest version (2022) can be found on the NDTI website www.ndti.org.uk/resources/green-light-toolkit

The Green Light Toolkit supports mental health services to provide effective care for:

- Autistic people
- People with learning disabilities
- Autistic people with learning disabilities

It briefly acknowledges that people living with other kinds of neurodiversity, such as attention deficit hyperactivity disorder, dyspraxia, dyscalculia or Tourette's syndrome may need mental healthcare too; they may also be autistic and/or have learning disabilities. Because the approach taken by the Green Light Toolkit is based on human rights and access to reasonable adjustments, it is applicable to all.

Advocated by the Care Quality Commission the Green Light Toolkit is seen as a good practice resource. As a framework of standards, it includes an online audit to effectively benchmark services and make informed decisions about where to make improvements. The Green Light Toolkit standards enhance the NHS England Learning Disability Improvement Standards, which pay particular attention to data collection related to the Building the Right Support programme and the Learning Disabilities Mortality Review. NHS England [59] have four improvement standards which concern:

- Respecting and protecting rights
- Inclusion
- Engagement
- Workforce

Some mental health services have used the Green Light Toolkit alongside the Improvement Standards so that the detailed work on reasonable adjustments for autistic people and people with learning disabilities is then enriched by the wider comparisons generated through use of the Improvement Standards.

Autistic people and people with a learning disability should expect high-quality care across NHS services, people should be able to live ordinary lives and access mainstream services, including mental health services wherever possible. The Autism Act 2009 [49] and its accompanying autism strategy [60] and Implementation plan [60] shapes what is offered to autistic people, while people with learning disabilities are included in the National Disability Strategy [61]. The Mental Capacity Act 2005 [62], Equality Act 2010 [63], Health and Social Care Act 2021 [64], Care Act 2014 [65] and Accessible Information Standards 2016 [66] are all influential in ensuring equitable services too.

This means that there is a clear duty and expectation for the advanced practitioner to have the skills to meet the needs of individuals with a learning disability and autistic individuals should they access the services where they are working, with support from specialist colleagues and the multidisciplinary team.

The Green Light Toolkit ensures mental health services provide fair access, make reasonable adjustments and work jointly with learning disability services. This can reduce anxiety and lack of confidence among staff, which have been found to be barriers to fair access to services for people with learning disabilities or autistic people. Completing the audit annually allows services to determine how well they meet the needs of these groups and identify areas requiring improvement.

The toolkit advocates for a Green Light Facilitator to be employed to coordinate activity across the mental health organisation while Green Light Champions in every team will be focus on this area of work alongside their other duties.

Within an organisation, Green Light Champions are responsible for completing the audit in their team; this can be done by the champions themselves or collectively in team meetings. The purpose is to obtain a collective picture of each team's performance, rather than individual views, as managers and frontline staff often have differing views on how the team is doing. The role should be taken up by a staff member who has prior training or experience in working with autistic people or people with learning disabilities, or by someone who is simply interested in learning. Due to their unique skill set Advanced Practitioners in Mental Health are ideally placed to be Green Light Champions.

The audit contains 27 standards and a Likert score of where individuals feel the team is graded. The standards include topics such as staff attitudes and values, buildings and environments, healthcare records, care plans, therapies, eligibility and access and leadership. All the standards are based on a human rights approach to provide the best possible care. Once benchmarked, the submission to the NDTI will produce an organisational report to provide an opportunity to develop and improve on the scores and in turn the delivery of care to individuals.

Mental health services should make adjustments to what they do so that autistic people, people with learning disabilities and autistic people with learning disabilities can obtain effective help when they need it. As a result, environments will become quieter, communication clearer and staff will provide more person-centred care.

The NDTI [58] state that the refreshed Green Light Toolkit will help mental health communities to consider what they can do. It offers more choice and control than before, so everyone can work together. Good solutions will be coproduced, since expertise comes from life and research. Families can be involved in taking stock too, as they are keenly aware of what is working and what is not. Together, mental health communities will be able to celebrate the best of what they do every day and then bravely name the difficulties that remain and plan to overcome them. In these busy times, addressing the Green Light agenda is not easy. Despite the challenges, it reduces discrimination, serves the whole community and improves outcomes in line with government expectations. Most importantly, it provides the kind of service that autistic people and people with learning disabilities deserve. We hope that mental health services will rise to the challenge.

A best practice example of how the Green Light Toolkit can be used can be found here:

https://webarchive.nationalarchives.gov.uk/ukgwa/20200501110649/https://improvement.nhs.uk/resources/learning-disability-improvement-guides

GOOD PRACTICE IN MENTAL HEALTH SERVICES – REASONABLE ADJUSTMENTS

Small changes, based on an understanding of the needs of the individual, can have big impacts on care outcomes. It is worth considering how you can adapt environments to ensure that people with learning disabilities and autistic people can better access mental health services. For instance, familiarising people with the environment with a visit, photos or videos before the assessment/admission; meeting the clinician beforehand; ensuring that waiting time is limited (the first appointment of the day or after lunch perhaps); and holding the assessment in a quiet, calm environment can all contribute to a successful outcome.

The use of alternative communication methods, such as social stories and simple (perhaps easy read for some) written information to prepare for a visit can be helpful.

Using pictures, signs and symbols can help people who have a learning disability and autism to understand what is being asked of them. Body maps are a useful tool to aid people in pinpointing and communicating pain. Information from carers and family can be particularly useful, in order to determine what reasonable adjustments are needed, and also generally in the individual's care.

Finally, the environment in which the assessment is undertaken should be carefully considered in relation to the sensory processing issues that autistic people experience. Busy, noisy, smelly, cluttered, bright environments are likely to be overwhelming and lead to additional stress, making assessment harder for the clinician and very unpleasant or even painful for the patient. Consider making simple changes to the environment, such as shutting doors or blinds to eliminate noise or glare or find a quiet spot. Double appointments to allow extra time, and appointments at the beginning of a clinic where there will be little waiting could be arranged. All these things would be considered reasonable adjustments under the Equality Act [54].

In line with Nursing and Midwifery Council guidelines regarding confidentiality, the cases below do not identify any individual person or their family [67].

CLINICAL LEARNING EVENT 1

Emily is a 15-year-old female who was seen by the advanced practitioner in mental health due to family concerns of continued weight loss and food restriction. Emily's BMI is 18. Currently her diet consists of green apples, salt and vinegar crisps from a green packet, rice cereal and milk. Emily reports feeling anxious most of the time and finding school difficult. She achieves good grades, but she is known to have issues with making and maintaining friendships. Emily will not eat, drink or use the toilet at school. Emily presents as nervous and finds it hard to sit still. She is a quiet girl but responds politely to any questions. She is often tearful, and her parents report that she increasingly spends time alone in her room where she likes to draw anime cartoons. Emily is part of an online community of anime enthusiasts and seems to draw support from her online friends.

Personal History

Antenatal and intrapartum complication – No complications
　　Development Milestones – Hit all milestones at right ages, but struggled with the social element of secondary school
　　Childhood environment – Lived with mum and dad. No brothers or sisters
　　Childhood trauma – Was severely bullied in years 7 and 8 at school and eventually moved to a new school.

- ***What does this presentation suggest?***
- ***What differential diagnoses should be considered?***

CLINICAL LEARNING EVENT 2 – (STOMP)

Amy is a 38-year-old woman who had two children in care due to safeguarding concerns around her mental health. Amy lived alone and frequently self-harmed due to the voices telling her to rid herself of demons. Amy was prescribed several antipsychotic medications by both her GP and her psychiatrist.

She was not aware of all the medications she took daily but did take her medication as prescribed. There have been no improvements in her mental health since your last visit. Her social worker felt that Amy's presentation was behavioural rather than mental health. Upon your visit, you felt there were several red flags. On review of the medications there were several contra-indications, and you were concerned that she was being over-medicated.

Personal History

Development Milestones – Hit all milestones at right ages until adolescence. Diagnosed with a learning disability and autism and went to a mainstream school and supported by a classroom assessment but failed to obtain any qualifications.

Childhood environment – Lived with mum, father absent. One sibling who has no contact.

Childhood trauma – There was a history of sexual abuse in childhood. In adolescence Amy had many inappropriate sexual relationships including with two older men resulting in two pregnancies.

- *What are the red flags in this situation?*
- *What would you do in this scenario?*

Case Study 16.1

David was referred to the MH service five times but never attended an appointment. David had bi-polar disorder and struggled with bouts of mania and depression. He lived on his own and there were safeguarding concerns raised by the GP due to self-harming and suicidal ideation. David used recreational drugs to self-medicate, he felt this helped ease his depressive moods when in fact, they heightened his depressive thoughts and his mental health was deteriorating.

When a mental health staff member called on him at home, he said he did not receive any letters about his appointments. Upon further discussion, it was evident that he could not read. He told the staff member that he would scoop up all his post and put it in the bin. The worker, concerned by the lack of support he received and deterioration in his mental health, offered to send future appointment letters in Easy Read format and in a blue envelope so that when it landed on his doormat, he knew to open it. The team sent an easy read appointment letter which included a photograph of the staff member that David was meeting, thus helping to relieve his anxiety when attending his appointments. The blue envelope worked, David engaged in services, underwent assessment and treatment and has been discharged.

Consequently, the organisation sends easy read letters in blue envelopes to people who require these reasonable adjustments. This is an example of best practice.

Case Study 16.2   Physical health (LEDER) highlight red flags and safeguarding

Ali is a 38-year-old man with a mild learning disability and autism. He has a history of dysthymia and anxiety. Ali has been complaining of chest pain and tightness, and says he feels out of breath all the time. He has been to the GP, who told him that everyone gets out of breath sometimes, and that there is nothing wrong with him. On talking to Ali, it does not seem that the GP undertook any other investigations/observations.

> Ali's support worker was concerned that Ali seemed distressed when he came back from the GP and had been dismissed without further investigation, and with Ali's consent, contacted the GP to ask what the next steps should be. The GP again seemed dismissive and said she would make a referral to the LD psychiatry team. The support worker is confused as Ali's mental health seems stable, but the GP insists that Ali does not need a follow up GP appointment. The GP tells the support worker that these are clearly anxiety symptoms associated with Ali's autism, and that he needs support with his mental health not his physical health. Over the weekend while visiting his mother, Ali develops a fever, and the breathlessness worsens. Ali's mother calls an ambulance and he is admitted to hospital with pneumonia.
>
> - *What are the potential risks/red flags here?*
> - *Why is the GP not making appropriate physical health checks?*
> - *Did you want this to be another clinical learning event? Or is there an organisational outcome?*

CONCLUSION

Research tells us that autistic people, people with learning disabilities and autistic people who have learning disabilities continue to experience physical and mental health inequalities. This injustice needs to be viewed by all healthcare practitioners as a priority for change. Advanced practitioners in mental health, with their unique knowledge and skill set, are well placed to address these inequalities, through increasing their understanding of the ways in which mental illnesses affect these populations and ensuring that individuals receive the appropriate and timely healthcare interventions that they deserve.

REFERENCES

1. NHS England (2022). Mental Health advanced practice area specific capability and curriculum framework.
2. AbleLight (2024). Why the autism wheel is replacing the spectrum. https://ablelight.org/blog/why-the-autism-wheel-is-replacing-the-spectrum/ (accessed 07 Jan 2025).
3. Posserud, M.B., Skretting Solberg, B., Engeland, A. et al. (2021). Male to female ratios in autism spectrum disorders by age, intellectual disability and attention-deficit/hyperactivity disorder. *Acta Psychiatrica Scandinavica* 144 (6): 635–646.
4. McCrossin, R. (2022). Finding the true number of females with autistic spectrum disorder by estimating the biases in initial recognition and clinical diagnosis. *Children* 9 (2): 272.
5. Lockwood Estrin, G., Milner, V., Spain, D. et al. (2021). Barriers to autism spectrum disorder diagnosis for young women and girls: a systematic review. *Review journal of autism and developmental disorders* 8 (4): 454–470.
6. Hull, L., Petrides, K.V., and Mandy, W. (2020). The female autism phenotype and camouflaging: a narrative review. *Review Journal of Autism and Developmental Disorders* 7: 306–317.
7. Alaghband-Rad, J., Hajikarim-Hamedani, A., and Motamed, M. (2023). Camouflage and masking behavior in adult autism. *Frontiers in Psychiatry* 14: 1108110.
8. Livingston, L.A. and Happé, F. (2017). Conceptualising compensation in neurodevelopmental disorders: reflections from autism spectrum disorder. *Neuroscience and Biobehavioral Reviews* 1 (80): 729–742.

9. Lai, M.C., Kassee, C., Besney, R. et al. (2019). Prevalence of co-occurring mental health diagnoses in the autism population: a systematic review and meta-analysis. *The Lancet Psychiatry* 6 (10): 819–829.
10. Zheng, Z., Zheng, P., and Zou, X. (2018). Association between schizophrenia and autism spectrum disorder: a systematic review and meta-analysis. *Autism Research* 11 (8): 1110–1119.
11. Brede, J., Cage, E., Trott, J. et al. (2022). 'We have to try to find a way, a clinical bridge'-autistic adults' experience of accessing and receiving support for mental health difficulties: a systematic review and thematic meta-synthesis. *Clinical Psychology Review* 93: 102131.
12. Hudson, C.C., Hall, L., and Harkness, K.L. (2019). Prevalence of depressive disorders in individuals with autism spectrum disorder: a meta-analysis. *Journal of Abnormal Child Psychology* 47: 165–175.
13. WHO (2024). Anxiety disorders (Internet). Place unknown: WHO. https://www.who.int/news-room/fact-sheets/detail/anxiety-disorders#:~:text=Anxiety%20disorders%20interfere%20with%20daily,an%20anxiety%20disorder%20(1).
14. Dell'Osso, L., Cremone, I.M., Nardi, B. et al. (2023). Comorbidity and overlaps between autism Spectrum and borderline personality disorder: state of the art. *Brain Sciences* 13 (6): 862.
15. McQuaid, G., Strang, J., and Jack, A. (2022). Borderline personality and late, missed, and misdiagnosis in female autism: a review of the literature. *PsyArXiv*. https://doi.org/10.31234/osf.io/t37vj.
16. Bentz, M. (2023). Autism Spectrum Conditions and Eating Disorders. In: *Eating Disorders: An International Comprehensive View* (ed. P. Robinson, T. Wade, B. Herpertz-Dahlmann, et al.), 1–15. Springer Nature.
17. Parsons, M.A. (2023). Autism diagnosis in females by eating disorder professionals. *Journal of Eating Disorders* 11 (1): 73.
18. Bouzy, J., Brunelle, J., Cohen, D., and Condat, A. (2023). Transidentities and autism spectrum disorder: a systematic review. *Psychiatry Research* 323: 115176.
19. Murphy, J., Prentice, F., Walsh, R. et al. (2020). Autism and transgender identity: implications for depression and anxiety. *Research in Autism Spectrum Disorders* 69: 101466.
20. Dunn, K., Rydzewska, E., Fleming, M., and Cooper, S.A. (2020). Prevalence of mental health conditions, sensory impairments and physical disability in people with co-occurring intellectual disabilities and autism compared with other people: a cross-sectional total population study in Scotland. *BMJ Open* 10 (4): e035280.
21. NHS Digital (Internet) England: NHS Health and Care of People with Learning Disabilities Experimental Statistics 2020 – 2021 (2021). https://digital.nhs.uk/data-and-information/publications/statistical/health-and-care-of-people-with-learning-disabilities/experimental-statistics-2020-to-2021/autism#:~:text=The%20percentage%20of%20patients%20with,rise%20of%208.8%20percentage%20points
22. Cooper, S.A., McLean, G., Guthrie, B. et al. (2015). Multiple physical and mental health comorbidity in adults with intellectual disabilities: population-based cross-sectional analysis. *BMC Family Practice* 16: 1–1.
23. Emerson, E. and Hatton, C. (2007). Mental health of children and adolescents with intellectual disabilities in Britain. *British Journal of Psychiatry* 191 (6): 493–499.
24. Hatton, C., Emerson, E., Robertson, J., and Baines, S. (2017). The mental health of British adults with intellectual impairments living in general households. *Journal of Applied Research in Intellectual Disabilities* 30 (1): 188–197.
25. Sheerin, F., Carroll, R., Mulryan, N. et al. (2017). Mental health, well-being, vitality and life events. In: *Health, wellbeing and social inclusion: Ageing with an intellectual disability in Ireland*, 87. The Intellectual Disability Supplement to The Irish Longitudinal Study on Ageing.
26. Perera, B., Audi, S., Solomou, S. et al. (2020). Mental and physical health conditions in people with intellectual disabilities: comparing local and national data. *British Journal of Learning Disabilities* 48 (1): 19–27.

27. Jahoda, A., Dagnan, D., Hastings, R. et al. (2024). Adapting psychological interventions for people with severe and profound intellectual disabilities: a behavioural activation exemplar. *Journal of Applied Research in Intellectual Disabilities* 37 (2): e13199.
28. Buckley, N., Glasson, E.J., Chen, W. et al. (2020). Prevalence estimates of mental health problems in children and adolescents with intellectual disability: a systematic review and meta-analysis. *Australian and New Zealand Journal of Psychiatry* 54 (10): 970–984.
29. Scheirs, J.G., Muller, A., Manders, N.C., and Van der Zanden, C.D. (2023). The prevalence and diagnosis of depression in people with mild or borderline intellectual disability: multiple instrument testing tells us more. *Journal of Mental Health Research in Intellectual Disabilities* 16 (1): 54–66.
30. Sheerin, F., Fleming, S., Burke, E. et al. (2023). Exploring mental health issues in people with an intellectual disability. *Learning Disability Practice* 26 (6).
31. Mazza, M.G., Rossetti, A., Crespi, G., and Clerici, M. (2020). Prevalence of co-occurring psychiatric disorders in adults and adolescents with intellectual disability: a systematic review and meta-analysis. *Journal of Applied Research in Intellectual Disabilities* 33 (2): 126–138.
32. Morgan, V.A., Leonard, H., Bourke, J., and Jablensky, A. (2008). Intellectual disability co-occurring with schizophrenia and other psychiatric illness: population-based study. *British Journal of Psychiatry* 193 (5): 364–372.
33. Mental Health Taskforce (2016). The five year forward view for mental health. NHS England.
34. Allabyrne, C., Chaplin, E., and Hardy, S. (2020). Advanced nursing practice in mental health: towards parity of esteem. *Nursing Times* 116 (12): 21–23.
35. White A, Sheehan R, Ding J et al. (2023). Learning from lives and deaths-people with a learning disability and autistic people (Leder) report for 2022. King's College London. Nov 30.
36. Lee, A.C., Herrieven, E., and Harrower, N.A. (2024). Health inequalities for people with learning disabilities: why it matters and what emergency physicians need to know. *British Journal of Hospital Medicine* 85: 1–7.
37. Pena-Salazar, C., Arrufat, F., Santos, J.M. et al. (2020). Underdiagnosis of psychiatric disorders in people with intellectual disabilities: differences between psychiatric disorders and challenging behaviour. *Journal of Intellectual Disabilities* 24 (3): 326–338.
38. Mantell, A.R. and Jennings, M. (2016). 'Nosey parkers? Professional curiosity in nursing and social work', 22nd International Network for Psychiatric Nursing (NPNR) Research Conference, Nottingham Trent University, UK, 15 September 2016. London South Bank University. Available at: https://openresearch.lsbu.ac.uk/item/87233
39. Phillips J, Westaby C, Fowler A, Ainslie S. (2022). Putting professional curiosity into practice. HM Inspectorate of Probation.
40. Bakken, T.L., Kildahl, A.N., Ludvigsen, L.B. et al. (2023). Schizophrenia in autistic people with intellectual disabilities: symptom manifestations and identification. *Journal of Applied Research in Intellectual Disabilities* 36 (5): 1076–1091.
41. Dalhaug, K.C., Storvik, K., and Kildahl, A.N. (2023). Undiagnosed psychotic disorder in autistic individuals with intellectual disabilities and suspected obsessive-compulsive disorder: an explorative, clinical study. *Journal of Mental Health Research in Intellectual Disabilities* 16 (3): 226–252.
42. Kildahl, A.N., Ludvigsen, L.B., Hove, O., and Helverschou, S.B. (2023). Exploring the relationship between challenging behaviour and mental health disorder in autistic individuals with intellectual disabilities. *Research in Autism Spectrum Disorders* 104: 102147.
43. Rosen, T.E., Mazefsky, C.A., Vasa, R.A., and Lerner, M.D. (2018). Co-occurring psychiatric conditions in autism spectrum disorder. *International Review of Psychiatry* 30 (1): 40–61.
44. Angel, L., Ailey, S.H., Delaney, K.R., and Mohr, L. (2023). Presentation of depressive symptoms in autism spectrum disorders. *Western Journal of Nursing Research* 45 (9): 854–861.

45. Wittkopf, S., Stroth, S., Langmann, A. et al. (2022). Differentiation of autism spectrum disorder and mood or anxiety disorder. *Autism* 26 (5): 1056–1069.
46. Allely, C.S., Woodhouse, E., and Mukherjee, R.A. (2023). Autism spectrum disorder and personality disorders: how do clinicians carry out a differential diagnosis? *Autism* 27 (6): 1847–1850.
47. Luciano, C.C., Keller, R., Politi, P. et al. (2014). Misdiagnosis of high function autism spectrum disorders in adults: an Italian case series. *Autism* 4 (2): 1–8.
48. Breau, L.M., Finley, G.A., PJ, M.G., and Camfield, C.S. (2002). Validation of the non-communicating children's pain checklist–postoperative version. *The Journal of the American Society of Anesthesiologists* 96 (3): 528–535.
49. Voepel-Lewis, T., Shayevitz, J.R., and Malviya, S. (1997). The FLACC: a behavioral scale for scoring postoperative pain in young children. *Pediatric Nursing* 23 (3): 293–297.
50. Lotan, M., Moe-Nilssen, R., Ljunggren, A.E., and Strand, L.I. (2009). Reliability of the non-communicating adult pain checklist (NCAPC), assessed by different groups of health workers. *Research in Developmental Disabilities* 30 (4): 735–745.
51. Raghavan, R. and Patel, P. (2005). Appendix 1: assessment tools. In: *Learning Disabilities and Mental Health* (ed. R. Raghavan and P. Patel). Wiley.
52. Helverschou, S.B., Bakken, T.L., and Martinsen, H. (2009). The psychopathology in autism checklist (PAC): a pilot study. *Research in Autism Spectrum Disorders* 3 (1): 179–195.
53. Royal College of Psychiatrists (2014). Report CR190: the risks and benefits of high-dose antipsychotic medication © 2023 The Royal College of Psychiatrists.
54. Branford, D., Gerrard, D., Saleem, N. et al. (2019). Stopping over-medication of people with intellectual disability, autism or both (STOMP) in England part 1 – history and background of STOMP. *Advances in Mental Health and Intellectual Disabilities* 13 (1): 31–40.
55. NHS (2018). NHS England (Internet) England. https://www.england.nhs.uk/learning-disabilities/improving-health/stomp-stamp
56. Mazza, M., Rossetti, A., Crespi, G., and Clerici, M. Prevalence of co-occurring psychiatric disorders in adults and adolescents with intellectual disability: a systematic review and meta-analysis. *Journal of Applied Research in Intellectual Disabilities* 33 (2): 126–138.
57. NHS England (Internet) England: NHS (2018). About LeDeR. https://leder.nhs.uk/about
58. National Development Team for Inclusion (2022). Green Light Toolkit.
59. NHS England (2018) The learning disability improvement standards for NHS trusts. https://www.england.nhs.uk/learning-disabilities/about/resources/the-learning-disability-improvement-standards-for-nhs-trusts/
60. Autism Act (2009). HMSO.
61. National Disability Strategy (2021). National Disability Strategy: Forewords, about this strategy, action across the UK, executive summary, acknowledgements. GOV.UK. https://www.gov.uk/government/publications/national-disability-strategy/forewords-about-this-strategy-action-across-the-uk-executive-summary-acknowledgements#executive-summary.
62. Mental Capacity Act (2005). HMSO.
63. Equality Act (2010). HMSO.
64. Health and Social Care Act (2021). HMSO.
65. Care Act (2014). HMSO.
66. NHS England (2016). Accessible Information Standard.
67. Nursing and Midwifery Council (2023). The Code: Professional Standards of Practice and Behaviour for Nurses, Midwives and Nursing Associates. https://www.nmc.org.uk/standards/code/

CHAPTER 17

Advanced Risk Assessment and Forensic Mental Health

Elizabeth Hearn

St George's, Epsom, and St Helier University Hospitals and Health Group, London, UK

Aim

The aim of this chapter is to provide an advanced overview of what constitutes a risk, how this can be assessed and what mitigations might be put in place to try and manage the risk with a particular focus on forensic mental health. The chapter will also review the role of the patient themselves in their own risk assessment and how risk priorities and assessments can be different in a range of contexts and subgroups.

LEARNING OUTCOMES

After reading this chapter, the reader will be able to:

1. Understand the different types of risk.
2. Gain the knowledge to complete a thorough risk assessment and formulation in forensic mental health.
3. Know how to approach risk management in practice.
4. Have an awareness of defensible decision-making and therapeutic risk taking
5. Understand the role of the advanced practitioner mental health (APMH) in risk assessment and management.

This chapter will embrace the following competences within the curriculum and capabilities framework of advanced clinical practice in mental health [1] (see Table 17.1).

The Advanced Practitioner in Mental Health, First Edition. Edited by Clare Allabyrne.
© 2026 John Wiley & Sons Ltd. All rights reserved, including rights for text and data mining and training of artificial intelligence technologies or similar technologies. Published 2026 by John Wiley & Sons Ltd.

TABLE 17.1 How this chapter meets the APMH curriculum and capabilities framework.

Clinical practice

1. Work autonomously within professional, ethical codes and legal frameworks, being responsible and accountable for their decisions, actions and omissions at this level of practice.
2. Demonstrate the underpinning psychological, biological and social knowledge required for advanced practice in mental health.
3. Demonstrate comprehensive knowledge of, and skills in, systematic history taking and clinical examination of patients who are culturally diverse and/or have complex needs in challenging circumstances, to develop a co-produced management plan.
4. Utilise clinical reasoning and decision-making skills to make a differential diagnosis and provide rationales for person-management plans, through critically reflecting on and evaluating their own role in relation to challenging traditional practices, new ways of working and the impact on the multidisciplinary team.
5. Initiate, evaluate and modify a range of interventions, which may include therapies, medicines, lifestyle advice and care.

Leadership and management

2. Exercise professional judgement and leadership to effectively promote safety in the presence of complexity and unpredictability.
3. Demonstrate team working, leadership, resilience and determination, managing situations that are unfamiliar, complex or unpredictable

Education

3. Effectively utilise a range of evidence-based educational strategies/interventions to support person-centred care with individuals, their families and carers and other healthcare colleagues.

Research

1. Critically appraise and apply the evidence base in influencing engagement, recovery, shared decision-making, transference and safeguarding.

INTRODUCTION

All types of healthcare settings will have safety standards to adhere to; however, it has been found that patient safety within mental health settings is much more complex, with unique challenges such as an increased risk of self-harm [2]. Caring for mentally ill offenders can be a fine balance of therapy, managing risk and maintaining safety; however, the emphasis on risk management and offence-related therapeutic work can often overshadow the personal traumas of the patients and the interrelationship of trauma and mental health [3]. Mental health care in forensic settings is subject to additional standards due to working across healthcare systems and criminal justice, this can include additional legal influences and input from the Ministry of Justice. Secure mental health units provide care to those with mental illness, personality disorders, learning disabilities (LDs) and autism, who are deemed to pose a risk to others and often themselves. Three levels of security exist which differ in their provision of physical, procedural and relational measures. Patients may come to be treated within the secure treatment pathway though a number of routes, including admission directly from the criminal justice system (CJS), a step up from other services or directly from the community, and can move up and down between the security levels as necessary [4, 5].

The Royal College of Nursing created a guidance document for the expected competencies of nursing staff working within forensic systems, and this includes the expectations and responsibilities for Advanced Practitioners (APs) [6]. Some of the competencies identified for advanced practice include risk assessment and management, as well as assessing dangerousness and providing therapeutic interventions. Currently this seems to be the only profession-specific guidance available; the Royal College of Occupational Therapists (OTs) produced a guidance document in 2012; however, they automatically withdraw publications after 10 years and this has not been replaced (personal communication). The colleges of pharmacists, allied health professionals (AHPs) and paramedics have all confirmed they do not have AP guidance in place (personal communication).

> **Learning Event: This gap in guidance presents a fantastic opportunity for an APMH to use their research and clinical skills to create some relevant publications.**

TYPES OF RISK

Risk can be categorised into three types, and it is important to assess for all three when completing a risk assessment.

Risk to self: this area includes self-harming behaviours, suicide, disordered eating and also self-neglect.

Suicide is the leading cause of death for men aged under 50 in the United Kingdom, with men accounting for approximately three quarters of all suicides [7]. Despite this, risk assessment tools for suicide have been found to be lacking in quality and have less than 5% predictive value for future suicide or repetition of self-harm, meaning they are wrong in 95% of cases [8]. A review looking at suicides over a 10-year period found that in almost half of cases the person had been in contact with services within the week leading up to their death, and 80% were considered to be 'low risk' [9]. Due to this, national guidelines now state that clinicians should 'not use risk assessment tools and scales to predict future suicide', and that risk stratification of high/medium/low should not determine whether treatment is offered or not [10]. Instead, service users should be involved in collaborative safety planning, with a formulation for risk management and identified harm reduction interventions [11].

Risk to others: this area is most commonly associated with physical violence and aggression, however, can also include other risks such as sexual violence or manipulation.

This area is the most prominent type in legislation and will often lead to negative portrayals of mental health in the media. It can be perceived to have worse outcomes and can lead to practitioners overlooking the other two areas [3].

Risk from others: e.g. violence, sexual and financial. Patients are also at risk of violence from others on a mental health ward or in the community [12] and witnessing violence could make them vulnerable to vicarious trauma [13]. Up to 91% of patients with serious mental illness (SMI) have been exposed to at least one episode of trauma in their lifetime [14]. If a person is identified to be at risk from others the healthcare practitioner should consider a safeguarding referral.

These are all discussed in more detail later in the chapter.

Research suggests that when discussing with patients about what risks they are aware of, they list a wider range than professionals and in particular mention risks from treatments or interventions, such as injury from restraints, medication-induced side effects and impacts on physical health [15]. In Ireland the best practice guidance lists risk under six categories: risk to self, risk to others, risk from others, risk from care planning, iatrogenic risk and risk of social exclusion [16].

ASSESSMENT OF RISK

In order to have a thorough risk assessment and management plan, it is crucial to have numerous disciplines involved [17] and the advanced practitioner mental health (APMH) can be the central point to liaise between different organisations and healthcare professionals (HCPs) to bring all available information together.

Risk assessment can be approached in different ways, and this can be grouped into three main categories:

- Unstructured: information is gathered as part of the clinical assessment; it is not restricted to a particular interaction and is an ongoing process. This can mean that the information found isn't captured in a consistent way and can be missed later when trying to formulate a full picture. This approach carries the highest likelihood of being subject to bias from the clinician.
- Actuarial: the focus here is on statistical risk factors that have been identified through large samples of people and confirmed as statistically correct. This approach is research evidenced and can be useful to bear in mind when forming a formulation, however, should not be applied to individual cases as it does not take into consideration individual differences and the influence of current context.
- Structured professional judgement (SPJ): this approach combines a few different areas including the service user's views, clinical knowledge of the service user and a set of specific factors to be assessed which are based on prior research and proven useful for a set population [18].

There are a variety of tools and scales available that can be utilised to structure risk assessment. These can vary depending on the type of risk, location of assessment, and the person involved. The use of a tool does not provide an assessment in itself but should be used in conjunction with a systematic and thorough clinical assessment.

The screening tools in Table 17.2 are examples of tools for different contexts and with different goals, some of these are not specifically risk assessment tools but can be useful in the formulation of risk presentations. There is also a tool used to assess the presence of protective factors which is one of the key areas in formulation. If using an assessment tool, it is important to consider:

- A person's age, language skills and cognitive capabilities.
- Whether the person is part of the populations that the tool has been validated for.
- Any factors that might affect the reliability and validity of the tool.
- If training is needed to use the tool and if so if it has been completed.

TABLE 17.2 Examples of assessment tools listed alphabetically.

Name of tool	Assesses for	Suitability/How to use
Beck hopelessness scale	Suicide	Self-report scale of 20 items to be identified as true or false to create a measure about the patients' negative expectations of the future. [19]
Broset violence checklist	Predictor for short-term violence within 24 hrs.	The BVC measures six behavioural areas with a score of 1 for each area that is identified as present. Absent areas score 0. The behaviours are confusion, irritability, boisterousness, verbal threats, physical threats and attacks on objects. A total score of 0 indicates low risk, 1–2 is moderate and 3–6 is high. [20]
Dynamic Appraisal of Situational Aggression (DASA)	Imminent aggression	A seven-item risk instrument most often used by inpatient nurses assessing each item being present or absent in the preceding 24 hrs. [21].
Dangerousness Understanding Recovery and Urgency Manual (DUNDRUM) -1	Level of security needed	A scale used to establish level of environmental security needed and whether the patient can be managed on an open ward or needs low/medium/high secure hospital stay. 11-item scale with each item being scored 0–4 based on severity; the items include factors such as seriousness of risk, immediacy, legal process and public confidence. This is one of four SPJs which together make up the DUNDRUM Quartet. [22]
Historical Clinical Risk-20 (HCR-20 – Version 3)	Violence	20 items with three main areas for risk subcategorised as historical, clinical and risk management. Each item is determined as present or absent and relevant or not relevant. This tool is normally completed with a team rather than an individual clinician and should be led by someone trained to use it. [23]
Health of the Nation Outcome Scale (HoNOS)	Scales measuring health and social functioning of people with SMI	A set of scales to measure behaviour, impairment, symptoms and social functioning. All scales measure severity on a 5-point scale of 0 for no problem to 4 for severe or very severe. There are different variations designed for the specific subgroup they are being used for: HoNOS for Working Age Adults, HoNOS 65+, HoNOSCA (Children and Adolescents), HoNOS-Secure, HoNOS-LD (Learning Disability), HoNOS ABI (Acquired Brain Injury). The HoNOS is not a risk assessment tool itself; however, it supports the clinician to rate the need for risk management procedures. [24]

(Continued)

TABLE 17.2 (Continued)

Name of tool	Assesses for	Suitability/How to use
Risk for Sexual Violence Protocol (RSVP)	Sexual violence	Designed for convicted sex offenders to predict the risk of recidivism. 20-item scale to assess psycho-social factors, sexual offences and future planning. Helps to develop risk management plans based on the identified areas. Should be used by someone with relevant training. [25]
Structured Assessment of Protective Factors (SAPROF)	Protective Factors	Produces an overall score from 17 items across three subscales looking at internal factors, external factors and motivational factors. Each item is scored 0–2, and the higher overall score indicates a high level of protective features. [26]
Scale for Suicide Ideation (SSI)	Suicide	21-item scale that should take about 10 min. to complete, can be via interview or self-completed by the service user. Designed to assess attitude, behaviours and plans to complete suicide and history of previous attempts. [27]

This list is not exhaustive and different localities may have policy guidance on which templates/tools they use. There can also be locally developed risk assessment templates that are site specific.

Assessment tools for suicide risk should not be used as a predictor of future suicide [10, 28, 29], with research having found that 80% of all assessments will categorise a person as no or low-risk and have a predictive value of less than 20% accuracy [30]. In assessments for suicide and self-harm there needs to be a much higher emphasis on clinical competence and inclusion of service user perspectives [31].

This move away from stratifying risk with a static assessment and instead moving towards dynamic, co-produced outcomes is also supported by Royal College of Psychiatrists [32] who highlight the dynamic nature of risk and that assessments need to have frequent reviews. They also recommend the creation of a formulation, with a plan that describes the current situation and mitigations for future risks.

One approach to formulation is to use the five Ps model [33].

The five Ps consist of:

- **Presenting issues**: a summary of the current difficulties being experienced by the person that has led to them accessing care, or other problems identified during the assessment process.
- **Predisposing factors:** issues in the persons past that could contribute to them experiencing mental health issues. This includes family history, significant events, social or cultural issues and adverse childhood experiences.
- **Precipitating factors:** events that have contributed or triggered the current situation, including substance misuse, interpersonal or physical stressors.
- **Perpetuating factors:** issues that are maintaining the current difficulties in the person's life, beliefs, substance misuse, avoidance or safety behaviours.
- **Protective factors**: individual and systemic strengths alongside the presenting problem and add to a person's resilience and resources. Social support, skills, interests and personal characteristics.

Collaborative Risk Assessment

The therapeutic alliance with patients is a crucial part of recovery and essential for recovery planning; however, there is a need to balance caring with restricting possible risk behaviours. It has been reported that health care professionals (HCPs) can struggle to create this alliance if the risk assessments are only focused on past negative behaviour and do not incorporate skills and protective factors. Patients have reported limited involvement, feeling powerless and that disagreeing with staff views can be perceived to have negative consequences in their own recovery pathway. Patients are often aware of having had a risk assessment, but not clear on the content or what the goals are for them to be able to move forwards, this can then contribute to a lack of responsibility for their own progression and a lack of drive to change [34].

When risk is assessed collaboratively, it can have a higher level of accuracy for prediction of violence and better management plans. One study found that after implementing a shared tool there was a decrease in the number of seclusions and restraints by more than half [35]. Another study found that when reviewing DUNDRUM scores collaboratively, the level of concordance between clinician and patient views increased significantly as the patient progressed through from high to medium to low-secure settings, indicating a higher level of insight as the patient becomes less acutely unwell [36]. When patients are moving into the community and facing discharge, they have been found to be able to more accurately assess their own vulnerabilities and strengths and therefore have better predictive value of recidivism [37].

Differences in Assessment Depending on Location

Inpatient

In inpatient environments the interpersonal relationships of patients can both provoke and reduce risk behaviours. DASA scores have been looked at to see how an individual who is deemed a high risk of violence behaves when they are on an unsettled ward and hypothesised that having high-risk patients together would increase the likelihood of violence. However, the opposite was found and high-risk individuals were more likely to be violent on settled wards. This could be due to an awareness of their own vulnerability and a fear of potential retaliation from a peer that they see as violent, whereas in a settled ward they may feel safer to act without consequences, there are also often lower staffing ratios on settled wards which could have an impact on how some patients act [21].

Emergency Department

The Care Quality Commission (CQC) has produced guidance on assessing those with mental health issues who present to the emergency department [38]. The guidance document covers areas such as environment, collaborative working with liaison and ED staff, ensuring risk to self is assessed and what risks may be present when the person is discharged. They stipulate there needs to be a specific plan in place for risk assessments for those under the age of 18 and reasonable adjustments made for those with LDs and autism. If an APMH is working in liaison psychiatry, they should be aware of their own competencies and limitations in this area to ensure they are not working beyond their own scope of practice.

Health-Based Place of Safety (HBPoS)

The use of Section 136 of the Mental Health Act (MHA 2007) [39] allows the police to remove someone from a public place and take them to an identified place of safety due to concerns around their mental health. It has been found that 92% of detentions under S136 are due to self-harm and suicidal behaviour, with a further 3% identifying suicide as a secondary factor [40]. Findings also suggest that there is a subset of patients who are detained multiple times under S136, with one study finding that within South East England 13% of the individuals detained accounted for a third of all S136 uses and two patients had a total of 44 detentions between them within a 12-month period [41]. There is a link between individuals who are repeatedly detained under S136 and the diagnosis of borderline personality disorder; this carries a higher likelihood of a trauma background and an increase in risk of suicide by up to 20 times. If an APMH is working within an HBPoS, it is therefore imperative that they are capable of formulating risk around suicide and ensuring this is factored into the decision about whether the person warrants a stay within inpatient services or what support they might need in the community.

One NHS trust trialled having a joint approach with the police and having a mental health nurse working alongside the police. Over a 6-month period, they found a 38% reduction in the use of S136, this demonstrates the benefits of having a mental health professional being there to advise and guide the police which could be a perfect role for an APMH [42].

RISK-SPECIFIC ISSUES

Confidentiality

Healthcare staff have a duty of confidentiality when handling patient information, this includes information disclosed by service users in interactions or assessments. Many staff will find it clear that if someone discloses intent to hurt someone else during an assessment that they need to escalate these concerns and potentially alert other agencies such as the police. Similarly, if a person discloses that they are being victimised or at risk from others then appropriate action will be taken. In either of these situations, a safeguarding alert/referral might need to be made.

In the case of harm to self, this line of when to share information can be harder to define and if a person discloses plans to hurt themselves or suicidal feelings, these can go unshared, especially when the person is deemed to have capacity. DoH [43] created a guideline around working collaboratively with service users to gain consent to share, and how/when to breach confidentiality if needed. It places emphasis on family involvement and ensuring there is a space for family to provide information and be involved in care planning.

Conlon et al. [44] found that confidentiality rules are not always well understood, and practitioners use their clinical intuition to assess risk and escalation plans, rather than relying solely on scores from an assessment tool. It is important for practitioners to understand local policy around confidentiality and consult colleagues for advice if they are not sure about when to disclose or escalate information given during an assessment.

Demographic Subgroups

Many risk assessment tools have only been tested with certain population groups and have not been proven to be accurate when used with women, ethnic minority groups and those driven by extreme religious or political views [45–47]. Some research has found that tools can have poor accuracy when not applied correctly, and excessively high scoring can be common in minority ethnic groups [45, 46].

Race

Black people are more likely to be stopped and searched by the police when compared to white people by 9-fold [48] and black children are up to five times more likely to be arrested than their white counterparts [49]. Systemic racism is present in the CJS and healthcare [50], and patients who come through these systems are likely to already have complex trauma histories due to a correlation between the degree of childhood adversity and serious offending [51]. Forensic formulation should take this into account and not simply accept that higher numbers of arrests are equal to a higher risk of re-offending and instead think about the needs of the person, what led them to that point and what support they might need. The Power Threat Meaning Framework is strongly linked with trauma-informed care and can be used to aid culturally informed formulation in forensic populations. This framework highlights that those with the fewest resources available are more likely to respond in ways that could be considered antisocial [52].

Racial stereotypes and unconscious bias can affect the clinician and the patient. Young offenders were found to self-report higher risk to others when they were asked about their racial identity in advance of their risk assessment when compared to those who were not asked or asked after the risk questions. Adults in the CJS have been found to increase their nonverbal responses due to fear of confirming a negative stereotype, which can be interpreted as implied guilt [53]. Due to these reasons, it is vitally important that when working with cultural minorities the appropriate risk assessment tool or approach is used [45].

Sexual Orientation

Lesbian, gay and bisexual (LGB) individuals have approximately twice the rates of poor mental health when compared to the heterosexual population [54]. This is thought to be due in part to discrimination; however, when looked at cross-nationally, it was found that there's no significant difference in rates of mental health between countries despite how socially acceptable homosexuality is [55].

This increased risk is particularly noted in lesbian and bisexual woman and is thought to be due to a decreased level of openness with their family. When seeing this population, it's important to check their support network and reflect this accurately in any safety planning [54].

Poor mental health has also been seen in transgender (T) people, due to stigma and discrimination [56], this is seen more extremely in individuals who are unable to access gender-affirming care [57].

It has been recorded that there are much higher rates of self-harm, suicidal ideation and suicide attempts in LGBT youth. One intervention that was found to have significant impact was interventions to improve their experience at school. Practitioners working with this group should ensure to include the school and other key stakeholders in building a collaborative support package [58].

Neurodiversity

A report published by the Equality and Human Right Commission warned that people with LDs and autistic people were being failed by the CJS and not getting a fair trial [59].

Most of the available literature suggests that autistic individuals are either less likely or have equal likeliness to commit a criminal offence than the general population. There are studies looking at likelihood within particular areas; however, these are unconclusive due to the differing findings [60]. Despite that, the rates of autistic patients within forensic mental health units and prison settings are higher than the population average [61]. This could be due to the likelihood of self-incriminating behaviour such as their style of communication, misunderstanding a question or a lack of recognition of important facts [62]. For those with attention deficit hyperactivity disorder (ADHD), they were found to be much more likely to say 'I don't know' when being questioned and have a higher rate of false confessions due to weakened resilience under pressure [63].

The Police and Criminal Evidence Act (PACE) 1984 stipulates that any vulnerable adult, or those under 18, suspected of a criminal offence must be offered an appropriate adult during questioning to safeguard their rights [64]. However, for this to take place, the person must be identified as having these additional needs, and this identification happens less than 40% of the time [65] which could lead to an increased risk in incorrect convictions. An APMH working in the CJS can complete a full assessment before court for any special measures to support communications, provide sensory or environmental adaptions, prepare the person to understand the process and provide autism awareness training for colleagues.

Evidence suggests HCR-20 and RSVP-V2 tools both have limited use with autistic individuals as it can lead to over- or under-estimation of level of risk, currently there are no validated risk assessment tools for use in autistic spectrum disorder (ASD) [66]. There are lower rates of recidivism in neurodiverse individuals when compared to the general population; however, risk assessment scores have been found to be insignificant for predicting this in this population [60].

Learning Disability (LD)

As aforementioned, it has been found that people with an LD are being failed by the CJS, and in the United Kingdom people with LD are overrepresented compared to in the general population [59] and face longer detentions [67]. This due to the lack of adjustments made, not identifying the individuals and legal professionals not having the required training [59]. Secure ward environments can pose a risk to the physical health and mental health for those with LD due to an inability to access appropriate support [68].

People with LD can have difficulties learning and analysing information as well as communicating their needs, this can lead to them processing risk differently and negatively affect their safety decision-making and possibly lead to risky behaviours [69].

Assessments for risk need to be dynamic and address situational triggers as well as try to understand how they may be perceived differently by the person. LDs and risk have a wider breadth of research than that of neurodiversity and there are some risk assessment tools have good validity for those with LD, such as Current Risk of Violence (CuRV) and Short Dynamic Risk Scale (SDRS) for predicting violence within community settings [70]. The Dynamic Risk Assessment and Management System (DRAMS) is an assessment for dynamic risk factors in people with LD which can be useful to create a formulation and support plan [71].

Age

Children and Young People (CYP)

There has been a 65% increase in the number of CYPs admitted to acute medical wards over a 10-year period to a lack of mental health beds and an increase in demand [72]. Between 2009 and 2019 the number of ED attendances for under 18 seconds increased × 5 [73]. If a CYP presents to ED in crisis, they may be initially triaged by a non-MH professional such as an ED nurse before being signposted on, especially as only 20% of paediatric liaison teams have 24/7 coverage for Child and Adolescent Mental Health Services (CAMHS) despite NHS England recommendations [73]. CQC stipulate there should be a specific plan in place for risk assessment for under 18 s [38]. Any APMH working in these areas should check what their local procedures are, as well as up to date national guidelines to ensure they are providing the best possible care.

For CYPs coming into Youth Offender Institutions (YOI) NHSE recommends the use of the Comprehensive Health Assessment Tool (CHAT), although this is not currently compulsory for individuals and may be refused. This is validated holistic tool including physical health, substance misuse, mental health, neurodivergence, traumatic brain injury and learning difficulties. This tool can also be a useful indicator for areas that might need further assessment [74].

The Violence Risk Assessment Checklist for Youth has been found to be a useful tool for predicting future violence within psychiatric units and giving staff a greater opportunity to intervene and prevent these from happening [75]; however, it has not been found useful within social care settings. One study is currently looking into the development of a tool specifically looking at identifying self-harm and suicide risk; however, the results for this are not yet available [76].

Older Adults

Risk and recidivism rates lower after a person enters their 60s; however, 90% of staff in long-term care are regularly exposed to violence and aggression. In a Canadian study, a homicide rate of 7 per 100,000 was found in long-term care which is significantly higher than the national homicide rates in England and Wales of 11.7 per million [77].

Research is lacking into the trajectory of violence and how this develops over the lifespan. Changes in cognition and executive functioning can be a key risk factor for aggression, and these can also be impacted by polypharmacy [78]. Individuals with dementia are 5x more likely to display aggressive behaviour compared to controls, with 96% of patient with dementia displaying at least one occasion of severe aggressive behaviour following their diagnosis. Observational tools such as the Aggressive Behaviour Risk Assessment Tool for Long-Term Care can be used to record incidents of aggression but they have been found to have variable results, and further research is needed to determine their ability to indicate future occasions [79].

Gender

Women

Over half of female offenders have been victims of serious crime and abuse, including childhood abuse and domestic violence. Up to 80% of women in prison with mental health issues have experienced domestic violence and 66% experienced childhood sexual abuse [80]. This affects their ability to engage with many other health services due to trauma, causing a lack of trust, increased stress sensitivity, emotional dysregulation and reduced self-control [81]. Evidence shows that the experience of traumatic adverse childhood events (ACEs) can predict the level of violence exhibited, the extremes of self-harm behaviours [81], impact the length of stay in hospital [82] and the likelihood to reoffend [83].

Working with female patients is more resource intensive due to higher levels of observations needed around self-harm risk, more frequent assaults and use of violence and high rates of staff turnover and burnout [84]. As an APMH it would be important to lean on the leadership pillar to support staff wellbeing in this environment.

Implementing a TIC approach can improve outcomes and empower these women to progress with their lives. (Please see Chapter 7 for more detailed information on trauma-informed care.)

There is not enough capacity within this chapter to list all demographics or factors to consider within different groups. It is also important to remember that an individual might be affected by many of these aspects if they fit into more than one subgroup, this could compound their risk and affect the ability of the APMH to fully address all factors. In all subgroups APMHs should use their research pillar to ensure they are following latest updates and best practice guidance.

PHARMACOLOGICAL CONSIDERATIONS

Antipsychotics, mood stabilisers and other mental health medications are prescribed widely for patients with psychiatric disorders in many different countries. However, none of these are specifically licenced to reduce risk and in some cases can even increase risk, for example one of the known possible side effects of aripiprazole is an increased risk of impulsive gambling [85]. However, despite this, there is precedent for prescribing to try and reduce risk, with certain medications found to be effective in some cases. Clozapine has been found to be effective in reducing violence and aggression [86] and can help to reduce the use of additional PRN medication [87]. This is especially noticed in forensic psychiatric patients with high levels of violence, that haven't responded to other antipsychotics. In a subgroup of service users who do not respond to clozapine, it has been found that the addition of amisulpride can enhance the therapeutic response and reduce aggression levels [86].

Benzodiazepines are frequently prescribed for rapid tranquilisation and the minimisation of aggression and agitation in inpatient service users. Evidence of their efficacy is mixed, with some research indicating they have equal efficacy as a placebo in the short-term and may even increase aggression in the long-term [88]. Paradoxical effects of benzodiazepines such as increased agitation and sleep disturbances are thought to occur in less than 1% of the population, but rates for this are increased in older adult populations [89]. Research suggests that the combination of haloperidol with promethazine or olanzapine as a monotherapy can be a more effective treatment for psychomotor agitation [88, 90].

When working with sexual offenders, there is limited evidence that pharmacological interventions provide any significant benefit [91].

Forensic mental health patients are often subject to polypharmacy and have more than one antipsychotic prescribed, as well as being more likely to receive High Dose Antipsychotic Therapy (HDAT) [92]. The prevalence of polypharmacy in this cohort of patients can vary across different settings but has been found to be 35%–55% [93, 94]. One study found the average patient's antipsychotic dosage was more than 1.5 times the recommended amount [92]. However, despite these high rates of increased treatment regimens, a review of literature found there currently isn't evidence to suggest polypharmacy is any more effective than single treatment within forensics, [95] as well as not being able to establish the best strategies for pharmaceutical treatment of violence risk in these settings [96]. Those who are on higher doses are more likely to have higher risk scores on HCR-20 and have poorer functioning in daily life [97].

Long-term antipsychotic treatment has been found to greatly increase the risks of metabolic conditions and is linked to lower mortality. Although a literature review found that on balance the risk of reducing dosages of antipsychotics in stabilised patients carries a higher risk to their mental state and recovery, than the benefit it would bring to their physical health [98].

The side-effects of antipsychotic medications are well documented, and these risks increase with polypharmacy and HDAT. HDAT greatly increased the risks of physical health complications and as such requires more frequent monitoring including ECGs and blood biochemistry [99, 100]. There is an expectation for all patients on HDAT to have a clear plan for reviewing treatment regularly, monitoring side effects and safety of the treatment [101].

Best practice is to review prescribing decisions with a multi-disciplinary assessment when considering using medication to target medium- or long-term risk of violence [100]. The presence of an APMH within this MDT assessment can bring additional pharmaceutical knowledge and utilise the four pillars to present the latest research on the topic and lead the team in discussion. APs have been found to be effective at significantly reducing the number of times medication is administered in long-term care [102].

A Special Note on Substance Misuse in Prison

It has been found that half of those residing in prisons and secure settings have misused drugs [56], a third actively use drugs during their incarceration [103] and up to 93% of those in prison have access to illicit substances [104]. This provides further complications for prescribers, and it is recommended that practitioners follow national and local guidance and procedures for how to prescribe in these circumstances to avoid risk of interactions and possible overdose.

Pharmacological Interventions for Risk to Self

Lithium has been established to have a significant effect on lowering mortality risk through self-harm, and there is a plethora of research documenting its anti-suicidal effects since the 1970s, with some studies even suggesting there can be a positive effect on reducing suicide risk in the general population in areas where there is a higher level of lithium in the drinking water [105]. This appears to be the case across wide groups of people and is not impacted by gender or age; however, different studies have found different levels of efficacy ranging from 1.5 to 28 x reduced risk, the reasons for these differences would need to be studied further. Lithium toxicity can have potentially fatal adverse effects, so its use needs to be monitored efficiently with physical health assessments being completed before initiation and at regular intervals during treatment [106].

A Cochrane review looked at multiple trials to assess the efficacy of medications on reducing the act of self-harm. It found that there was a slightly lower likelihood of repeat self-harm when using antipsychotics compared to placebo; however, there was no difference between placebos and antidepressants, anxiolytics, mood stabilisers or natural remedies such as omega-3 fatty acids [107]. This is further supported by a meta-analysis that found on average an 8% reduction in self-harming thought and behaviours for psychotropic medications, but this increased to a 20% reduction for antipsychotics [108]. Interestingly, it was also found that citalopram could lead to a reduction of up to 40% despite other antidepressants being non-significant or in the case of paroxetine even increasing risk [108].

Unfortunately, neither of these reviews looked at the efficacy of naltrexone which has a growing evidence base for reducing self-harm. Naltrexone is an opiate antagonist and is commonly used in opiate and alcohol abuse to reduce dependence and relapse. It was first documented to be effective for self-harm in someone with borderline personality disorder in 1997, and although there is a presence of research including case studies and larger reviews, it is still not commonly used outside of substance use treatment [109]. In a review of the current research available incorporating animal studies (as self-harm behaviours are mirrored in certain monkeys), naltrexone has been successful at either decreasing or eliminating self-harm behaviours, although it is recognised that a larger trial is needed [110]. Naltrexone has also been found to be effective at reducing self-harming behaviours in people with LDs and can reduce the severity of the harm as well as the frequency of occurrences [111].

> ### RED FLAGS
>
> DoH identified a list of risk factors for different events including 27 risk factors for violence and 25 for suicide. These factors are grouped into demographic factors, background, clinical history, psychological and psychosocial factors and the current context and include things such as lack of social support, violence at a young age, substance abuse, self-harm and relationship instability. Each service user should be treated as an individual, and the team should work with the patient to collate a list of signs and triggers that are indicative of an increase in risk [7].

> **Learning event:** Which of these factors can you identify in some of the cases you have worked with directly? Are these things you have considered previously?

RISK MANAGEMENT

Violence to Other

WHO [112] separates risk interventions into three stages:

> Primary: aimed at preventing aggression before it occurs
> Secondary: preventing imminent aggression
> Tertiary: responding when aggression is occurring and needs to be controlled

Tertiary responses such as a restraint and seclusion should only be used as a last resort when all other approaches have failed [113]. It has been found that without a systematic approach to risk management ward staff can lack consistency, not use a person-centred approach and its absence can often lead to the use of reactive and/or restrictive practices [114]. This can be counterproductive as it has been found that aggression can be caused by irritability at the restrictions imposed by staff. This is especially present in forensic populations as it has been found that the more violent patients are more likely to have dominant, coercive or hostile interpersonal styles which are often associated with aggression and the desire to regain control over their environment [115].

> **Learning Event:** There are specific assessment tools and management guides for subcategories of violence to others such as fire setting, stalking and sex offending. Find out if any of these apply to the patient group you work with, and see what the latest research recommends.

Recidivism

Approximately 27% of prison leavers will re-offend in a year; however, this increases to 57% for those who have abused drugs [104]. This requires careful, thoughtful planning in how to support people upon their release with specific targeted support. The UK government published a 10-year strategy around the use of drugs; however, the efficacy of this has been called into question and practitioners are encouraged to personalise their care plans to the individual needs of those they work with [116].

The difference in re-offending rates for those with and without a mental illness is not so clear cut; different studies suggest the presence of mental illness might increase [117] or have no impact on the chances of re-offending [118]. It has also been found that when relying on arrest rates alone this may only capture a quarter of actual committed violence when compared to self-report as well as staff and carer collateral [119].

Research has been able to identify certain factors that may positively or negatively influence offending. This includes higher rates in those who are discharged at tribunal against clinical advice [120] and higher rates of violence in those who experience command hallucinations, threat-control-override symptoms and Capgras Syndrome [121]. Lower rates of re-offending have been found as a direct correlation to the amount of support offered [122], as well as when there is contact within the first 30 days of release [123].

Therapeutic Risk Taking

The HCR-20 is widely used as part of risk assessment, management and future planning [124]; however, its validity for predicting re-offending has been called into question, with some studies finding it a good predictor of future offending [125], while others finding it failed to predict future violence regardless of setting or timescale [126]. These extreme variations in findings could be down to the skill of the clinician using the tool and the amount of information available to them at the time [126]. The difference could also be due to the level of patient involvement in their own care planning, as discussed earlier in the chapter, collaborative risk assessments are proven to have better outcomes for prediction and are more likely to be followed by the patients themselves when they have a trusting therapeutic relationship with their HCP.

This variation highlights that risk can never be completely eradicated, but with the support of experienced and skilled clinicians, including APMHs and the use of continuous assessment, evaluation, thorough formulation and patient collaboration, it can be reduced to a minimum [17]. The use of protective factors within formulation of risk can help practitioners to think about risk management on discharge and bring a more balanced view than traditional assessments which only look at the presence of negative features. A person might be seen as high risk, but if they also have a high level of protective factors that could alleviate some of the ongoing risk and make someone less likely to commit risk behaviours or re-offend, especially when compared to someone with the same high-risk profile but low or no protective factors. Patients in forensic settings have significantly lower levels of protective factors when compared to non-forensic or community mental health patients [26].

Therapeutic risk taking involves professionals taking risks to support a person's development and moving forward in their recovery, while supporting the patient to feel empowered in making decisions about their own level of safety [15]. It can be around large or small decisions and involve restrictive interventions such as Community Treatment Orders (CTO) to discharge someone while still under strict controls or therapeutic approaches and care planning [15], such as transferring to a lower level of security, reducing the level of enhanced observations, granting unescorted or overnight leave, unsupervised visits or attendance to college or work in the community. One example is the use of electronic monitoring to be able to track patients while on leave which was found to have an increase in the granting of leave and a decrease in leave violations [127]. APMHs from an occupational therapy background are particularly valuable in risk taking and discharge risk management as the use of occupation has been linked to reduction of reoffending [128]. Some of the key areas identified in this area include:

- formulation
- integration into the community
- realignment of volition
- increasing protective factors
- developing a prosocial identity

Supporting the patient to create a new identify and activities of living that aren't associated with previous criminal enterprises can help them to stay away from possible triggers that might cause them to re-engage with offending [128]. All these areas require a level of coproduction and collaboration between the professional team and the patient and ensuring the patient is actively included and involved within risk discussions [129]. The APMH can bring together research in this area as well as their clinical expertise and knowledge of the patient to help MDT discussions when reviewing next steps and discussions around taking risks. Some of the factors that may be considered could be whether the patient has completed a specific therapy programme or achieved a certain amount of time without exhibiting risk behaviours. There is still a long way to go until all services are truly co-produced; however, there has been drastic improvement. One example of this is the Mental Health Secure Care Programme which was established in 2016 as part of the 5 Year Forward View. Within this programme was the start of Specialist Community Forensic Teams which were a co-produced model of care to try and reduce length of stays and work collaboratively with patients in the community, using therapeutic risk taking as a large part of their model [130]. One systemic area to be aware of when implementing and supporting a therapeutic risk-taking approach is to consider when things go 'wrong'. Hindsight can suggest an outcome was more predictable than it appeared at the time and it is important to support staff when decisions do not turn out as expected and instead turn these into positive learning experiences [15].

CONCLUSION

Only 15% of mental health patients within prisons are transferred within the 28-day period recommended by NHSE, with some waiting up for 462 days. This causes the patients' health to deteriorate as they rely on staff who do not have the appropriate training and may not have access to the correct treatment and medication, this can further perpetuate a negative stereotype around mental health patients being violent and risky [131]. Discrimination and stigma greatly affect this group due to negative portrayal in the media [132] but also due to the backgrounds and experiences of the patients themselves [53, 54, 59] and pre-existing bias within the health practitioner working with them [133]. The role of the APMH needs to not only address the clinical issues present for the patient but also use their leadership pillar to role model to others and address the presence of bias.

There are many areas of risk that have not been covered in this chapter, and it is imperative to know local protocols and have best practice guidance for the area the APMH is working in. Some of the takeaway messages that can be applicable to all areas are:

- Check the assessment tool is relevant and applicable to the person/group you are working with.
- 'Risk' as a concept is not just about violence to others but also addresses risk to self, risk from others and the iatrogenic harm people might receive.
- Working across systems can complicate matters, and having to navigate different professional groups with different priorities can delay the journey and negatively impact the patient experience.
- Risk should not be stratified; it is not static. Risk can change in minutes and should be assessed using dynamic formulation with attention paid to triggers and protective factors.
- As in all other areas, collaborative working is vitally important to ensure the person has a voice in their own care and can form a trusting, therapeutic relationship with the APMH they are working with.

FURTHER READING

NHS England Trauma Informed Care. Available at: https://www.e-lfh.org.uk/programmes/trauma-informed-care/

DoH Risk guide. Available at: https://assets.publishing.service.gov.uk/media/5a8020a840f0b62302691adf/best-practice-managing-risk-cover-webtagged.pdf

NHSE stratifying risk: NHS England. Staying safe from suicide: Best practice guidance for safety assessment, formulation and management. Available at: https://www.england.nhs.uk/publication/staying-safe-from-suicide/

REFERENCES

1. The Centre for Advancing Practice (2025). *Mental health advanced practice area specific capability and curriculum framework*. NHS England. https://advanced-practice.hee.nhs.uk/wp-content/uploads/sites/28/2025/01/Mental-health-advanced-practice-area-specific-capability-and-curriculum-framework-NHSE.pdf
2. Thibaut, B., Dewa, L.H., Ramtale, S.C. et al. (2019). Patient safety in inpatient mental health settings: a systematic review. *BMJ Open* 9: e030230. https://doi.org/10.1136/bmjopen-2019-030230.
3. Markham, S. (2021). The totalising nature of secure and forensic mental health services in England and Wales. *Frontiers in Psychiatry* 8. https://doi.org/10.3389/fpsyt.2021.789089.
4. Ryland, H., Davies, L., Kenney-Herbert, J. et al. (2022). Advancing research in adult secure mental health services in England. *Medicine, Science and the Law* 62 (3): 225–229. https://doi.org/10.1177/00258024211066981.
5. NHS England. *Service specification high secure mental health services*. Service Specification Number: 1752. 2021. Available from: https://www.england.nhs.uk/wp-content/uploads/2021/02/service-specification-high-secure-mental-health-services-adult.pdf
6. NHS England. *Competence Framework: Health & Justice Sector*. 2017. Available from: https://www.england.nhs.uk/south/wp-content/uploads/sites/6/2017/03/health-justice-competence-framework.pdf
7. Department of Health (2022). *Press Release: Men urged to talk about mental health to prevent suicide*. Available from: https://www.gov.uk/government/news/men-urged-to-talk-about-mental-health-to-prevent-suicide
8. Healthcare Quality Improvement Partnership (2018). *The assessment of clinical risk in mental health services*. National confidential inquiry into suicide and safety in mental health. https://documents.manchester.ac.uk/display.aspx?DocID=38466
9. Healthcare Quality Improvement Partnership. *National Confidential Inquiry into Suicide and Safety in Mental Health*. 2022. https://documents.manchester.ac.uk/display.aspx?DocID=60521
10. National Institute for Health and Care Excellence (NICE) (2022). Self-harm: assessment management and preventing recurrence: NICE Guideline [NG225]. www.nice.org.uk/guidance/ng225
11. Hawton, K., Lascelles, K., Pitman, A. et al. (2022). Assessment of suicide risk in mental health practice: shifting from prediction to therapeutic assessment, formulation, and risk management. *Lancet Psychiatry* 9 (11): 922–928. https://doi.org/10.1016/S2215-0366(22)00232-2.
12. Christ, C., Have, M.T., de Graaf, R. et al. (2020). Mental disorders and the risk of adult violent and psychological victimisation: a prospective, population-based study. *Epidemiological Psychiatric Sciences* 29 (13). https://doi.org/10.1017/S2045796018000768: e13.
13. Atwoli, L., Platt, J., Williams, D.R. et al. (2015). Association between witnessing traumatic events and psychopathology in the south African stress and health study. *Social Psychiatry and Psychiatric Epidemiology* 50 (8): 1235–1242. https://doi.org/10.1007/s00127-015-1046-x.
14. Floen, S.K. and Ellkit, A. (2007). Psychiatric diagnoses, trauma, and suicidality. *Annals of General Psychiatry* 6 (12). https://doi.org/10.1186/1744-859X-6-12.
15. Felton, A., Wright, N., and Stacey, G. (2017). Therapeutic risk-taking: a justifiable choice. *BJPsych Advances* 23 (2): 81–88. https://doi.org/10.1192/apt.bp.115.015701.
16. Higgens A, Morrissey J, Doyle L, Bailey J, Gill A. *Best Practice Principles for Risk Assessment and Safety Planning for Nurses Working in Mental Health Services*. 2015. https://www.drugsandalcohol.ie/25683/1/Best_Practice_Principles_for_Risk_Assessment.pdf
17. Ayhun, F. and Ustun, B. (2021). Examination of risk assessment tools developed to evaluate risks in mental health areas: a systematic review. *Nursing Forum* 56: 330–340.

18. Department of Health (2009). Best practice in managing risk. https://assets.publishing.service.gov.uk/media/5a8020a840f0b62302691adf/best-practice-managing-risk-cover-webtagged.pdf.
19. Beck, A.T. (1998). *Beck Hopelessness Scale*. Chicago: Harcourt Brace Jovanovich.
20. Almvik, R., Woods, P., and Rasmussen, K. (2000). The Brøset violence checklist: sensitivity, specificity, and interrater reliability. *Journal of Interpersonal Violence* 15 (12): 1284–1296.
21. Simmons, M.L., Maguire, T., Ogloff, J.R.P. et al. (2023). Using the dynamic appraisal of situational aggression (DASA) to assess the impact of unit atmosphere on violence risk assessment. *Journal of Psychiatric and Mental Health Nursing* 30 (5): 942–951. https://doi.org/10.1111/jpm.12913.
22. Kennedy, H.G., O'Neill, C., Flynn, G. et al. (2013). *Dangerousness Understanding, Recovery and Urgency Manual (the DUNDRUM Quartet) V1. 0. 26 (01/08/13) Four Structured Professional Judgement Instruments for Admission Triage, Urgency, Treatment Completion and Recovery Assessments*. Dublin, Ireland: Trinity College Dublin.
23. Douglas, K.S., Hart, S.D., Webster, C.D., and Belfrage, H. (2013). *HCR-20V3: Assessing Risk of Violence – User Guide*. Burnaby: Mental Health, Law, and Policy Institute, Simon Fraser University.
24. Royal College of Psychiatrists (2024). Health of the nation outcome scales. www.rcpsych.ac.uk/improving-care/ccqi/health-of-nation-outcome-scales
25. Hart, S.D. and Boer, D.P. (2010). Structured professional judgment guidelines for sexual violence risk assessment: The sexual violence Risk-20 (SVR-20) and risk for sexual violence protocol (RSVP). In: *Handbook of Violence Risk Assessment* (ed. R.K. Otto and K.S. Douglas), 269–294. Routledge/Taylor & Francis Group.
26. Haines, A., Brown, A., Javaidi, S.F. et al. (2018). Assessing protective factors for violence risk in UK general mental health services using the structures assessment of protective factors. *International Journal of Offender Therapy and Comparative Criminology* 62 (12): 3965–3983.
27. Beck, A.T., Maria, K., and Arlene, W. (1979). Assessment of suicidal intention: the scale for suicide ideation. *Journal of Consulting and Clinical Psychology* 47 (2): 343–352. https://doi.org/10.1037//0022-006x.47.2.343.
28. Royal College of Psychiatrists (2023). *Press Release: inaccurate suicide risk assessments could be putting lives at risk says RCPsych*. www.rcpsych.ac.uk/news-and-features/latest-news/detail/2023/09/10/inac.urate-suicide-risk-assessments-could-be-putting-lives-at-risk-says-rcpsych
29. NHS England (2025). Staying safe from suicide https://www.england.nhs.uk/long-read/staying-safe-from-suicide/#:~:text=Suicide%20prediction%20tools%2C%20scales%20and,widespread%2C%20but%20it%20is%20unacceptable.
30. Carter, G. and Spittal, M.J. (2018). Suicide risk assessment: risk stratification is not accurate enough to be clinically useful and alternative approaches are needed. *Crisis: The Journal of Crisis Intervention and Suicide Prevention* 39 (4): 229–334. https://doi.org/10.1027/0227-5910/a000558.
31. Fedorowicz, S.E., Dempsey, R.C., Ellis, N. et al. (2023). How is suicide risk assessed in healthcare settings in the UK? A systematic scoping review. *PLoS One* 18 (2). https://doi.org/10.1371/journal.pone.0280789: e0280789.
32. Royal College of Psychiatrists (2016). Assessment and management of risk to others. www.rcpsych.ac.uk/docs/default-source/members/supporting-you/managing-and-assessing-risk/assessmentandmanagementrisktoothers.pdf
33. Macneil, C.A., Hasty, M.K., Conus, P., and Berk, M. (2012. Published Online, https://doi.org/10.1186/1741-7015-10.111). Is diagnosis enough to guide interventions in mental health? Using case formulation in clinical practice. *BMC Medicine* 10.

34. Nyman, M., Hofvander, B., Nilsson, T., and Wijk, H. (2022). You should just keep your mouth shut and do as we say. Forensic psychiatric inpatients experiences of risk assessments. *Issues in Mental Health Nursing* 43 (2): 137–145.
35. Ray, I. and Simpson, A.I.F. (2019). Shared risk formulation in forensic psychiatry. *The Journal of the American Academy of Psychiatry and the Law* 47 (1): 22–28. https://doi.org/10.29158/JAAPL.003813-19.
36. Davoren, M., Hennessy, S., Conway, C. et al. (2015). Recovery and concordance in a secure forensic psychiatry hospital the self-rated DUNDRUM-3 programme completion and DUNDRUM-4 recovery scales. *BMC Psychiatry* 15 (61). https://doi.org/10.1186/s12888-015-0433-x.
37. van den Brink, R.H.S., Troquete, N.A.C., Beitema, H. et al. (2015). Risk assessment by client and case manager for shared decision making in outpatient forensic psychiatry. *BMC Psychiatry* 15 (120). https://doi.org/10.1186/s12888-015-0500-3: 120.
38. Care Quality Commission (2022). Brief guide: assessing mental health care in the emergency department (ED). Available at: www.cqc.org.uk/sites/default/files/2022-09/Brief_Guide_Assessing_mental_health_in_the_emergency_department.odt
39. Mental Health Act (2007). www.legislation.gov.uk/ukpga/2007/12/contents.
40. Warrington, C. (2019). Repeated police mental health act detentions in England and Wales: trauma and recurrent suicidality. *International Journal of Environmental Research and Public Health* 16 (23): 4786. https://doi.org/10.3390/ijerph16234786.
41. Bendelow, G., Warrington, C.A., Jones, A.M., and Markham, S. (2019). Police detentions of mentally disordered persons. A multi-method investigation of section 136 use in Sussex. *Medicine, Science and the Law* 59 (2): 95–103. https://doi.org/10.1177/0025802419830882.
42. Jenkins, O., Dye, S., Obeng-Asare, F. et al. (2017). Police liaison and section 136: comparison of two different approaches. *BJPsych Bulletin* 41 (2): 76–82. https://doi.org/10.1192/pb.bp.115.052977.
43. Department of Health (2021). Share: consent, confidentiality & information sharing in mental healthcare & suicide prevention. https://assets.publishing.service.gov.uk/media/6124b7098fa8f53dce96067b/zero-suicide-alliance-share.pdf
44. Conlon, D., Raeburn, T., and Wand, T. (2019). Disclosure of confidential information by mental health nurses, of patients they assess to be a risk of harm to self or others: an integrative review. *International Journal of Mental Health Nursing* 28 (6): 1235–1247. https://doi.org/10.1111/inm.12642.
45. Shepherd, S.M. (2016). Violence risk instruments may be culturally unsafe for use with indigenous patients. *Australasian Psychiatry* 24 (6): 565–567. https://doi.org/10.1177/1039856216665287.
46. Shepherd, S.M. and Lewis-Fernandez, R. (2016). Forensic risk assessment and culture diversity – contemporary challenges and future directions. *Psychlogy, Public Policy and Law* 22 (4): 427–438. https://doi.org/10.1037/law0000102.
47. Shepherd, S.M. and Sullivan, D. (2017). Covert and implicit influences on the interpretation of violence risk instruments. *Psychiatry, Psychology and Law* 24 (2): 292–301. https://doi.org/10.1080/13218719.2016.1197817.
48. Home Office (2020). Police powers and procedures, England and Wales, year ending 31 March 2020 second edition. https://assets.publishing.service.gov.uk/media/5faea42d8fa8f55defe432a9/police-powers-procedures-mar20-hosb3120.pdf
49. Youth justice Board for England and Wales (2021). Youth justice statistics: 2021 to 2022. https://www.gov.uk/government/statistics/youth-justice-statistics-2021-to-2022

50. Lammy, D. (2017). The Lammy review. https://assets.publishing.service.gov.uk/media/5a82009040f0b62305b91f49/lammy-review-final-report.pdf

51. Burke, C., Ellis, J.D., Peltier, M.R. et al. (2023). Adverse childhood experiences and pathways to violent behavior for women and men. *Journal of Interpersonal Violence* 38 (3–4): 4034–4060. https://doi.org/10.1177/08862605221113012.

52. Wilmot, P. (2023). Working towards more culturally informed formulation using the power threat meaning framework. *Forensic Update* 1 (144): 20–24. https://doi.org/10.53841/bpsfu.2023.1.144.20.

53. Andretta, J., Worrel, F., Watkins, K.M. et al. (2019). Race and stereotypes matter when you ask about conduct problems: implications for violence risk assessment in juvenile justice settings. *Journal of Black Psychology* 45 (1): 26–51. https://doi.org/10.1177/0095798418821278.

54. Sandfort, T.G.M., de Graaf, R., ten Have, M. et al. (2014). Same-sex sexuality and psychiatric disorders in the second Netherlands mental health survey and incidence study (NEMESIS-2). *LGBT Health* 1 (4): 292–301. https://doi.org/10.1089/lgbt.2014.0031.

55. Gmelin, J.-O.H., De Vries, Y.A., Baams, L. et al. (2022). Increased risks for mental disorders among LGB individuals: cross-national evidence from the world mental health surveys. *Social Psychiatry and Psychiatric Epidemiology* 57 (11): 2319–2332. https://doi.org/10.1007/s00127-022-02320-z.

56. Tordoff, D.M., Wanta, J.W., Collin, A. et al. (2022). Mental health outcomes in transgender and nonbinary youths receiving gender-affirming care. *JAMA Network Open* 5 (7). https://doi.org/10.1001/jamanetworkopen.2022.29031.

57. Tan, K.K.H., Byne, J.L., Treharne, G.J., and Veale, J.F. (2023). Unmet need for gender-affirming care as a social determinant of mental health inequities for transgender youth in Aotearoa/New Zealand. *Journal of Public Health* 45 (2): e225–e233. https://doi.org/10.1093/pubmed/fdac131.

58. Jadva, V., Guasp, A., Bradlow, J.H. et al. (2023). Predictors of self-harm and suicide in LGBT youth: the role of gender, socio-economic status, bullying and school experience. *Journal of Public Health* 45 (1): 102–108. https://doi.org/10.1093/pubmed/fdab383.

59. Equality and Human Rights (2020). Inclusive justice: a system designed for all. https://www.equalityhumanrights.com/sites/default/files/ehrc_inclusive_justice_a_system_designed_for_all_june_2020.pdf.

60. Woodhouse, E., Hollingdale, J., Davies, L. et al. (2024; https://doi.org/10.1186/s12916-024-03320-3). Identification and support of autistic individuals within the UK criminal justice system: a practical approach based upon professional consensus with input from lived experience. *BMC Medical* 22: 157.

61. Blackmore, C.E., Woodhouse, E.L., Gillan, N. et al. (2022). Adults with autism spectrum disorder and the criminal justice system: an investigation of prevalence of contact with the criminal justine system, risk factors and sex differences in a specialist assessment service. *Autism* 26 (8): 2098–2107. https://doi.org/10.1177/136246132210.1343.

62. Slavny-Cross, R., Allison, C., Griffiths, S., and Baron-Cohen, S. (2022). Autism and the criminal justice system: an analysis of 93 cases. *Autism Research* 15 (5): 904–914. https://doi.org/10.1002/aur.2690.

63. Anns, F., D'Souza, S., MacCormick, C. et al. (2023). Risk of criminal justice system interactions in young adults with attention-deficit/hyperactivity disorder: findings from a national birth cohort. *Journal of Attention Disorders* 27 (12): 1332–1342. https://doi.org/10.1177/10870547231177469.

64. Police and Criminal Evidence Act (1984). www.legislation.gov.uk/ukpga/1984/60/contents

65. Crane, L., Maras, K.L., Hawken, T. et al. (2016). Experiences of autism Spectrum disorder and policing in England and Wales: surveying police and the autism community. *Journal of Autism and Developmental Disorders* 46 (6): 2028–2041. https://doi.org/10.1007/s10803-016-2729-1.

66. Girardi, A., Hancock-Johnson, E., Thomas, C., and Wallang, P.M. (2019). Assessing the risk of inpatient violence in autism spectrum disorder. 47 (4): 427–436. https://doi.org/10.29158/JAAPL.033864-19.

67. Chester, V., Vollm, B., Tromans, S. et al. (2018). Long-stay patients with and without intellectual disability in forensic psychiatric settings: comparison of characteristics and needs. *BJPsych Open* 4 (4): 226–234. https://doi.org/10.1192/bjo.2018.24.
68. Quinn, S., Rhynas, S., Gowland, S. et al. (2022). Risk for intellectual disability populations in inpatient forensic settings in the United Kingdom: a literature review. *Journal of Applied Research in Intellectual Disabilities* 35 (6): 1267–1280. https://doi.org/10.1111/jar.13030.
69. Martí-Agustí, G., García-Largo, L.M., Martin-Fumadó, C. et al. (2019). Intellectual disability: criminality, assessment and forensic issues. *Spanish Journal of Legal Medicine* 45 (4): 155–162. https://doi.org/10.1016/j.remle.2019.03.002.
70. Lofthouse, R.E., Golding, L., Totsika, V. et al. (2020). Predicting aggression in adults with intellectual disability: a pilot study of the predictive efficacy of the current risk of violence and the short dynamic risk scale. *Journal of Applied Research in Intellectual Disabilities* 33 (4): 702–710. https://doi.org/10.1111/jay.12665.
71. Matthews, M. and Bell, E. (2020). Assessment of Risk of Violent Offending for Adults with Intellectual Disability and/or Autism Spectrum Disorder. In: *The Wiley Handbook of What Works in Violence Risk Management* (ed. J.S. Wormith, L.A. Craig, and T.E. Hogue). https://doi.org/10.1002/9781119315933.ch17.
72. Ward, J.L., Vazeuz-Vazquez, A., Phillips, K. et al. (2025). Admission to acute medical wards for mental health concerns among children and young people in England from 2012 to 2022: a cohort study. *The Lancet Child and Adolescent Health* 9 (2): 112–120. https://doi.org/10.1016/S2352-4642(24)00333-X.
73. Royal College of Emergency Medicine (2022). A survey of children and adolescent mental health (CAMH) Services in the Emergency Department. https://rcem.ac.uk/wp-content/uploads/2022/08/CAMHS_ED_Survey_August_2022.pdf.
74. Chitasbesan, P., Lennox, C., Theodosiou, L. et al. (2014). The development of the comprehensive health assessment tool for young offenders within the secure estate. *The Journal of Forensic Psychiatry and Psychology* 25 (1): 1–25. https://doi.org/10.1080/14789949.2014.882387.
75. Laake, A.L., Roaldset, J.O., Husum, T.L. et al. (2025). Predictive accuracy of the violence risk assessment checklist for youth in acute institutions: a prospective naturalistic multicenter study. *European Psychiatry* 68 (1). https://doi.org/10.1192/j.eurpsy.2025.3.
76. Manning, J.C., Walker, G.M., Carter, T. et al. (2018). Children and Young people-Mental health safety assessment tool (CYP-MH-SAT) study: protocol for the development and psychometric evaluation of an assessment tool to identify immediate risk of self-harm and suicide in children and young people (10-19 years) in acute paediatric hospital settings. *BMJ Open* 8 (4). https://doi.org/10.1136/bmjopen-2017-020964.
77. Allen, G., Mansfield, Z. (2023). Homicide statistics. [House of Commons Library Research Briefing]. Available at: https://researchbriefings.files.parliament.uk/documents/CBP-8224/CBP-8224.pdf.
78. Mamak, M. and Chaimowitz, G. (2022). Violence risk assessment of older adult. *International Journal of Risk and Recovery* 5 (1): 1–4.
79. Ravyts, S.G., Perez, E., Donovan, E.K. et al. (2022). Measurement of aggression in older adults. *Aggressive and Violent Behavior* 51. https://doi.org/10.1016/j.avb.2020.101484.
80. Walker, T., Shaw, J., Gibb, J. et al. (2021). Lessons learnt from the narratives of women who self-harm in prison. *Crisis* 42 (4): 255–262.
81. Fosse, R., Eidhammer, G., Selmer, L.E. et al. (2021). Stong associations between childhood victimization and community violence in male forensic mental health patients. *Frontiers in Psychiatry* 11. https://doi.org/10.3389/fpsyt.2020.628734.

82. Ryland, H., Cook, J., Yukhnenko, D. et al. (2021). Outcome measures in forensic mental health services: a systematic review of instruments and qualitative evidence synthesis. *European Psychiatry* 64 (1). https://doi.org/10.1192/j.eurpsy.2021.32: 1–40.
83. Messina, N., Calhoun, S., and Braithwaite, J. (2014). Trauma-informed treatment decreases PTSD among women offenders. *Journal of Trauma & Dissociation* 15 (1). https://doi.org/10.1080/15299732.2013.818609: 6–23.
84. Somers, N. and Bartlett, A. (2014). Women's secure hospital care pathways in practice: a qualitative analysis of clinicians views in England and Wales. *BMC Health Services Research* 14. https://doi.org/10.1186/1472-6963-14-450.
85. Wolfschlag, M. and Hakansson, A. (2023). Drug-induced gambling disorder: epidemiology, neurobiology, and management. *Pharmaceutical Medicine* 37 (1): 37–52. https://doi.org/10.1007/s40290-022-00453-9.
86. Hotham, J.E., Simpson, P.J.D., Brooman-White, R.S. et al. (2014). Augmentation of clozapine with amisulpride: an effective therapeutic strategy for violent treatment-resistant schizophrenia patients in a UK high-security hospital. *CNS Spectrums* 19 (5): 403–410. https://doi.org/10.1017/S1092852913000874.
87. Cavaliere, V.S., Glassman, M., BA, D.P. et al. (2022). Anti-aggressive effects of clozapine in involuntarily committed black patients with severe mental illness. *Schizophrenia Research* 243: 163–169. https://doi.org/10.1016/j.schres. 2022.03.006.
88. Hirsch, S. and Steinart, T. (2019). The use of rapid tranquilization in aggressive behavior. *Dtsch Arztebl International* 116: 445–452. https://doi.org/10.3238/arztebl.2019.0445.
89. Valdivieso-Jiminez, G. (2018). Paradoxic effect of benzodiazepines in geriatric population. *MOJ Gerentology & Geriatrics* 3 (3): 219–220.
90. Bak, M., Weltens, I., Bervoets, C. et al. (2019). The pharmacological management of agitated and aggressive behaviour: a systematic review and meta-analysis. *European Psychiatry* 57: 78–100. https://doi.org/10.1016/j.eurpsy.2019.01.014.
91. NICE (2017). NG66 Overview|Mental health of adults in contact with the criminal justice system|Guidance|NICE. https://www.nice.org.uk/guidance/ng66
92. Margetic, B., Margetic, B.A., Ivanec, D., and Palijan, T.Z. (2017). What leads to high antipsychotic dosing in forensic patients with schizophrenia? *CNS Spectrums* 22 (6): 435–438. https://doi.org/10.1017/S1092852916000675.
93. Lassen, S., Heintz, T., Pederson, T. et al. (2023). Nationwide study on antipsychotic polypharmacy among forensic psychiatric patients. *International Journal of Circumpolar Health* 82 (1). https://doi.org/10.1080/22423982.2023.2218654.
94. Farrell, C. and Brink, J. (2020). The prevalence and factors associated with antipsychotic polypharmacy in a forensic psychiatric sample. *Frontiers in Psychiatry* 11. https://doi.org/10.3389/fpsyt.2020.00263.
95. Howner, K., Andine, P., Engberg, G. et al. (2020). Pharmacological treatment in forensic psychiatry – a systematic review. *Frontiers in Psychiatry* 10: 10. https://doi.org/10.3389/fpsyt.2019.00963.
96. Reisegger, A., Slamanig, R., Winkler, H. et al. (2022). Pharmacological interventions to reduce violence in patients with schizophrenia in forensic psychiatry. *CNS Spectrums* 27 (4): 388–398. https://doi.org/10.1017/S1092852921000134.
97. Waqar, M.U., Amin, H., Ni Mhuircheartaigh, E. et al. (2023). Prevalence of treatment resistant psychoses in a complete national forensic mental health service: a Dundrum forensic redevelopment evaluation study (D-FOREST). *European Psychiatry* 66 (S1): 431–432. https://doi.org/10.1192/j.eurpsy.2023.928.

98. Correll, C.U., Rubio, J.M., and Kane, J.M. (2018). What is the risk-benefit ratio of long-term antipsychotic treatment in people with schizophrenia. *World Psychiatry* 17 (2): 149–160. https://doi.org/10.1002/wps.20516.
99. Buston, G., Kay, H., Nwibe, I. et al. (2022). Prescribing and monitoring of high dose antipsychotic therapy (HDAT) in the acute inpatient setting. *BJPsych Open* 8 (S1). https://doi.org/10.1192/bjo.2022.452.
100. Royal College of Psychiatrists (2023). The risks and benefits of high-dose antipsychotic medication. https://www.rcpsych.ac.uk/docs/default-source/improving-care/better-mh-policy/college-reports/college-report-cr190.pdf?sfvrsn=54f5d9a2_2
101. Royal College of Psychiatrists (2017). Prescribing high dose and combined antipsychotics on adult psychiatric wards. https://www.elft.nhs.uk/sites/default/files/2022-03/POMH-UK%2BTopic%2B1g%2Band%2B3d%2Breport%2B-Trust%2B12.pdf
102. Bergman-Evans, B. (2020). A nurse practitioner led protocol to address polypharmacy in long-term care. *Geriatric Nursing* 41 (6): 956–961. https://doi.org/10.1016/j.gerinurse.2020.07.002.
103. Austin, A., Favril, L., Craft, S. et al. (2023). Factors associated with drug use in prison: a systematic review of quantitative and qualitative evidence. *International Journal of Drug Policy* 122: 104248. https://doi.org/10.1016/j.drugpo.2023.104248.
104. van de Baan, F.C., Montanari, L., Royuela, L., and Lemmens, P.H.H.M. (2022). Prevalence of illicit drug use before imprisonment in Europe: results from a comprehensive literature review. *Drugs: Education, Prevention and Policy* 29 (1): 1–12. https://doi.org/10.1080/09687637.2021.1879022.
105. Lewitzka, U., Severus, E., Bauer, R. et al. (2015). The suicide prevention effect of lithium: more than 20 years of evidence – a narrative review. *International Journal of Bipolar Disorder* 3: 32. https://doi.org/10.1186/s40345-015-0032-2.
106. Sarai, S.K., Mekala, H.M., and Lippmann, S. (2018). Lithium suicide prevention: a brief review and reminder. *Innovations in Clinical Neuroscience* 15 (11–12): 30–32.
107. Witt, K.G., Hetrick, S.E., Rajaram, G. et al. (2021). Pharmacological interventions for self-harm in adults. *Cochrane Database of Systematic Reviews* 2021: 1. https://doi.org/10.1002/14651858.CD013669.pub2.
108. Huang, X., Harris, L.M., Funsch, K.M. et al. (2022). Efficacy of psychotropic medications on suicide and self-injury: a meta-analysis of randomized controlled trials. *Translational Psychiatry* 12: 400. https://doi.org/10.1038/s41398-022-02173-9.
109. Moghaddas, A., Dianatkhah, M., Ghaffari, S., and Ghaeli, P. (2017). The potential role of naltrexone in borderline personality disorder. *Iranian Journal of Psychiatry* 12 (2): 142–146.
110. Karakula-Juchnowicz, H., Banaszek, A., and Juchnowicz, D. (2024). Use of the opioid receptor antagonist-naltrexone in the treatment of non-suicidal self-injury. *Psychiatria Polska* 58 (4): 605–618. https://doi.org/10.12740/PP/OnlineFirst/161954.
111. Rana, F., Gormez, A., and Varghese, S. (2013). Pharmacological interventions for self-injurious behaviour in adults with intellectual disabilities. *Cochrane Database of Systematic Reviews* 2013: 4. https://doi.org/10.1002/14651858.CD009084.pub2.
112. Krug, E.G., Dahlberg, L.L., Mercy, J.A. et al. (2022). *World Report on Violence and Health*. Geneva Switzerland: WHO https://www.who.int/publications/i/item/9241545615.
113. National Institute for Health and Care Excellence (2015). Violence and Aggression: Short-Term management in mental health, health and community settings. [London] Clinical Guidelines NG10. Available at: www.nice.org.uk/guidance/ng10.

114. Maguire, R., Daffern, M., Bowe, S.J., and McKenna, B. (2018). Risk assessment and subsequent nursing interventions in a forensic mental health inpatient setting: associations and impact on aggressive behaviour. *Journal of Clinical Nursing* 27: 971–983.

115. Holley, J., Tapp, J., and Draycott, S. (2021). How do forensic inpatients' interpersonal sensitivity to dominance and perceptions of staff coercion impact upon anger and rates of aggression? *The Journal of Forensic Practice* 25 (2): 90–105.

116. Holland, A., Stevens, A., Harris, M. et al. (2023). Analysis of the UK government's 10-year drugs strategy – a resource for practitioners and policymakers. *Journal of Publish Health* 45 (2): 215–224. https://doi.org/10.1093/pubmed/fdac114.

117. Yukhenenko, D., Blackwood, N., Lichtenstein, P., and Fazel, S. (2023). Psychiatric disorders and reoffending risk in individuals with community sentences in Sweden: a national cohort study. *The Lancet* 8 (2): 119–129. https://doi.org/10.1016/S2468-2667(22)00312-7.

118. Zgoba, K.M., Reeves, R., Tamburello, A., and Debilio, L. (2020). Criminal recidivism in inmates with mental illness and substance use disorders. *The Journal of the American Academy of Psychiatry and Law* 53 (1). https://doi.org/10.29158/JAAPL.003913-20.

119. Hardin, K. and Scurich, N. (2022). The dark figure of violence committed by discharged psychiatric inpatients. *Journal of Forensic Practice* 24 (3): 229–240. https://doi.org/10.1108/FJP-11-2021-0058.

120. Nagtegaal, M.H. and Boonmann, C. (2016). Conditional release of forensic psychiatric patients consistent with or contrary to behavioral experts' recommendations in the Netherlands: prevalence rates, patient characteristics and recidivism after discharge from conditional release. *Behavioural Sciences and the Law* 34 (2–3): 257–277. https://doi.org/10.1002/bsl.2224. PMID: 27256002.

121. Chan, B. and Shehtman, M. (2019). Clinical risk factors of acute severe or fatal violence among forensic mental health patients. *Psychiatry Research* 275: 20–26. https://doi.org/10.1016/j.psychres.2019.03.005.

122. Adily, A., Albalawi, O., Sara, G. et al. (2023). Mental health service utilisation and reoffending in offenders with a diagnosis of psychosis receiving non-custodial sentences: a 14-year follow-up study. *The Australian and New Zealand Journal of Psychiatry* 57 (3): 411–422. https://doi.org/10.1177/00048674221098942.

123. Adily, A., Albalawi, O., Karaminia, A. et al. (2020). Association between early contact with mental health services after an offense and reoffending in individuals diagnosed with psychosis. *JAMA Psychiatry* 77 (11): 1137–1146. https://doi.org/10.1001/jamapsychiatry.2020.1255.

124. de Vogel, V., De Beuf, T., Shepherd, S., and Schneider, R.D. (2022). Violence risk assessment with the HCR-20V3 in legal contexts: a critical reflection. *Journal of Personality Assessment* 104 (2): 252–264. https://doi.org/10.1080/00223891.2021.2021925.

125. Gray, N.S., Taylor, J., and Snowden, R.J. (2018). Predicting violent reconvictions using the HCR-20. *The British Journal of Psychiatry* 192 (5): 384–387. https://doi.org/10.1192/bjp.bp.107.044065.

126. Tully, J. (2017). HCR-20 shows poor field validity in clinical forensic psychiatry settings. *Evidence-Based Mental Health* 20 (3): 95–96. https://doi.org/10.1136/eb-2017-102745.

127. Murphy, P., Potter, L., Tully, J. et al. (2016). A cost comparison study of using global positioning system technology (electronic monitoring) in a medium secure forensic psychiatric service. *The Journal of Forensic Psychiatry & Psychology* 28 (1): 57–69. https://doi.org/10.1080/14789949.2016.1261172.

128. Connell, C. (2016). Forensic occupational therapy to reduce risk of reoffending: a survey of practice in the United Kingdom. *Journal of Forensic Psychiatry & Psychology* 27 (6): 907–928. https://doi.org/10.1080/14789949.2016.1237535.

129. Ahmed, N., Reynolds, L., Barlow, S. et al. (2024). Barriers and enablers to shared decision-making in assessment and management of risk: a qualitative interview study with people using mental health services. *PLOS mental Health* 1 (6). https://doi.org/10.1371/journal.pmen.0000157.

130. NHS England (n.d.). Mental health secure care programme. Available at: https://www.england.nhs.uk/mental-health/adults/secure-care/#:~:text=The%20Mental%20Health%20Secure%20Care,a%20stronger%20focus%20on%20recovery.
131. HM Prison and Probation Service (2025). HMPPS response: A thematic review of delays in the transfer of mentally unwell prisoners. Policy Paper. https://assets.publishing.service.gov.uk/media/682736d4010c5c28d1c7e732/HMPPS_and_NHSE_response_to_the_thematic_review_of_delays_in_the_transfer_of_mentally_unwell_prisoners.pdf.
132. Zhang, H. and Firdaus, A. (2024). What does media say about mental health: a literature review of medica coverage on mental health. *Journal Media* 5 (3): 967–979. https://doi.org/10.3390/journalmedia5030061.
133. Crapanzano, K.A., Deweese, S., Pham, D. et al. (2023). The role of bias in clinical decision-making of people with serious mental illness and medical co-morbidities: a scoping review. *The Journal of Behavioral Health Services & Research* 50 (2): 236–262. https://doi.org/10.1007/s11414-022-09829-w.

CHAPTER 18

Substance Use – Including Co-occurring Mental Health and Drugs and Alcohol (COMHAD)

Lois Dugmore

Leicestershire Partnership NHS Trust, Leicester, UK

> **Aim**
>
> The aim of this chapter is to review the fundamental principles of collaborating with clients with substance use and being able to understand co-occurring mental health, alcohol and drugs (COMHAD) issues, focusing on assessment and treatment for both groups in line with the Advanced Practice Mental Health Curriculum and Capabilities Framework [1]. This will enable advanced practitioners in mental health (APMHs) to work confidently and effectively with individuals and both educate and lead staff groups to understand the principles of working with substance use and COMHAD. The chapter will include an understanding of the complex nature of COMHAD and current service delivery models. It will review how stigma and inequalities and cultural competence are explored and challenged in the context of substance use at an advanced level. The chapter will also highlight the importance of framing interventions and service development at an advanced level to improve outcomes for substance use and COMHAD individuals in relation to their health and well-being.

LEARNING OUTCOMES

After reading this chapter, the reader will be able to:

1. Demonstrate advanced skills in working with substance use in line with national and local guidance.
2. Have an enhanced knowledge of frameworks and demonstrate skills in line with NICE guidance.

The Advanced Practitioner in Mental Health, First Edition. Edited by Clare Allabyrne.
© 2026 John Wiley & Sons Ltd. All rights reserved, including rights for text and data mining and training of artificial intelligence technologies or similar technologies. Published 2026 by John Wiley & Sons Ltd.

3. Evidence advanced skills in working with substance use.
4. Utilise these skills to develop the nursing workforce using evidence-based good practice.
5. Provide advice and guidance in the assessment and treatment of substance use by demonstrating advanced clinical skills and be able to develop advanced clinical policy.
6. Initiate and deliver evidence-based knowledge to enhance good practice within the wider mental health team to reduce stigma.
7. Contribute to organisational learning including cultural competence.
8. Work within different commissioning positions in substance use services and facilitate senior joint working with other agencies.

ADVANCED PRACTICE MENTAL HEALTH CURRICULUM AND CAPABILITIES FRAMEWORK [1]

This chapter will meet capabilities from across the four pillars; see the following examples in Table 18.1.

TABLE 18.1 Examples from the four pillars.

Clinical practice	
Initiate, evaluate and modify a range of interventions, which may include therapies, medicines, lifestyle advice and care.	Interventions should include: Solution-focused therapy Motivational interviewing Harm minimisation advice Relapse prevention Patient safety advice
Leadership and management	
Identify, critically evaluate and reformulate understanding of professional boundaries to support new ways of working within the context of organisational and service need.	Develop key relationships within substance use services. Sharing of key information regarding substance use and other commissioned services including opiate prescribing, alcohol and drug detoxification and rehabilitation.
Education	
Effectively utilise a range of evidence-based educational strategies/interventions to support person-centred care with individuals, their families and carers and other healthcare colleagues.	Work with all staff groups to develop skills in relation to substance use. Facilitate inter-professional working and use evidence-based models.
Research	
Critically appraise and apply the evidence base in influencing engagement, recovery, shared decision-making, transference and safeguarding.	Lead on the development of research within substance use. Provide clinical supervision for substance use. Promote safety and work within statutory responsibilities related to substance use.

Source: Adapted from [1].

Clinical Practice

Substance use and COMHAD encompass demonstrating compassion, understanding and delivering clinical care underpinned by research-based practice and accredited tools in both substance use and mental health to include Assist-Lite [2]. Assist-Lite is a World Health Organisation (WHO) tool developed as an assessment tool for substance use and adapted for mental health settings. It records the patient's current self-reported substance use and signposts to appropriate services. Using appropriate tools provides the advanced practitioner with the equipment to formulate management plans for substance use, when working with an ever-changing portfolio of substances. It also requires in-depth knowledge in working across multi-agency groups. There is a need to deliver a range of substance use therapeutic interventions including pharmacology, psychosocial interventions, motivational interviewing, harm minimisation and relapse prevention based on trauma-informed care to improve outcomes. It is essential to have knowledge of and understand local service provision and interagency working within clinical practice to develop links with and co work with other agencies providing substance use services; ensuring protocols are in place for transition of individuals between mental health and substance use services.

Leadership and Management

It is vitally Important within leadership and management to participate and work within the professional boundaries across and outside of the organisations involved. This has more bearing for substance use and COMHAD services due to the separate commissioning streams; meaning more co-working, co-location and information sharing agreements need to be in place. It is requisite to be a role model and offer leadership and promote safe care in complex cases, with the ability to lead by example and be able to demonstrate skills in engagement of complex individuals.

Education

Deliver evidence-based practice in substance use by implementing and training others to use recognised tools in assessment and treatment of substance use. Develop inter-professional learning and development opportunities within substance use by creating networks for discussion and education across multi-agencies. Identify new developments in practice and share across networks. Development of training programmes both face to face and e learning to enhance workforce skills. Developing relationships with substance use agencies to develop training on substance use for mental health services and enabling other agencies to join local training as part of partnership working. The mainstreaming of discussions in education regarding the needs of drug and alcohol using individuals as part of core needs assessment.

Research

The APMH will evidence quality improvement by implementing evidence-based practice. Promoting and delivering new treatments and evidence-based practice within the role of APMH can lead to organisational change and improvement in clinical outcomes. An example of this could be the implementation for supply and use of naloxone for those at risk of overdose. The APMH will be able to respond to patient safety notices and adapt individual care needs as a response. Working with others on research projects across the organisation as an opportunity to collaborate and lead in research enables the cross fertilisation of ideas between agencies. Undertaking small projects involving quality improvement, being a principal investigator on local/national studies develops the portfolio and sets an example for good research led practice.

INTRODUCTION

Across the United Kingdom, 9.6% (3.1 million) of the population uses drugs [3] between the ages of 18 and 50, with the most common drug being cannabis followed by cocaine. Those using alcohol equate to 57% (29.2 million) adults in the United Kingdom [4]. Drug and alcohol use can be viewed as mainstream with statistically representative numbers of the population using drugs and alcohol [5]. In recent times the surge in the media's portrayal of drug and alcohol use as 'the norm' brings the issues into homes and highlights the increasing impact on individuals' lives with an element of acceptance of substance use [6]. This leads to the need for a greater understanding of how drug and alcohol use impacts on individuals and how this then impacts on management within clinical care. Within mental health settings alcohol, cocaine and cannabis use are widespread [7]; this could lead to individuals finding the challenge of disclosure more difficult and for clinicians being able to hear such disclosure. Training and education of staff are key to making this change. An empathetic voice that recognises the experiences of COMHAD individuals and the complex nature of change can help to engage and change the outcome.

Substance use encompasses alcohol use, any form of drug use, both illicit use and the misuse of prescribed or over-the-counter medication. This would include:

Alcohol, heroin, cocaine, ketamine, codeine, dihydrocodeine, amphetamines, cannabis, edibles, khat, benzodiazepines, gabapentin and pregabalin.

For the APMH it is essential to understand and be able to complete risk assessments for those at greater risk of suicide within this group and be able to work with others to implement these plans [8]; however, often these clients with co-occurring issues fall between the gaps [9] and can seek to self-medicate with substances. Many will have experienced trauma and have complex multiple needs [10, 11]. Working with clients who have co-occurring issues requires APMHs to support recovery journeys that include hope, as well as prescribing, talking therapy-based interventions and compassion to engage this client group in a non-judgemental way. There are significant challenges around stigma and experience of working with diverse cultures in this client group and clinical supervision is key to managing thoughts, feelings and emotions that can be generated from working with co-occurring mental health, alcohol and drugs issues. The services that are commissioned to provide substance services are measured on treatment outcomes under the National Drug treatment monitoring system [12]. These outcomes include the length of time in treatment, completion of treatment, substance use, quality of life, crime, and health and injecting risk. For APMHs this can lead to greater complexity when managing care episodes due to the number of agencies and commissioning groups involved in the patients care.

SPECIFIC CONSIDERATIONS IN SUBSTANCE USE AND COMHAD

It is quite common for people to experience problems with their mental health and alcohol/drug use (co-occurring conditions) at the same time [9, 13].

Research shows that mental health problems are experienced by the majority of drug (70%) and alcohol (86%) users in community substance misuse treatment. Death by suicide is also common, with a history of alcohol or drug use being recorded in 54% of all suicides in people experiencing mental health problems. Those individuals with co-occurring conditions have a heightened risk of other health problems and early death. We also know that despite the shared responsibility, the National Health Service (NHS) and local authority commissioners must provide treatment, care and support for people with co-occurring conditions who are often excluded from health services [13].

Stigma

Whilst stigma remains an issue across mental health, stigma for individuals with COMHAD has played a significant role in individuals finding the resilience to enter treatment systems [14]. For substance users, stigma and negative attitudes from staff can delay individuals seeking treatment for their substance use and lead to poorer outcomes [15].

Organisations including the NHS and substance use agencies can inadvertently create barriers within services that can exclude individuals from accessing treatment services [16]. These include exclusion criteria based on non-engagement, staff attitude, access to services, times of appointment for working adults and the venues of services.

Specifically for women, stigma arises from gendered judgements around female substance use and especially for women who have children [17] that can lead to disengagement with services. Women feel judged in services and are concerned they will lose custody of their children and are therefore more likely to underplay or not seek help with substance use.

Populations who use drugs to enhance sex (chem sex) can often feel excluded from services when seeking help with mental health, and a greater understanding of chem sex is required [18, 19]. Being more flexible with service provision and understanding the needs of individuals that are poor engagers with services can reduce stigma and enable acceptance of services.

Cultural Competence

Cultural competence within healthcare is key to ensuring safe care and reducing health inequalities [20]. Cultural competence within the healthcare setting can be seen as a process [21, 22] to facilitate understanding of cultural need within healthcare delivery. For migrant populations culture and language can be an extremely specific barrier to engaging in COMHAD care. Cultural competence in mental healthcare settings has a role to play within these settings to engage all populations within treatment. For many, COMHAD are wrapped in stigma within the individual's culture, which leads to a reduction in help seeking [23]. Ensuring staff are trained to meet the needs of this complex client group is essential in engaging clients within treatment specific to their cultural needs [24].

Inequalities

'Health inequalities are unfair and avoidable differences in health across the population, and between different groups within society. These include how long people are likely to live, the health conditions they may experience and the care that is available to them' [25, p. 1]. Inequalities in health are present in individuals who use alcohol in relation to early deaths and increased poor health [26]. Individuals accessing treatment report stigma and prejudice. For substance users they are likely to enter many healthcare settings where structural stigma plays a part in services that are underfunded; so, accessing several different elements of healthcare based on both physical and mental health need can lead to more difficulties in access because of substance use [27, 28]. Additional difficulties arise in more marginalised groups, for example, those with sexual dysphoria or who identify with LGBTQIA are less likely to access substance use services and therefore have increasing need [29, 30]. For ethnic minority groups there exist cultural issues related to substance use that need to be addressed to engage this population within treatment systems [31] Health inequalities in substance use occur due to the language used to describe substance users, lack of compassion as substance users can be viewed as the instigators of their own problems and political rhetoric that criminalises some forms of substance use leading to a lack of uptake within services [32, 33]. Digitalisation to some extent can also lead to inequalities in service provision as many substance users have no credit for phones or access to a computer; this can be because of poor socioeconomic factors or substance use. Diagnostic overshadowing can also play its part (this is discussed in more detail in Chapter 1), when clients are not diagnosed or incorrectly diagnosed because their substance use overshadows the recognition of other explanations for presenting symptoms or they are asked to manage substance use before they can access other healthcare settings, for example mental health.

Legal Issues

It is important to recognise the need for treatment and acceptance of the consequence of the legislation regarding the supply of drugs. The process for assessment of treatment for substance use in mental health settings can be complex due to commissioning streams.

Understanding current local drug trends and change in drug supplies enables clinicians to ask appropriate questions of individuals in an informed way. Although we have a good understanding of drugs that include heroin, cocaine and cannabis, recent market changes include new strains of Synthetic Cannabinoid Receptor Agonist (SCRA), like spice and mamba, nitazines, synthetic opioids, nitrous oxide and home-produced substances such as Lean which can include some or all of these ingredients: codeine, boiled sweets, codeine linctus, promethazine, paracetamol, dextromethorphan and soft drinks. Understanding these trends and drug interactions with prescribed other drugs can lead to safer service provision when being able to identify the risks of substance use and when prescribing. See Table 18.2 for implications.

ASSESSMENT AND TREATMENT

The advanced practice mental health framework [1] provides a basis on which to focus advanced complex skills within assessment and treatment. Table 18.3 demonstrates how this can be delivered in practice with substance use clients.

A: PERSON-CENTRED THERAPEUTIC ALLIANCE

Developing and engaging individuals with substance use or COMHAD can be challenging when this group struggle to access services. Proiding clear policies and procedures for acceptance and access to services is a starting point to training staff to work with this group through evidence-based practice. When engaging and developing a therapeutic alliance, it is essential to meet on the individuals' terms. Finding the right setting, time, language and their acceptance of use provide the individual with a starting point that allows them to make choices and for the APMH to identify inequalities and work towards therapeutic alliances with individuals which are based on collaborative thinking and shared decision-making.

This can start with:

- My name is: what would you like me to call you?
- Can you tell me about why you are here?

TABLE 18.2 Legal issues and implications.

Class A
- cocaine
- crack cocaine
- ecstasy (MDMA)
- heroin
- LSD
- magic mushrooms
- methadone
- methamphetamine (crystal meth)

Class B
amphetamines
- barbiturates
- cannabis
- codeine
- gamma hydroxybutyrate (GHB)
- gamma-butyrolactone (GBL)
- ketamine
- methylphenidate (Ritalin)
- synthetic cannabinoids
- synthetic cathinones (for example mephedrone, methoxetamine)

Class C
anabolic steroids
- benzodiazepines (diazepam)
- khat
- nitrous oxide (laughing gas)
- piperazines (BZP)
- gabapentin
- pregabalin

Classification refers to perceived harm, severe penalties for possession, trafficking and supply. A carries highest penalty.

Drugs are classed in 3 categories based on the risk to the individual and whether the drug use also includes supply to others.
Penalties by class of drug are
Class A between 7 years and life imprisonment
Class B between 5 and 14 years
Class C between 5 and 14 years
All classes include possibility of an unlimited fine or both a fine and sentencing.

Source: Adapted from [34].

TABLE 18.3 Capabilities in practice for substance use.

A: Person-centred therapeutic alliance	B: Assessment and investigations	C: Formulation
D: Collaborative planning	E Intervention and evaluation	F: Leadership, management, education and research

Source: Adapted from [1].

- What do you feel is your main issue and what you would like help with?
- Can you tell me about your drug and alcohol use?
- Explore carers role and views.
- Explore trauma and sensitive and complex subjects with compassion and remain non-judgemental.
- Time slots that meet the needs of service users.
- Identify if there is a role to offer joint service clinics.
- Would the client benefit from an outreach programme if engagement is challenging?
- Review how the service views missed appointments, and bring the focus on those that are attended.
- Explore mental health, physical health, housing and parental responsibilities alongside substance use.
- Listen to the service user – engage on their terms.
- What does recovery look like from service user perspective?
- Share information, as necessary.

The importance of identifying wider health determinants and social aspects of an individual's life enable a more integrated approach to care, which enables the individual to make an informed choice about service use. Being involved in decision-making around care increases hope, choice and engagement. Clear care planning conducted with the individual promotes inclusivity and acceptance. Avoid making assumptions including that the individual wants to stop using.

B: ASSESSMENT AND INVESTIGATIONS

Clinical Assessment in Substance Use

Clinical assessment for substance misuse should include information from the individual, the referrer, carers and other agencies. Referral to substance use services should always be with individual consent. Check if the individual has the capacity to consent and are willing to discuss their substance use as part of their referral. The assessment should include the completion of the Assist-Lite tool and then additional questions that include:

Questions Concerning Substance Use

What substances are currently used?
The route taken for each substance, for example smoking, snorting, eating and injecting?
First age of using substances and type?
Previous periods of not using?
Any injuries related to substance use?
Who do they use substances with?
Any debts related to substance use or contact with criminal justice system?
Exploited by anyone in relation to obtaining substances (prostitution, sex trafficking)?
Impact on mental and physical health?
Is anyone else worried about the individuals use?
What is it that you are seeking today?

Service Expectations

What does the individual expect to gain from the assessment? This could include referral into substance services, just for information, risks with prescribed medication, overdose advice, harm minimisation advice, prescribing, psychosocial interventions or physical investigations (bloods, urine, drug/alcohol screening). It is important to establish if the individual is currently in treatment with a substance agency or private prescribing.

Substance Use Screening Tools

Substance use screening tools give us a starting point for a conversation and can be incorporated into existing assessment frameworks. There is an array of screening tools for drug and alcohol use. Each screening tool needs to be agreed by the individual organisation and may be subject to licencing agreements. Within mental health settings there has been a move towards using Assist-Lite [35] in a shortened version adapted for mental health settings.

Assist-Lite Adapted for Mental Health Settings

Assist-Lite is a tool created by the WHO [2] for use within mental health settings by clinicians. The tool screens for tobacco, alcohol, illicit drugs and over-the-counter and prescribed medication. The tool takes 5–10 minutes to complete, and the completed tool recommends appropriate psychosocial interventions and/or referral into commissioned substance services [2]. This tool fits with the National Institute of Clinical Excellence (NICE) recommendations in:

- NICE guidance CG51 'Drug misuse in over 16s: psychosocial interventions' [36].
- Nice guidance CG100 'Alcohol-use disorders: diagnosis and management of physical complications' [37].
- NICE guidance CG115 'Alcohol-use disorders: diagnosis, assessment and management of harmful drinking (high-risk drinking) and alcohol dependence' [38].
- Nice guidance NG58 2016 – quality statement people aged fourteen and over with suspected or confirmed severe mental illness are asked about their use of alcohol and drugs [39].
- Nice guidance CG120 – coexisting mental illness (psychoses and substance misuse) [40].
- The national clinical guidelines on drug misuse and dependence (known as the Orange Book) [41].

For more comprehensive assessment of a specific substance, the following assessments can be applied.

AUDIT– Alcohol Use Disorders Identification Test [42]
SADQ – Severe Alcohol Detection Questionnaire [43]
DAST – Drug Abuse Screening Tool [44]
GMAWS – Glasgow Modified Alcohol Withdrawal Scale [45]
CIWA-AR – Clinical Institute Withdrawal Assessment for Alcohol [46]
COWS – Clinical Opiate Withdrawal Scale [47]

Assessment of Alcohol

When Assessing for Alcohol or Drugs, Always Asks About Both; Poly Substance Use is Common

Complete Assist-Lite, Audit and SADQ [43] depending on the severity of use.
Ask additional questions about family and friends views on the individuals alcohol use.
Ask about previous treatment episodes and outcomes.
If currently intoxicated assess for withdrawal using GMAWS or CIWA – AR [4, 46].
Ask if the individual is currently open to a substance service; if yes, liaise with substance agency regarding treatment.

Are there complicating factors including history of:

- seizures
- alcohol-related liver disease
- alcohol-related pancreatitis
- Korsakoffs syndrome
- Wernicke's encephalopathy
- Decompensated liver disease

Are there any concerns regarding housing, social care or medical history?
Signs of withdrawal include:

- Tremor
- Sweating
- Nausea
- Anxiety
- Delirium tremens
- Disorientation
- Hallucination
- Motor incoordination

Current government recommendations for drinking alcohol are:

Limit to 14 units of alcohol a week.
Drink over more than 3 days.
Pregnant women should not drink at all.
Have 2 days with no alcohol each week [48].
Alcohol use is measured in two forms of risk: harmful and hazardous drinking.

Harmful drinking (high risk)

Alcohol consumption that is leading to mental and physical concern.
Drinking 35 units a week or more for women and 50 units and over for men.

Hazardous (increasing risk)

Alcohol use above recommended levels and risk of harm to the individual both mentally and physically.
Drinking 14–35 units a week for women and for men 14–50 units a week [48].

Physical Investigations

Blood tests specifically when using alcohol:

Bloods for Alcohol Use
U & E – Urea & electrolyte
FBC – Full blood count
LFT – Liver function test
INR – Internationalised normalised ratio
SF – Synthetic function
GGT – Gamma-glutamyl transferase
TFT – Thyroid function tests
Lipid profile
Vitamin B12 and folate
Calcium magnesium
Phosphate glucose
ECG – Electrocardiogram
Repeat as necessary

Source: Adapted from [49].

Risk Assessment

Risk assessment is key to fully understanding the individual's needs in regard to substance use and an essential element of any substance use and mental health assessment. The risk assessment should be conducted in line with organisational policies.

Substance use comes with an array of risks and with the additional complexity of mental health issues can lead to concerns by service providers. These risks may include:

Increased risk of suicide and suicidal ideation
Risk of overdose
Physical health BBV, Hep B, C, STI
Violence: perpetrator and victim
Vulnerable
Self-harm
Non-compliance around treatment
Poorer outcomes
Risk of needle stick injuries/abscess
Sexual exploitation/trafficking/prostitution
Lack of housing
Safeguarding vulnerable adults and children
Financial debt
Elevated risk pregnancies
More likely to be in contact with criminal justice
Risk of falls/accidents due to intoxication
Withdrawal seizures

Source: Adapted from [46].

Individuals with COHMAD are more likely to have complex needs including trauma. Therefore, risk profiles present as elevated risk and need comprehensive risk assessments to meet the needs. This will include multiple agencies and the need for closer working relationships with key lead providers. These may include housing, social care, probation, criminal justice settings and voluntary sector support agencies.

C: FORMULATION

Formulation relies on the evidence gathered to make an informed choice for care options. By using the 5Ps framework [50]
Identify the problem: in this case substance use and mental health.

1. **Predisposing factors:** life experiences, trauma, parent substance use, mental health, exploitation and coping strategy.
2. **Precipitating factors:** triggers for substance use may include low mood, change in type of drug/alcohol use, psychoses, suicidal ideation, financial hardship and relationship breakdown.
3. **Presenting:** low mood, change in coping strategies, increased substance use, changes in home life, difficulties in managing thoughts and feelings, inability to sleep, recently come off prescribing or reduced alcohol use and breakdown in support networks.
4. **Perpetuating factors:** continued substance use, lack of support networks and social acceptance of substance use. Stigma.
5. **Protective factors:** family support, access to treatment, acceptance of substance use causal effects on mental health, coping abilities and social prescribing.

Using validated screening tools and physical intervention tests e.g. drug/alcohol screening, blood/urine tests, enable the decisions to be formed based on current evidence-based service specifications and local policies for treatment provided.

D: COLLABORATIVE PLANNING

Collaborative planning is key to working with COMHAD individuals due to commissioning arrangements and many third sector agencies providing this care element. Having robust information sharing agreements allow the cross sharing of information for the benefit of the individual. It is essential to manage the expectations of the individual when negotiating across agencies. Each organisation will work to its own specifications and time scales which may differ and cause confusion for the individual trying to access services. Working across multi professional agencies relies on developing robust policies to ensure the safety of those entering services across different organisational settings. Understanding who is holding the lead for care for the individual and who is responsible for care planning and risk assessment is an essential component for collaborative working.

E: INTERVENTION AND EVALUATION

Each intervention comes with its own risk, be it pharmacological or a psycho-social model of support. It is essential to share those risks with individuals when making choices for treatment and care. The development of care planning and the role of each individual within that process should be clear.

This should include management strategies for when the individual accesses out of hours services and how that information is shared. The care plans should be clear regarding prescribing and the re-issuing of prescriptions to ensure no duplication is made. When reduction regimes are in place these need to be care planned and clearly followed. Psychological interventions should be delivered through evidence-based interventions in line with local and national policy. For individuals with COMHAD there will be examples of social need related to housing, social care regarding interventions with individuals' children and being aware of other agency involvement is key. Outcome measures need to be applied based on substance use interventions. These need to be measured against the individuals experience and expectations.

Pharmacological Principles in Substance Use

The use of drug screening using urine and mouth swabs should be considered before prescribing to confirm drugs currently in the system. The aim of screening is to ensure individual safety, as due to contaminates in street purchased drugs individuals are not always aware of the substances they have taken or may have purchased items not correctly sold, for example being sold nitazines instead of heroin.

Offer access to blood-borne virus (BBV) testing and sexually transmitted infections (STI) screening as appropriate.

When first assessing the individual, it is essential that we recognise the signs of overdose and check for this at each appointment.

British National Formulary (BNF) and NICE guidance suggest using long-acting benzodiazepines, for example, chlordiazepoxide or diazepam to manage alcohol withdrawal symptoms whilst following local clinical guidance. This would be in conjunction with alcohol withdrawal scales to measure withdrawal symptoms.

Alcohol withdrawal protocols would normally occur for 7–10 days. This would entail using a reducing dose down to zero. Most alcohol reductions are conducted in inpatient settings or through community substance use agencies. The individual should be monitored daily for withdrawal symptoms.

When prescribing, this must be conducted within national, regional and local guidelines in relation to first line prescribing for clients with substance use. The drug dependence guidelines known as the orange guide [46] provide a concise guide to drug treatment.

Substance use services and mental health services commissioned to provide substance use do so on both a psychosocial and pharmacological interventions model.

Prescribing in substance use will include:
- Heroin stabilisation and moving towards abstinence
- Benzodiazepine withdrawal
- Alcohol withdrawal

Opiate prescribing things to consider:
Check if individual is open to local substance use service.
Check with dispensing pharmacy. Out of hours usually will be available.

Confirm:
Key worker/prescriber
Dose
Dispensing pharmacy including last date picked up

Consider:

- Use of heroin, diamorphine, methadone, other opiates (dihydrocodeine and buprenorphine, buvidal, naltrexone), benzodiazepines, amphetamines mamba/spice and alcohol. Other drugs including over the counter.
- Urine drug screen must be completed.
- Give written information on methadone treatment (e.g. methadone handbook).
- Physical examination: examine injection sites, BP, pulse, BM and ECG, full blood count, urea and electrolytes, liver function tests with gamma glutamyl transferase (GGT), offer hepatitis C testing and hepatitis B vaccination, advice on BBVs. Consider referral for HIV screening.
- Do not prescribe to those clearly intoxicated.
- If prescribed by local substance agency, continue regime.
- If new to prescribing:

If the client is not in withdrawal, then no methadone needs to be given and prescribing can wait until the next day when a discussion with local substance service can take place (use COWS to assess for withdrawal)

PRN Methadone Regimen [41]

DAY 1

- Initial dose of 30 mg can be given (20 mg if the individual has COPD, low weight or is alcohol dependent and being prescribed alcohol withdrawal meds). The individual can then be given 10 mg methadone PRN only once if continues to have withdrawal at 4 hours.
- The total dose from day 1 should be given on day 2 in the morning with 10 mg to be given once only if there are features of withdrawal (COWS) at 4 hours.
- This is repeated to day 3 to a max of 60 mg as needed or remains at lower dose if no further withdrawal noted.
- Doses above 60 mg may be required but should be discussed with clinical lead.

DAY 2 Onward

➤ STOP PRN dosing and give the total dose given on day one.
➤ Further dose increases should be no more than 5–10 mg on one day and no more than 30 mg in the first week.

Other Supportive Treatment

- **Diarrhoea:** Loperamide 4 mg immediately followed by 2 mg after each loose stool for up to 5 days.
  Usual dose 6–8 mg
  Maximum dose 16 mg/24 hours
- **Nausea/vomiting:** metoclopramide 10 mg tds
- **Stomach cramps:** hyoscine butyl bromide 20 mg qds

- **Agitation/insomnia:** promethazine 25–50 mg, max 100 mg/24 hours, at night for hypnotic effect. Z-hypnotics and benzodiazepines should be avoided for insomnia; however, if short courses of 3 days are used, they should be prescribed along with good sleep hygiene advice
- **Muscular pain/headaches:** paracetamol or NSAIDs

Other Prescribing for Opiates

Buprenorphine can be considered.

This is a partial agonist. The individual needs to be in withdrawal to start which is confirmed through urine testing and COWS (Clinical Opiate Withdrawal Scale).

Dose 4 mg, then 4 mg PRN if symptoms continue.

Prescribing can be increased up to 16–32 mg in 4 mg in increments.

Buvidal Prescribing Through Substance Agencies

Buprenorphine prolonged-release injection (buvidal, camurus) is an opioid partial agonist/antagonist.

It is administered as a weekly or monthly subcutaneous injection and must be given by a healthcare professional.

On Discharge from Hospital Settings

No take home opiate substitute prescribing. Transfer prescribing to local substance service.

Prescribe naloxone take home.

Other Drugs

Drugs such as cannabinoids and stimulants prescribing are only appropriate for risk of seizures in withdrawal or presenting with psychosis.

Benzodiazepines

Illicit use of benzodiazepines comes with risk when purchased on the street or through the internet. It is important to follow local and national guidelines on withdrawal.

For individuals with long-term benzodiazepine use, the starting point is to move from short acting benzodiazepines, for example, lorazepam to longer acting diazepam. It is important to recognise that long-term use can take extended periods of time to withdraw. Slow regimes for withdrawal are preferred. Usually reducing diazepam by 1–2 mg every 2–4 weeks within inpatient settings or by one tenth of the dose every 1–2 weeks. If withdrawals occur, slow down the reduction. Some individuals require reduction by as little as 500 micrograms. This withdrawal needs to be delivered with ongoing psychosocial support [43].

Risks

Prescribing without a full history.

Drugs that have QtC prolonging medication. Methadone is also a QtC prolonging medication (as are promethazine, some antidepressants and many antipsychotics). Before starting methadone, a pre- and post-prescription ECG to ensure that the QtC is not prolonged by the substance use or of another QtC prolonging agent. Consideration needs to be given when prescribing alongside mental health medication.

Conduct a review of any other over-the-counter medication, alcohol use and other illicit drug use prior to prescribing.

Signs of Opiate overdose [41]

This is not an exhaustive list. Each person's response to substances can be different based on experience of substances and type of substance taken. This is specifically for opiate overdose, and some people may not display any of the listed signs of an overdose.

Things to be aware of are:

- Nausea and vomiting
- Blue tinge around mouth, fingers and toes
- Severe stomach pain and abdominal cramps
- Diarrhoea
- Chest pain
- Dizziness
- Loss of balance
- Loss of co-ordination
- Being unresponsive but awake
- Rasping noise or snoring

Steps to Carry Out If You Are with Someone Who Overdoses

The first thing is to call for help. Ask someone else to call 999 for you so that you can stay with the person; if this is not possible, ensure they are positioned on their side, reducing the risk of inhaling their own vomit and then call 999.

Keep talking to them to try to keep them awake.

Use naloxone.

If you are not already aware, try to find out what they have taken. Keep hold of any that is left over.

Place the person in the recovery position.

Stay with the person. It is helpful if you are able to hand over to attending staff what you think the person has taken and hand over any that is left over. Police do not routinely attend call outs for a drug overdose, so do not worry about getting into trouble.

In the case of an opiate overdose – i.e. heroin, methadone or morphine, it is useful to know if the person you are with has a naloxone injection. Naloxone blocks the effects of opiates. It can be given by anyone using opioids without prescription through substance agencies.

Naloxone and Risk at Discharge

Overdose is elevated risk at the point of discharge and measures to prevent this risk should be taken based on local guidelines but can include:

Naloxone in mental health settings should be given to all know opiate users on discharge. Prescribing should be passed back to the local substance agency with no take home opiate substitute treatment given. Prescribing should commence from drug agency the next day.

Interventions

Interventions within substance use are evidence based and can be provided by anyone with training. From harm minimisation advice for individuals who are not ready to change to relapse prevention for individuals who are abstinent. Motivational interviewing provides support and guidance whilst decision-making remains with the individual [51]. Trauma-informed care [52, 53] provides the individual with input and ownership of their treatment pathway and allows for autonomous and shared decision-making. (There is more detail about trauma-informed care in Chapter 7.)

Harm Minimisation

Harm minimisation strategies are important in working with substance users to build better outcomes and give informed choice to individuals around their substance use [54]. The aim is to reduce harm. Stigma can play a part in service users being able to receive harm minimisation when not all agencies attended by individuals deliver harm minimisation [54]. The aim is to consider that individuals may return to use or just wish to cut down on use.

Types of advice given in harm minimisation include:

Alcohol harm minimisation
It is important not to tell someone to 'just stop' drinking. In a dependant, heavy drinker, this has the potential to lead to seizures and even death. Advice and information should be given to individuals based on local guidance. This advice should include.
Try to enjoy more alcohol-free days.
Drink alcohol later in the day. Alternate alcoholic drinks with non-alcoholic drinks.
Aim for lower strength drinks, or add a soft drink to dilute (shandy, wine spritzers, for example)
Do not drink in rounds; take limited cash/card out with you.
Do not mix with prescribed medication or any over-the-counter or purchased medication.
Eat before drinking alcohol.
Make a plan to mix less with friends who drink.
Drink more water to stay hydrated.
Try to drink later in the day.

Harm Minimisation Advice for Drugs [55]

Start low and grow.
Test dose.
Let others know you are using.
Carry naloxone.
Find a safe environment.

Seek help if you are struggling.
Risk of sharing needles.
Try not to mix with alcohol or other types of drugs [55].

Relapse Prevention

Relapse prevention aims to work with individuals who are currently not using and to enable them to remain abstinent. This includes support to manage cravings, to change thought processes and work towards maintaining change. This is supported through one-to-one counselling, group therapy and change strategies [55]. Follow local guidelines.

Motivational Interviewing

Motivational interviewing is recognised as being effective in working with change for COHMAD individuals. This form of counselling style works with the individual as the catalyst for change. The counsellor provides the role for reflection and works on inspiring change and encouraging change conversations. Solutions for change come from the individual [46]. Promoting the training and implementation of motivational interviewing across staffing groups is a key opportunity to improving access for individuals to explore change.

Trauma-Informed Care

Following the principles of trauma-informed care can lead to better outcomes for COHMAD individuals by understanding the dialogue of trauma that can lead to substance use and explore ways in which to enable the individual to create change [52]. As mentioned previously, Chapter 7 contains more detailed information on trauma-informed care.

Case Scenario
George is a 64-year-old Afro Caribbean man. He lives alone. He has little family support. There is a history of psychoses. He has a long history of substance use including use of heroin, crack and cannabis. He uses tobacco. George presents with the following symptoms: Delusional ideation Not eating Non-engagement with team Signs of recent drug use Please pause to think after each question before reading the proposed answer. You may also have answers of your own.

What would you consider the diagnosis and treatment to be?

Answer

Psychoses not necessarily related to drug use but could be considered.

Treat the psychoses.

Consider prescribing for opiate stabilisation following assessment of current drug use and liaison with local substance agency.

Smoking assessment and review with dietician regarding current noneating.

Build relationship.

What are the risks?

Answer

Risk of overdose

Needle stick injuries

Deterioration in mental health for psychoses

Impact of illicit drugs on prescribed drugs

Isolation

Malnutrition

Disengagement with services

What would your management plan be?

Answer

1. Exploration of psychoses in line with organisations protocol. Full drug and alcohol history needs to be taken using Assist-Lite. Assessment of physical health/nutritional and review with consent Review history via both mental health and substance use service notes. Contact local substance use service to discover if open to services and whether is on opiate substitute prescribing.
2. Risks would include needle stick and abscesses, nasal discharge and drug-induced psychoses. Risk to self and others whilst under the influence of illicit substances. Risk of mixing drug and alcohol. Impact of not eating whilst intoxicated. Deterioration in mental health.
3. Assess for prescribing opiate substitute medication following assessment and urine testing. Start opiate prescribing. Monitor for withdrawal from substance use, using appropriate tools COWS for opiates or GMAWS for alcohol. Monitor and evaluate mental health using validated tools within organisation.

Responses to assessment and investigations needs to be conducted in a timely and appropriate manner and in conjunction with the individual. Physical health issues can be referred on through the GP. Identification does not always need to service response especially for more complex specialist interventions and will require referral on to appropriate agencies. Review for admission/treatment order.

F: LEADERSHIP, MANAGEMENT, EDUCATION AND RESEARCH

Good leadership is essential to the delivery of good quality care [56]. In order to deliver good-quality healthcare, it is essential to understand how the management of staff and how staff are treated significantly influence care provision and organisational performance; so understanding how leaders can help ensure staff are cared for, valued, supported and respected is important. Working with all staffing groups and engendering good relationships can lead to improved healthcare delivery and outcomes. Understanding the needs of diverse groups and the stigma associated with both mental health and substance use can reduce the discrimination faced by the individuals presenting to services. Clinical supervision provides all staff with an opportunity to reflect on practice and evaluate the care they provide. Ensuring that time is available and staff feel valued as part of the process leads to improved outcomes from supervision. The APMH role provides an opportunity to deliver training in their specialist area and to lead/advise/inform on research led practice from their clinical practice areas.

Learning Events

World Hepatitis Day https://www.worldhepatitisday.org/

This is a yearly event to raise awareness and provide education about the risk of hepatitis.

World Aids Day https://worldaidsday.org/

Raising awareness of blood borne viruses.

International day against Drug Abuse

https://www.papyrus-uk.org/international-day-against-drug-abuse/#:~:text=Since%201989%2C%20it%20has%20been,on%2026%20June%20every%20year.

Promoting the integration of substance users within treatment and safer practice.

Alcohol Awareness Week

https://alcoholchange.org.uk/get-involved/campaigns/alcohol-awareness-week-1

Resources and information on raising awareness of alcohol use.

Overdose awareness day 31st August

https://www.overdoseday.com/#:~:text=International%20Overdose%20Awareness%20Day%3A%2031,family%20and%20friends%20left%20behind.

Information on drugs - Talk to frank [57]

CONCLUSION

COMHAD individuals require robust mental health assessments that incorporate recognised drug and alcohol screening tools. As a minimum standard, APMHs should be offering assessment of substance use, referral into appropriate services and to be able to offer harm minimisation and relapse prevention advice to all clients entering services. The key aims of this chapter are to highlight the needs of this client group and enable advanced practitioners in mental health to understand the complexities and the need to work collaboratively with commissioned substance use agencies to enable clients to move towards recovery on their own terms. Multidisciplinary and co-working are essential in making this model of care effective and sustainable. The complex nature of substance use can lead to exclusion and services unintentionally not meeting needs based on mental health criteria. There is a long-term need to develop closer working networks and understand the substance use pathway for clients who are waiting for places in the substance system such as detox beds and rehab beds. The journey can be long and support in-between is essential in maintaining continuity of care. There remain health inequalities based on stigma, stereotypes, service division and non-engagement. These can be overcome with effective communication links and seamless pathways between services. Good practice for this marginalised group is based on honest, open communication, incorporating the clients' needs and understanding of their expectations; as well as knowing where service provision can be shared [51].

REFERENCES

1. Multi-professional framework for advanced clinical practice in England (2025). https://www.hee.nhs.uk/sites/default/files/documents/multi-professionalframeworkforadvancedclinicalpracticeinengland.pdf
2. How to use the Assist-lite screening tool to identify alcohol and drug use and tobacco smoking (2021). https://www.gov.uk/government/publications/assist-lite-screening-tool-how-to-use/how-to-use-the-assist-lite-screening-tool-to-identify-alcohol-and-drug-use-and-tobacco-smoking#:~:text=The%20process%20is%20made%20up%20of%20the,*%20Review%20risk%20at%20a%20future%20appointment.
3. Drug misuse in England and Wales: year ending March 2023. https://www.ons.gov.uk/peoplepopulationandcommunity/crimeandjustice/articles/drugmisuseinenglandandwales/yearendingmarch2023#:~:text=1.,%20around%201.1%20million%20pe
4. Drug use alcohol and smoking (2023). https://www.ons.gov.uk/peoplepopulationandcommunity/healthandsocialcare/drugusealcoholandsmoking
5. Hanson, G.R., Venturelli, P.J., and Platteborze, P. (2024). *Drugs and society*. Jones & Bartlett Learning.
6. Motyka, M.A. and Al-Imam, A. (2021). Representations of psychoactive drugs' use in mass culture and their impact on audiences. *International Journal of Environmental Research and Public Health* 18 (11): 6000.
7. Drug misuse in England and Wales: year ending June 2022. https://www.ons.gov.uk/peoplepopulationandcommunity/crimeandjustice/articles/drugmisuseinenglandandwales/yearendingjune2022
8. National Confidential Inquiry into Suicide and Safety in Mental Health Annual Report 2024. https://nspa.org.uk/resource/national-confidential-inquiry-into-suicide-and-safety-in-mental-health-annual-report-2024-including-easy-read-version-2/
9. Metcalfe, B. (2024). Supporting people with co-occurring mental health issues, alcohol, and drug use. *Mental Health Practice* 27 (6): 34–42.
10. Hamilton, I. (2014). The 10 most important debates surrounding dual diagnosis. *Advances in Dual Diagnosis* 7 (3): 118–128.
11. Dugmore, L. and Bauweraerts, S. (2021). When policy fails try something different integrated practice improve outcomes for dual diagnosis co-occurring service users accessing mental health services. *Drugs and Alcohol Today* 21 (2): 157–170.

12. National Drug treatment monitoring system 2025. https://www.ndtms.net/
13. Better care for people with co-occurring mental health and alcohol/drug use conditions 2017. https://assets.publishing.service.gov.uk/media/5a75b781ed915d6faf2b5276/Co-occurring_mental_health_and_alcohol_drug_use_conditions.pdf
14. Wang, T.R., Moosa, S., Dallapiazza, R.F. et al. (2018). Deep brain stimulation for the treatment of drug addiction. *Neurosurgical Focus* 45 (2): E11.
15. Muncan, B., Walters, S.M., Ezell, J., and Ompad, D.C. (2020). 'They look at us like junkies': influences of drug use stigma on the healthcare engagement of people who inject drugs in New York City. *Harm Reduction Journal* 17: 1–9.
16. Schnyder, N., Panczak, R., Groth, N., and Schultze-Lutter, F. (2017). Association between mental health-related stigma and active help-seeking: systematic review and meta-analysis. *The British Journal of Psychiatry* 210 (4): 261–268.
17. Lee, N. and Boeri, M. (2017). Managing stigma: women drug users and recovery services. *Fusio: The Bentley Undergraduate Research Journal* 1 (2): 65.
18. Íncera-Fernández, D., Gámez-Guadix, M., and Moreno-Guillén, S. (2021). Mental health symptoms associated with sexualized drug use (Chemsex) among men who have sex with men: a systematic review. *International Journal of Environmental Research and Public Health* 18 (24): 13299.
19. Macfarlane, A. (2016). Sex, drugs, and self-control: why chemsex is fast becoming a public health concern. *The Journal of Family Planning and Reproductive Health Care* 42 (4): 291–294.
20. Capell, J., Veenstra, G., and Dean, E. (2007). Cultural competence in healthcare: critical analysis of the construct, its assessment, and implications. *Journal of Theory Construction & Testing* 11 (1): 30–37.
21. Campinha-Bacote, J. (2011). Delivering patient-centered care in the midst of a cultural conflict: the role of cultural competence. *Online Journal of Issues in Nursing* 16 (2): 1–8.
22. Betancourt, J.R., Green, A.R., Carrillo, J.E., and Park, E.R. (2005). Cultural competence and health care disparities: key perspectives and trends. *Health Affairs* 24 (2): 499–505.
23. Urbanoski, K., Pauly, B., Inglis, D. et al. (2020). Defining culturally safe primary care for people who use substances: a participatory concept mapping study. *BMC Health Services Research* 20: 1–2.
24. McGregor, B., Belton, A., Henry, T.L. et al. (2019). Improving behavioral health equity through cultural competence training of health care providers. *Ethnicity and Disease* 29 (Suppl 2): 359.
25. Equality, diversity and health inequalities 2017. https://ww.england.nhs.uk/about/equality/equality-hub/national-healthcare-inequalities-improvement-programme/what-are-healthcare-inequalities/
26. Boyd, J., Wilson, R., Elsenbroich, C. et al. (2022). Agent-based modelling of health inequalities following the complexity turn in public health: a systematic review. *International Journal of Environmental Research and Public Health* 19 (24): 16807.
27. Livingston, J.D. (2020). *Structural stigma in health-care contexts for people with mental health and substance use issues*. Ottawa: Mental Health Commission of Canada.
28. Glass, T.A. (2004). Health inequalities: lifecourse approaches. *American Journal of Epidemiology* 160 (5): 503–504.
29. Connolly, D. and Gilchrist, G. (2020). Prevalence and correlates of substance use among transgender adults: a systematic review. *Addictive Behaviors* 111: 106544.

30. Yensabai, R. and Kiatrungrit, K. (2021). Association between parental attachment, sexual and substance use problems among patients with gender dysphoria. *Journal of the Psychiatric Association of Thailand* 65 (4): 355–372.
31. Rübig, L.L., Fuchshuber, J., Köldorfer, P. et al. (2021). Attachment, and therapeutic alliance in substance use disorders: initial findings for treatment in the therapeutic community. *Frontiers in Psychiatry* 10: 730876.
32. Wogen, J. and Restrepo, M.T. (2020). Human rights, stigma, and substance use. *Health and Human Rights* 22 (1): 51.
33. Heaslip, V., Thompson, R., Tauringana, M. et al. (2022). Health inequity in the UK: exploring health inequality and inequity. *Practice Nursing* 33 (2): 72–76.
34. Drugs penalties 2025 Gov. UK. https://www.gov.uk/penalties-drug-possession-dealing
35. McRee, B., Babor, T.F., Lynch, M.L., and Vendetti, J.A. (2018). Reliability and validity of a two-question version of the World Health Organization's alcohol, smoking, and substance involvement screening test: the ASSIST-FC. *Journal of Studies on Alcohol and Drugs* 79 (4): 649–657.
36. NICE guidance CG51 (2017). Drug misuse in over 16s: psychosocial interventions.
37. Nice guidance CG100 (2017). Alcohol-use disorders: diagnosis and management of physical complications.
38. NICE guidance CG115 (2011). Alcohol-use disorders: diagnosis, assessment and management of harmful drinking (high-risk drinking) and alcohol dependence.
39. Nice guidance NG58 2016 quality statement people aged fourteen and over with suspected or confirmed severe mental illness are asked about their use of alcohol and drugs.
40. Nice guidance CG120 (2011). Coexisting mental illness (psychoses and substance misuse).
41. Department of Health. PHE -done Clinical Guidelines on Drug Misuse and Dependence Update (2017). *Independent Expert Working Group (2017) Drug misuse and dependence: UK guidelines on clinical management.* London: Department of Health.
42. Gov. UK Alcohol use disorders identification test (AUDIT) 2025. https://assets.publishing.service.gov.uk/media/6357a7af8fa8f557d85b7c44/Alcohol-use-disorders-identification-test-AUDIT
43. Nice - Alcohol-use disorders: diagnosis, assessment and management of harmful drinking (high-risk drinking) and alcohol dependence 2011. https://www.nice.org.uk/guidance/cg115/chapter/Recommendations
44. Skinner, H.A. (1982). The drug abuse screening test. *Addictive Behaviors* 7 (4): 363–371. https://doi.org/10.1016/0306-4603(82)90005-3. PMID: 7183189.
45. McPherson, A., Benson, G., and Forrest, E.H. (2012). Appraisal of the Glasgow assessment and management of alcohol guideline: a comprehensive alcohol management protocol for use in general hospitals. *QJM*. 105 (7): 649–656. https://doi.org/10.1093/qjmed/hcs020. Epub 2012 Feb 10. PMID: 22328545.
46. Sullivan, J.T., Sykora, K., Schneiderman, J. et al. (1989). Assessment of alcohol withdrawal: the revised clinical institute withdrawal assessment for alcohol scale (CIWA-Ar). *British Journal of Addiction* 84 (11): 1353–1357.
47. Wesson, D.R. and Ling, W. (2003). The clinical opiate withdrawal scale (COWS). *Journal of Psychoactive Drugs* 35 (2): 253–259.
48. K Chief Medical Officers' Low Risk Drinking Guidelines 2016. https://assets.publishing.service.gov.uk/media/5a80b7ed40f0b623026951db/UK_CMOs__report.pdf
49. Nice Alcohol Dependence April, 2017. https://bnf.nice.org.uk/treatment-summaries/alcohol-dependence/#assisted-alcohol-withdrawal

50. Northern Healthcare Understanding the 5 Ps Formulation in Mental Health and Supported Living Services 2025. https://www.northernhealthcare.org.uk/news-resources/understanding-the-5-ps-formulation-in-mental-health-and-supported-living-services/
51. Miller, W.R. and Rollnick, S. (2012). *Motivational interviewing: Helping people change*. Guilford Press.
52. Purkey, E., Patel, R., and Phillips, S.P. (2018). Trauma-informed care: better care for everyone. *Canadian Family Physician* 64 (3): 170–172.
53. Bartholow, L.A. and Huffman, R.T. (2023). The necessity of a trauma-informed paradigm in substance use disorder services. *Journal of the American Psychiatric Nurses Association* 29 (6): 470–476.
54. Strang, J. and Farrell, M. (1992). Harm minimisation for drug misusers. *BMJ: British Medical Journal* 304 (6835): 1127.
55. Drug wise – Promoting Evidence Based information on drugs alcohol and tobacco. 2022. https://www.drugwise.org.uk/harm-reduction-2/
56. Firth-Cozens, J. (2004). Organisational trust: the keystone to patient safety. *BMJ Quality and Safety* 13 (1): 56–61.
57. Honest information about drugs. https://talktofrank.com/

PART 4

THE ROLE OF THE ADVANCED PRACTITIONER IN MENTAL HEALTH

CHAPTER 19

Mapping the Role to the Four Pillars of Advanced Practice

Chloe Parkin[1,2]

[1] Cornwall Partnership NHS Foundation Trust, Cornwall, UK
[2] South West Clinical School, University of Plymouth, Plymouth, UK

Aim

To empower advanced practitioners in mental health (APMHs) by fostering a deep understanding and critical reflection of their role and clinical practice, with a focus on integrating the pillars of advanced practice (AP) to enhance professional development and effectiveness.

Learning Outcomes

After reading this chapter, the reader will be able to:

- Critically reflect on the APMH role, development and journey in the context of the pillars of AP.
- Critically examine the current individual APMH clinical practice with specific reference to the pillars.
- Enhance individual APMH practice by exploring potential opportunities for incorporating the pillars into practice.

To protect anonymity, all case studies used represent an amalgamation of cases.

INTRODUCTION

The four pillars underpinning advanced practice (AP) are clinical, leadership and management, education and research [1]; developing competence in each equips the APMH to autonomously lead in complex and unpredictable situations [2].

The Advanced Practitioner in Mental Health, First Edition. Edited by Clare Allabyrne.
© 2026 John Wiley & Sons Ltd. All rights reserved, including rights for text and data mining and training of artificial intelligence technologies or similar technologies. Published 2026 by John Wiley & Sons Ltd.

Whilst this chapter focuses on the four pillars of AP, these link with the AP in Mental Health Curriculum and Capabilities Framework which was developed in recognition of the unique value of AP in facilitation of holistic patient care within mental health services [3]. The AP in Mental Health framework outlines six additional domains: person-centred therapeutic alliance (A); assessment and investigations (B); formulation (C); collaborative planning (D); intervention and evaluation (E); leadership and management, education and research (F); see Box 19.1. The pillars of AP and domains of AP in mental health combine to form 103 competencies that the trainee AP must evidence within the advanced practitioner in mental health (APMH) master's pathway.

> **Box 19.1   Mapping the Pillars to the Capability Domains [1, 3]**
>
> | Pillar | Domains |
> |---|---|
> | Clinical practice | A, B, C, D, E |
> | Leadership and management | D, F |
> | Education | C, D, F |
> | Research | A, E, F |
>
> Source: Adapted from Health Education England [3].

There is a paucity of research reviewing AP in mental health settings. Broader studies into the impact of AP tend to focus on the clinical pillar, with a scarcity of evidence relating to AP and the other pillars, particularly research; this may reflect the predominant clinical focus of AP with challenges around dedicating time to work across the pillars, or perhaps research has not yet sought to evaluate the AP work in relation to non-clinical pillars [4–6]. Acknowledgement of the largely clinical focus of AP may relate to expectations of the role, lack of job planning or the prior experience of the practitioner which may mainly be clinical [7, 8].

The professional background of the APMH impacts how specific capabilities within pillars are demonstrated, despite this, all APMHs must work to the advanced level of practice. This level of practice is distinguished by significant autonomy and the ability to make complex decisions, underpinned by a master's level award or equivalent [1]. The transition towards multi-professional roles may contribute to trainee APMHs, APMHs and those working towards, or at, consultant-level practice, struggling with their professional identity [9]. In recognition of this challenge, emphasis is placed on the variable scope of the APMH which is associated with contextual factors: the patient group; the trust, service and setting; and the professional background and pre-existing experience of the APMH [10].

This chapter encourages APMHs to critically reflect on their practice and identify additional opportunities to incorporate the pillars to enhance patient care. Critical reflection is a fundamental aspect of AP, and this is explored in greater detail in Chapter 20. The main mechanism for this will be through specific examples of the pillars, enabling the reader to evaluate and consider translation into practice.

AP is founded on an autonomous level of practice that breaks down traditional workplace boundaries using creative methods to ensure high quality person-centred care [1]. Examples discussed within this chapter are not intended to be prescriptive; acknowledging this supports in avoiding unhelpful comparison.

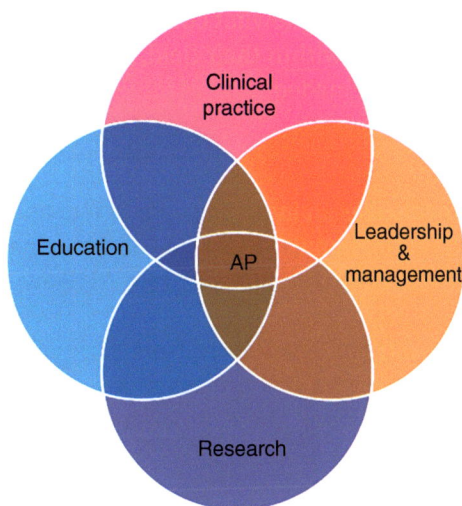

FIGURE 19.1 The Pillars: an intersecting view from above. Source: Adapted from HEE [1].

In the interest of mapping the APMH role to the AP pillars, this chapter artificially splits the pillars to enable analysis of examples. The concept of four AP pillars implies each area is clearly delineated; however, in practice the pillars are often interconnected; there could be scope to adapt the AP framework to demonstrate the interconnection of the clinical, leadership and management, research and educational AP elements (Figure 19.1).

CLINICAL PILLAR

What Is This Pillar?

Advanced clinical practice is underpinned by person-centred therapeutic alliance [11], collaborative working [12], advanced communication skills [13], patient advocacy [14], professional accountability [15, 16], cultural humility [17, 18] and self-reflection and awareness [19]. Self-awareness commands advanced understanding of ethical principles and values (personal, organisational and professional) [16, 20]. The APMH demonstrates in-depth knowledge of governance at a local and national level [1].

These contextual factors form the foundation of the APMH ability to work autonomously in complex and unpredictable clinical situations to systematically assess, risk assess, formulate, diagnose and develop collaborative integrative treatment plans [3]. The APMH uses proportionate clinical reasoning and decision-making skills to manage differentiated and undifferentiated complex clinical presentations [3]. APMH clinical practice is underpinned by evidence-based approaches and analytical reasoning; the APMH may use existing practice models or may foster new ways of working by adapting their own integrative models for clinical practice [1, 3].

Development of the Clinical Pillar

APMH demands high levels of clinical responsibility. Development of the clinical pillar may be accompanied by feelings of inadequacy as the learning process may place emphasis on analysis of actions that perhaps the APMH previously undertook intuitively (and expertly) towards deconstruction of the underpinning evidence. Consequently, and somewhat counterintuitively, APMH development demands the practitioner shift from being an expert within their field, perhaps reverting towards beginner stages, which may contribute towards feelings of inadequacy [21].

Professional Perspectives

Independent prescribing can be recognised as an important clinical function of AP, when appropriate [22, 23]; this does not preclude allied health professionals (AHPs) from advancing their practice. Studies exploring AP in AHPs are limited, though available research suggests AHPs working to AP level have positive influence on health services [7].

This chapter provides a rich tapestry of experiences from various professionals who have embraced the APMH role. Through their narratives and practice examples, the diverse pathways and unique challenges encountered can be explored. Reading these experiences will enable readers to gain valuable insights into the practical application of the AP pillars to enhance patient care.

Advanced Clinical Practice Examples

The following clinical practice examples intend to empower readers to thoughtfully consider translation into their own practice. As mentioned, these examples are designed to inspire, encouraging innovative and individualised approaches. Examples are linked to the multi-professional framework (MPF) aligned with the title of the chapter [1].

1. **Advanced Communication: Empowering Choice**

    Clinical setting: Older People's Mental Health (OPMH) – Community Mental Health Team (CMHT).

    Scenario: A 76-year-old with depression; the patient had taken amitriptyline for more than 50 years and had been unable to tolerate other antidepressants. Recently experiencing increasing cardiac issues. The patient wished to continue to take amitriptyline despite cardiac issues, the capacity of the patient to consent to treatment was in doubt [24].

    APMH role: Facilitated mental capacity assessment relating to the decision to remain on amitriptyline; underpinned by therapeutic alliance, including review of records and liaison with the cardiologist, consultant psychiatrist and pharmacist.

    Impact of AP intervention for patient and family: Promoted autonomy within complex decision-making. Without AP intervention, consultant or medically led mental capacity assessment may have been required.

    Key elements: Advanced communication; therapeutic alliance; person-centred care; equality, diversity and inclusion; patient advocacy; psychopharmacology; complex mental capacity assessment; parity of esteem.

    MPF pillar: 1.1–1.6, 1.9, 1.11

2. **Therapeutic Alliance: Parity of Esteem**

    Clinical setting: Child and Adolescent Mental Health Services (CAMHS) Crisis.

    Scenario: A 17-year-old presented with low mood and suicidality.

    APMH role: Conducted a holistic biopsychosocial assessment with an emphasis on physical health history, this enabled clinical and diagnostic reasoning; evidence of fatigue and low mood was found.

    Blood investigations requested by the APMH which identified deranged results requiring further investigation [25]; concurrent CAMHS intervention focused on building a therapeutic alliance, instilling hope, collaborative risk assessment, formulation and safety planning.

Impact of AP intervention for patient and family: Holistic mental and physical healthcare. Without AP intervention, physical health issues contributing to the presentation might have gone unidentified.

Key elements: Parity of esteem; diagnostic overshadowing; therapeutic alliance; comprehensive risk assessment and management.

MPF pillars: 1.1–1.6, 1.8, 1.9, 1.11

3. **Collaborative Working: Navigating Complex Care**

   Clinical setting: Inpatient Adult Acute Unit

   Scenario: An autistic female with a diagnosis of emotionally unstable personality disorder; detained under Section 3 of the Mental Health Act (MHA).

   Inpatient multidisciplinary team (MDT) included a psychologist, APMH, consultant psychiatrist, occupational therapist, pharmacist and the nursing team.

   Multi-agency in-reach included a positive behavioural support lead, speech and language therapist, social worker and CMHT key worker.

   APMH role: A person-centred approach to improve understanding of the patient's values, openly acknowledging the complex power dynamics associated with being detained under the MHA, to hear the voice of the patient, inform collaborative working and identify need for adaptations such as inpatient environmental changes.

   Collaborative work with the patient, family, MDT and multi-agency services to ensure personalised approaches to communication strategies; ensured strategies focused on personalised care planning and were consistently implemented.

   Critical awareness of complex relational dynamics and therapeutic boundaries, application of self-awareness to attend to own reactions and supported the MDT in managing their own responses to complex situations.

   Impact of AP intervention for patient and family: Consistency of care resulted in closer working relationships and potentially contributed to a reduction in self-harm. Without AP involvement, there may have been siloed working with uncoordinated meetings resulting in inconsistent communication, care approaches and goals.

   Key elements: Management of complex patients; lead complex clinical risk management; collaborative working; values-based care; equality, diversity and inclusion; shared decision making; least restrictive intervention; promote autonomy.

   MPF pillars: 1.1–1.11

4. **Person-Centred Care: Collaborative Planning**

   Clinical setting: Psychiatric Liaison Service (PLS)

   Scenario: An adult referred following an overdose and 'bizarre' presentation; no medical intervention required. No previous mental health history.

   APMH role: Comprehensive biopsychosocial assessment, risk assessment and collaborative formulation to inform clinical reasoning and intervention planning. Family involvement enabled understanding of premorbid presentation. A values-based approach allowed insight into the person's belief system and consideration around potential engagement in treatment [19].

   The patient presented with symptoms of psychosis, predominantly auditory hallucinations and paranoid ideation. With emphasis on shared decision-making, the patient agreed to referral to the Home Treatment Team (HTT); the least restrictive option and there was no reason to doubt his capacity to make this decision [24, 26, 27]. APMH intervention planning focused on integrative approaches: pharmacological, psychological, social, occupational, lifestyle, environmental, complementary and alternative medicine interventions; all reasonable treatment options were explored [28].

Impact of AP intervention for patient and family: Holistic assessment and intervention planning with the person and family. Without AP intervention there may have been less emphasis on integrative approaches to interventions and potential hospital admission.

Key elements: Management of complex patients; lead complex clinical risk management; values-based care; equality, diversity and inclusion; shared decision-making; least restrictive intervention; integrative treatment planning; analytical reasoning.

MPF pillars: 1.1–1.11

5. **Patient Advocacy: Inclusive Care**
   Clinical setting: CAMHS
   Scenario: Autistic young person with functional disorder, presented with symptoms of Complex PTSD.
   APMH role: Focused on therapeutic alliance with collaborative goal setting to develop trust. Trauma psychoeducation included focus on somatic symptoms alongside stabilisation work to ensure adequate grounding strategies. Facilitated trauma-focused cognitive behavioural therapy (TF-CBT) with reasonable adjustments for neurodiversity and mobility.

   Multi-agency liaison and collaboration with Children's Social Care due to safeguarding concerns, included advocating for the voice of the young person.

   Impact of AP intervention for patient and family: Promoted autonomy of the young person; supported the young person and family to feel heard. A safe space to explore the mental and physical impact of trauma. Without AP intervention, the approach to physical and mental health may have been less coordinated, with fewer adaptations for neurodiversity and less focus on the young person's voice.

   Key elements: Development of expert practice; person-centred care; therapeutic alliance; equality, diversity and inclusion; patient advocacy; trauma-focused care; management of complex patients; safeguarding; integrative treatment planning; shared decision-making; cultural awareness.

   MPF pillars: 1.1–1.11

Reflection

Critically reflect on the examples; how would you have enhanced APMH care delivery in the context of your professional background and experience?

Tips

- Undertake complex clinical reasoning e-learning programme: https://www.e-lfh.org.uk/programmes/complex-clinical-reasoning [29].
- Consider existing clinical interests; how can you advance these to become your expert practice?

Trainee Tips

- A helpful way to support reflective practice may be to ask yourself the question 'what would my considerations be if I were independently managing this episode of care as the APMH?'
- Reflect to APMH level by deconstructing previous intuitive practice to analyse the underpinning evidence base.

LEADERSHIP AND MANAGEMENT

What Is This Pillar?

The APMH is a visible, approachable and credible clinical role model [1, 3]. APMHs facilitate service development by identifying new ways of working to influence safe and person-centred transformation [3]. Advanced leadership can be separated into four domains: clinical leadership, professional leadership, health system leadership and health policy leadership (see Box 19.2) [30].

> **Box 19.2   Four Domains of Advanced Leadership**
>
> **Clinical leadership** – high-quality care including focus on collaborative working, role modelling and enhancing evidence-based practice.
>
> **Professional leadership** – role model learning and development culture, participation in peer review opportunities and participation in activities that influence organisational advanced practice development.
>
> **Health systems leadership** – focus on strategic approaches necessitating comprehensive knowledge of systems to influence organisational vision.
>
> **Health policy leadership** – shape practice and influence policy, contributions include ability to articulate the value of APMH.
>
> Source: Adapted from [31, 32].

DEVELOPMENT OF THE LEADERSHIP AND MANAGEMENT PILLAR

Self-awareness

Leadership is a relational process; to lead is to influence and therefore trust is integral [33, 34]. Accordingly, communication and relationship building are key; additionally, vision establishment and resilience are cornerstones of leadership development [35]. Given the relational nature of leadership, attention is drawn to the significance of emotional intelligence and self-awareness as an APMH leader.

Compassion

Compassionate leaders work to balance the head and heart to connect, influence and inspire others; they continually endeavour to understand and meet the needs of people they work alongside [36, 37].

Well-being including psychological safety, thriving and engagement of health practitioners is impacted by fundamental factors, categorised into three core needs set out in the ABC model which can be used in practice – see Figure 19.2 [36, 37]. Supporting these needs can help practitioners to improve their work lives, positively influencing care [37].

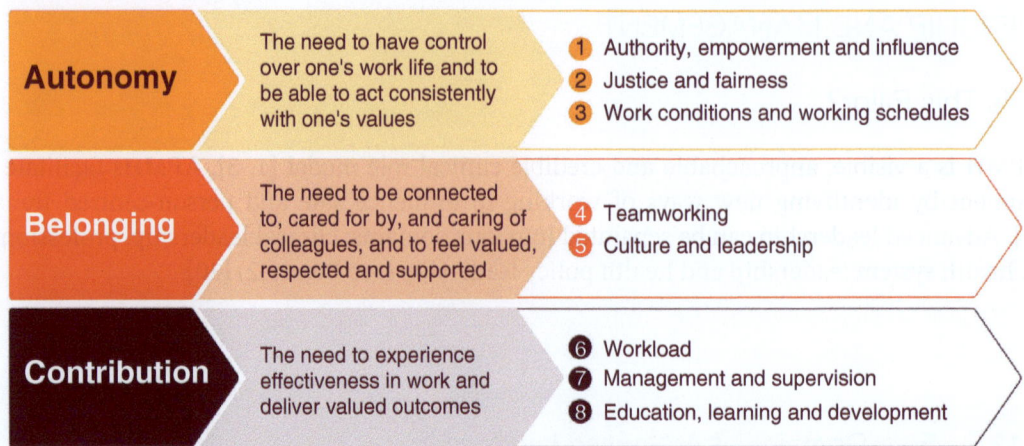

FIGURE 19.2 The ABC framework of nurses' and midwives' core needs. Source: Adapted from Kings Fund [37].

Advanced Leadership Examples

1. **Health Policy Leadership: Shaping National Practice**

   Scenario: Presentation at National AP conference.

   APMH role: Utilised trainee experience to provide ideas focusing on integrating the four pillars of AP directly in clinical care; the presentation centred around a case study whereby the patient provided unexpected feedback in relation to intervention from the team and the APMH consultation, enabling insight into lived experience.

   Opportunities: Influence APMH practice at a national level to support in shaping practice and articulate the value of APMH.

   Challenges: Due to unforeseen circumstances the patient was unable to be directly involved in delivery, though did provide consent for the case study to be presented.

   Key elements: Role model; shaping practice; person-centred approaches to service delivery and development; demonstrate the impact of APMH on service quality.

   MPF pillars: 2.1–2.3, 2.7, 2.8, 2.11

2. **Clinical Leadership: Uniting Forces**

   Scenario: CAMHS Multi-Agency Risk Management Forums.

   APMH role: Facilitation of multi-agency risk management forums through use of appropriate governance for complex young people underpinned by evidence-based models such as adolescent mentalisation-based integrative therapy to foster collaborative and systemic approaches to risk mitigation [38].

   Opportunities: Offering support to teams working with complex young people, where they feel all options have been exhausted. The panel establishes an agreed service wide plan of care for children and families; in turn, this enhances quality of decision-making by improving communication and collaboration.

   Challenges: Consent to share information across agencies poses barriers to integrated working; utilising established therapeutic relationships and clear communication around the intentions of the forum can help.

Key elements: Apply advanced clinical expertise in facilitatory ways to provide consultancy across professional and service boundaries; compassionate leadership; demonstrate leadership in managing complex and unpredictable situations.

MPF pillars: 2.1–2.5, 2.7, 2.8, 2.11

3. **Health Systems Leadership: Building Bridges**

   Scenario: National Specialist AP Networks.

   APMH role: Establishment of specialist APMH Networks in CAMHS, Urgent Care and OPMH, using existing links, social media and the National AP in Mental Health Network.

   CAMHS Network

   Opportunities: A supportive space to share good practice and service development.

   Challenges: Encouraging members to present, implementation of a rota to present ideas is being explored.

   Urgent Care Network

   Opportunities: Learn from others who work in crisis services and share ideas; it has been inspiring when case studies are presented.

   Challenges: Striking a balance between having a structured agenda yet flexibility to discuss 'hot topics' as they arise; however, this is navigated together.

   OPMH Network

   Opportunities: Networking has enabled formation of a national steering group to improve services for those living with dementia who identify as LGBT+.

   Challenges: Identification of rotational chairs has been challenging and is currently led by one region.

   Key elements: Broaden sphere of influence; sharing best practice; seek to build confidence in others; cultural awareness; equality, diversity and inclusion.

   MPF pillars: 2.1, 2.2, 2.5, 2.7, 2.8

4. **Professional Leadership: Pathway to Progress**

   Scenario: Development of pilot clinical care pathway within HTT.

   APMH role: Co-facilitated development of a clinical pathway for people with presentations consistent with complex emotional difficulties (CED) who are in crisis.

   With a team approach, comprised of HTT practitioners, the CED Team and operational management, and in consultation with Experts by Experience, the pathway development was underpinned by patient and staff feedback, available literature and clinical audit. This necessitated in-depth understanding of the scope of practice within legal, ethical, professional and organisational policy to ensure focus on managing risk and upholding safety.

   Emphasis placed on mentoring and supporting HTT practitioners throughout the process, fostering a culture of continuous learning and development. Incorporated peer review sessions to ensure quality and shared learning.

   Opportunities: Working in partnership with Experts by Experience to gain invaluable input. Influencing organisational practices and contributing to the development of advanced practice within the organisation.

   Challenges: Balancing the facilitation of development meetings where all attendees feel valued and heard whilst moving the project forward. Encouraging team members to actively participate in peer review sessions.

Key elements: Working with Experts by Experience; person-centred approaches to service development; peer review; influencing organisational practice; compassionate leadership; trauma-focused care; formulation and implementation of strategies to make improvements; lead service redesign solutions in response to feedback.

MPF pillars: 2.1–2.11

5. **Clinical Leadership: Ethical Leadership in Action**

    Scenario: Complex case team discussion quality improvement (QI) project.

    APMH role: Complex case team discussions underpinned by an adaptation of the action consequences model [39, 40]; this supports the team from a leadership perspective when working in complex and unpredictable situations.

    The model is indicated where practitioners are concerned a decision may be unhelpful, to offer a structured approach to weigh up complex ethical issues whilst keeping the patient and their family central [20]. Decisions are sensitively communicated with the patient, and their family, where appropriate.

    Opportunities: Patients have reported feeling listened to. Staff have reported feeling more confident with complex decisions and able to keep the patient central. The underpinning principles appear to be influencing broader clinical practice of practitioners to consider complex ethical issues even without direct use of the model [39, 40].

    Challenges: A development of this project would be to hold complex team discussions with the patient and family present; this currently remains aspirational.

    Key elements: Apply advanced clinical expertise in facilitatory ways to provide consultancy; demonstrate leadership in managing complex situations whilst seeking to build confidence; demonstrate person-centred approaches to service development; ethical decision-making; service evaluation; compassionate leadership; evidence-based practice.

    MPF pillars: 2.1–2.11

Reflection

What challenges do you anticipate as an APMH clinical leader? How will you demonstrate clinical leadership and credibility in contexts where there may not be a shared understanding of AP?

Tips

- Join/Attend the National APMH Network (formerly Community of Practice).
- Attend relevant specialist AP Networks, or implement one if none currently exist.
- Utilise relational leadership skills to establish and maintain links with other teams and services.

EDUCATION

Education Pillar

What Is This Pillar?

The educational pillar encompasses self-learning and facilitation of learning for others, including students, colleagues, patients and families. The APMH holds comprehensive understanding of the contemporary evidence-base, and applies this directly to facilitate safe, effective and high-quality care, and to influence a culture of organisational learning to inspire colleagues [1, 3].

Education

AP is reinforced by master's level education or equivalent that encompasses the four pillars of practice [1]. Some literature asserts the need for APs to be educated to a minimum of master's degree level relevant to their role [41]; though research indicates this has not been consistently adopted in practice [42]. Generally, APs would welcome standardised education and credentialing processes; equally there are concerns this could disadvantage practitioners in existing AP posts [5, 42].

Facilitating Learning

Whilst in training, the trainee APMH has a nominated coordinating education supervisor with whom they have regular focused AP supervision in line with the Health Education England (HEE) minimum standards for supervision [43].

Bloom's taxonomy of learning can be used to aid the continual learning process by using the six cognitive domains to underpin assessment (including self-assessment) of individual skillsets and abilities [44, 45] (see Figure 19.3 and Box 19.3).

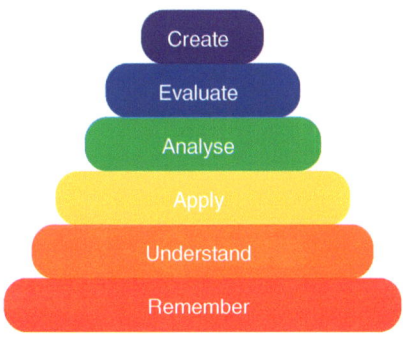

FIGURE 19.3 Taxonomy of learning. *Source:* Adapted from Bloom [44] and Anderson and Krathwohl [45].

Box 19.3 Revised Cognitive Domain

Stage	Name	Description	Associated verbs
1	Remember	Ability to recall information	Retrieve, recognise
2	Understand	Summarise stages in own words	Classify, explain
3	Apply	Use knowledge in new scenarios	Predict, demonstrate
4	Analyse	Examine the concepts in detail. Find supporting evidence	Research, appraise

(Continued)

Box 19.3 (Continued)

Stage	Name	Description	Associated verbs
5	Evaluate	Make a judgement. Present, defend, justify and critique.	Persuade, validate
6	Create	Build on learning. Transform knowledge to design new projects.	Develop, formulate

Source: Adapted from Bloom [44] and Anderson and Krathwohl [45].

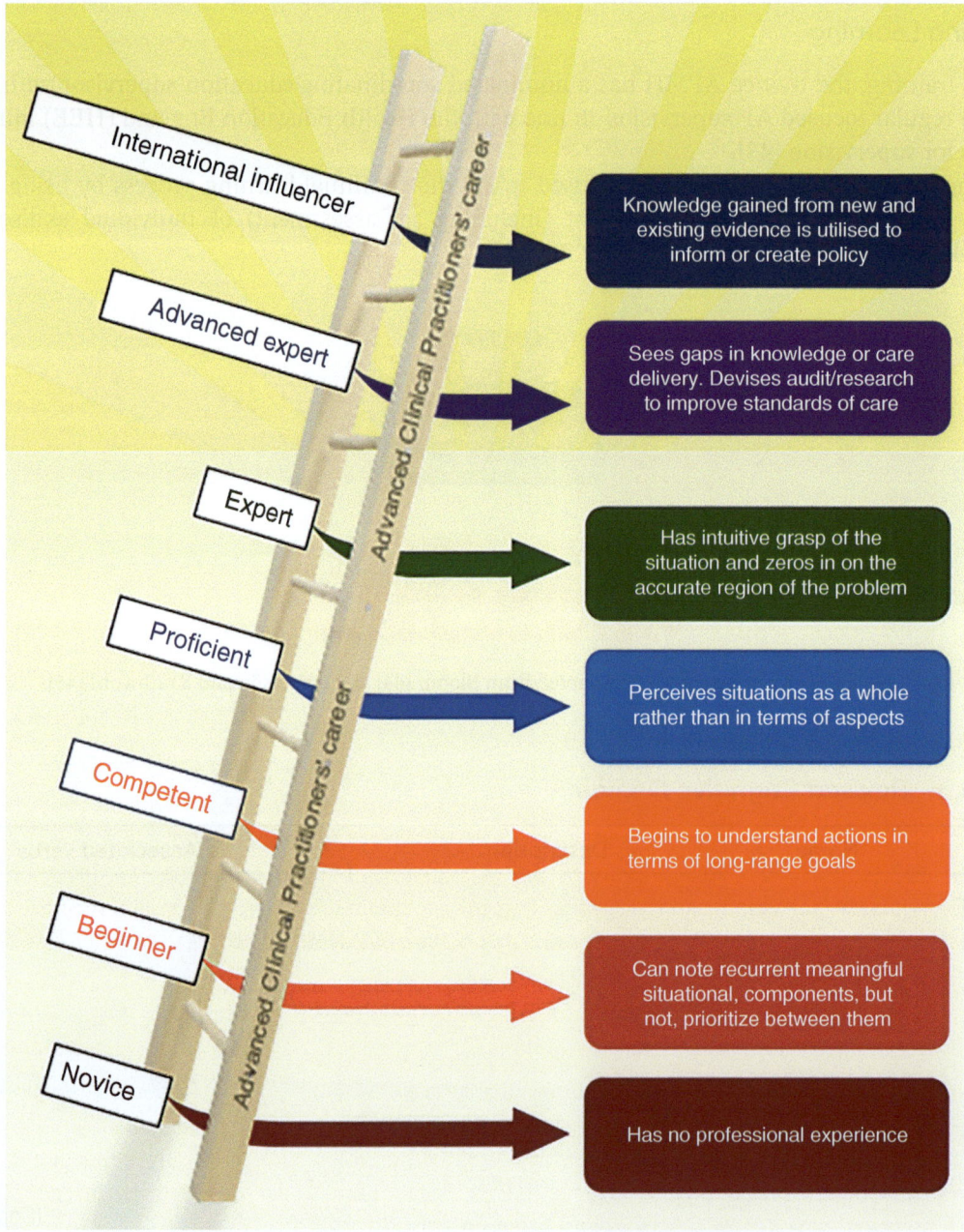

FIGURE 19.4 The Derby model. Source: [46] / with permission of MA Healthcare Ltd.

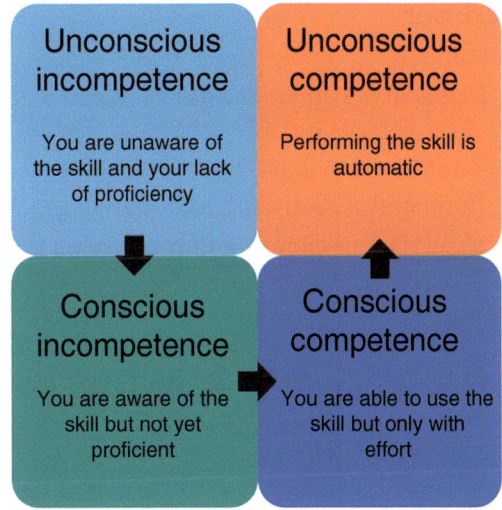

FIGURE 19.5 Four stages of competence. Source: Adapted from Howell [47].

The Derby model: '7 Levels of Practice Advancement' updates Benner's: 'From Novice to Expert' framework – Figure 19.4 [21, 46]. The Derby model suggests two additional levels of 'expert' which provides nuance and maps against advanced and consultant levels of practice [46]. Derby's model provides useful benchmarking of learning stages for the AP. Whilst APMHs may commence training identifying as experts in a particular field, on examination as part of comprehensive training, they may revert to a state of conscious incompetence (Figure 19.5) in relation to specific areas of development; therefore, it is suggested this model can provide a framework to support APMH to conceptualise and address this [46, 47].

Reflective Practice

Use of frameworks to facilitate learning such as Kolb, Gibbs and Driscoll aides in critical reflection [48–50]. Kirk's 'waves of reflection' model provides a social-realist basis that may enhance depth of reflection and integration of relevant theory to practice [51].

Examples of Advanced Facilitation of Learning

1. **Evaluate: Reflect, Grow, Inspire**
   Scenario: Clinical supervision.
   APMH role: Facilitation of clinical supervision that supports reflection focusing on clinical practice and professional development, and promotes equality, diversity and inclusion, by championing person-centred care, interrogation of biases and encouraging learning about cultures, ethnicities, religions and demographics [17, 18].
   Opportunities: Use of reflective models to facilitate critical examination of experiences and enhance learning. Supporting supervisees in development to achieve career progression.
   Challenges: Clinical pressures can result in omission of supervision; however, it remains essential to prioritise and reinforce a culture that encourages restorative clinical supervision.
   Key elements: Advocate for a culture of organisational learning to inspire colleagues; promote a culture of self-reflection and awareness; promote equality, diversity and inclusion; support in addressing development needs; act as a role model, educator, supervisor, coach and mentor.
   MPF pillars: 3.3, 3.4, 3.6–3.8

2. **Apply: Carer Empowerment**

   Scenario: Psychoeducation.

   APMH role: As part of clinical consultation, use of expert knowledge to facilitate support to carers in relation to suicide risk, focusing on:
   - Risk: tensions between short- and long-term risk management.
   - Consent, confidentiality, mental capacity and information sharing.
   - Self-care: carer burnout, self-compassion and implementing safe boundaries.

   Carer and family involvement is fundamental in improving mental healthcare and suicide prevention [52–54].

   Opportunities: Empowering family members, particularly around their rights; for instance, regardless of consent to share information arrangements, the carer still has the right to be listened to by practitioners.

   Challenges: Terminology can be a barrier, not everyone identifies as a 'carer', so it is important to explore this in more depth.

   Key elements: Empower individuals to maximise well-being; act as an educator; evidence-based practice.

   MPF pillars: 3.3, 3.8

3. **Create: Framework for Growth**

   Scenario: Implementation of Registered Mental Health Nurse (RMN) competence framework: a pilot project.

   APMH role: The APMH Nurse used the RMN Career and Competence Framework to develop a competence framework based on the four pillars of practice [3]. The framework can be used as part of supervision, is self-directed by the RMN, requiring sign off from the clinical supervisor. The framework has been presented at the trust clinical assurance group to ensure alignment with local governance.

   Opportunities: Enables RMN development by supporting: knowledge of the pillars; clarity around current level of practice; career development; effective utilisation of training budgets as emerging themes are analysed with the education department.

   Challenges: Potentially perceived as additional work; however, the framework intends to add structure to existing supervision discussions.

   Developments: The APMH Nurse has met with colleagues to consider translation across allied professions. The APMH has linked in with the trust appraisals lead to consider alignment.

   Key elements: Advocate for a culture of organisational learning; support in addressing development needs; act as a role model, educator, supervisor, coach and mentor; contribution of development of robust governance systems.

   MPF pillars: 3.3–3.8

4. **Understand: Inspiring Minds**

   Scenario: Guest Lecturing.

   APMH role: Facilitation of teaching sessions for undergraduate students focusing on areas of expertise including psychosocial assessment and formulation, care planning and suicide risk.

Opportunities: A social constructivist approach to encouraging engagement and learning [55, 56]. Facilitating learning develops APMH confidence whilst supporting learning for others.

Challenges: Confidence initially, though with support from the university, this has proved a learning experience with positive and constructive feedback.

Key elements: Advocate for a culture of organisational learning. Act as a role model and educator.

MPF pillars: 3.1, 3.4, 3.5, 3.8

5. **Apply: Cultivating Professional Development**

   Scenario: Facilitation of team continuing professional development (CPD) sessions.

   APMH role: Identification of opportunities for team development; facilitation of a CPD session about clinical supervision.

   Opportunities: Application of educational theory to increase engagement supported to enable rich discussion and understand current perceptions of clinical supervision in practice. CPD sessions inspire and result in identification of further areas for development.

   Challenges: Time pressures; future CPD will predominantly be 'bite sized' sessions.

   Key elements: Advocate for a culture of organisational learning. Act as a role model, educator and supervisor.

   MPF pillars: 3.3, 3.4, 3.6–3.8

6. **Evaluate: Shaping Career Paths**

   Scenario: Poster presentation about APMH at service-wide meeting.

   APMH role: The trainee APMH utilised opportunity to present to support understanding of APMH and potentially influence career progression for others.

   The presentation focused on the background to AP, the trainee experience and how APMH translates into practice.

   Opportunities: Questions raised by attendees, evidencing interest in APMH.

   Challenges: Accurately representing the autonomy of the level of practice, and conveying that APMH may look different dependent on contexts.

   Key elements: Advocate for a culture of organisational learning to inspire colleagues; act as a role model and educator.

   MPF pillars: 3.1–3.4, 3.6, 3.8

7. **Analyse: Building Expertise**

   Scenario: Professional portfolio development.

   APMH role: Training to be an APMH necessitates development of a specific AP portfolio; development of this portfolio lays the foundation for deconstructing and analysing practice to critically examine the evidence-base and compels the APMH to scrutinise previous intuitive actions.

   Opportunities: Supports development to AP level; enables opportunity for the trainee APMH to critically reflect on development.

   Challenges: Volume of evidence for competencies, though with use of organisational skills, this can be managed to distribute pressure.

   Key elements: Critical assessment of own learning needs; engagement in critical reflection.

   MPF pillars: 3.1, 3.2

> **Reflection**
>
> How do you foster a culture where learners actively contribute as part of the learning process? What educational theory underpins your facilitation of learning in practice?
>
> **Tips**
>
> - Use themes from clinical supervision to identify areas for CPD.
> - Develop links with local universities to identify teaching opportunities.
> - Utilise opportunities to present and promote AP.
>
> **Trainee Tips**
>
> - Gain exposure to different teams and services.
> - Consider supervision with a range of professionals to support your learning needs.

RESEARCH

What Is This Pillar?

Research aims to expand knowledge and drive the transformation of services, ultimately improving outcomes and fostering innovation in practice. National strategies for nurses and for AHPs place emphasis on their roles in driving forward high-quality and evidence-based innovation [57, 58]. Despite this, the inspirational element of advancing practice through research can be overlooked. AP research capability development is fundamental to achieving high quality patient care and advancing services [6]. This pillar encompasses various components that collectively contribute to advancing practice (Figure 19.6).

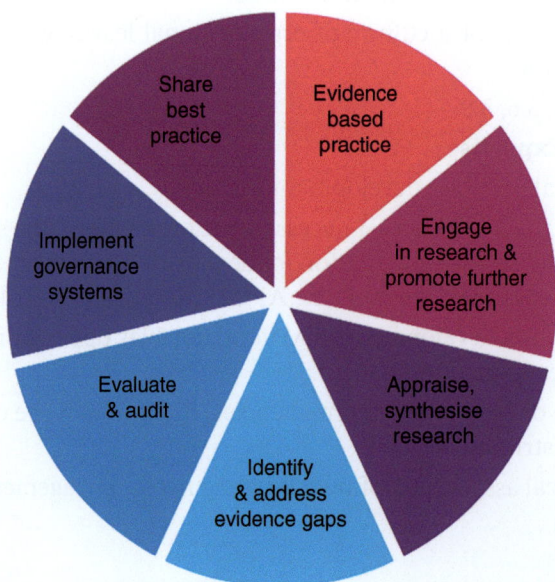

FIGURE 19.6 Core research pillar domains. Source: Adapted from Health Education England [1].

Development of the Research Pillar

Trainee APMHs on the master's degree pathway will undertake at least one specific research module; this module is designed to enhance critical appraisal skills and familiarise practitioners with essential research terminology.

Studies into AP and the research pillar are scarce [4–6]; this may demonstrate limited practitioner confidence and time pressures in practice [5]. It is suggested the research pillar may be disadvantaged in practice until it becomes mandatory [6]. Recognising the barriers to engaging in research, the AP Research Pillar Toolkit has been developed to support trainee and qualified APs [59, 60]. The toolkit provides essential guidance and resources to help APs initiate research projects and identify key research priority areas; by offering structured support, the toolkit aims to overcome common obstacles, enabling APs to contribute effectively to evidence-based practice and improve patient outcomes [59, 60].

Advanced Research Examples

1. **Engage in research and promote further research: DIAMONDS**

   Scenario: Principal investigator for a randomised control trial, diabetes and mental illness, improving outcomes and self-management (DIAMONDS programme), focusing on type 2 diabetes for people with severe mental illness (SMI).

   APMH role: Working closely with the research team to lead the trial in our area.

   Opportunities: People with SMI often have poorer physical health than the general population, with their lives 15–20 years shorter mostly from preventable physical illnesses [61, 62]. It is a privilege to be involved in advancing practice that aims to improve the physical health of people with SMI.

   Challenges: Recruitment to the study; the APMH and research team have worked together to address this.

   Key elements: Contribute to research activity; facilitate collaborative links between clinical practice and research; promote equality, diversity and inclusion; parity of esteem.

   MPF pillars: 4.1, 4.4, 4.5, 4.7, 4.8

2. **Evaluate and Audit: Elevating Healthcare Standards**

   Scenario: Service Accreditation Involvement. Meeting the national service accreditation standards evidences the quality of the healthcare service.

   APMH role: The APMH supported evidencing standards by undertaking clinical record audit.

   Opportunities: Enabled a critical approach to identify existing good practice and to identify areas for service development.

   Challenges: Audit data is reliant on documentation; accuracy may be impacted by record keeping systems and/or user inconsistencies.

   Key elements: Evaluate and audit practice.

   MPF pillars: 4.1–4.3

3. **Evidence-Based Practice: Transforming Care Through QI**

   Scenario: Crisis planning QI project. Personalised crisis planning should be offered to all HTT patients [63].

APMH role: Working with a small team, review of available literature and development of an audit tool. The audit tool reviewed data including presence of personalised crisis planning.

Underpinned by Plan, Do, Study, Act (PDSA) cycles, the objective was for all people engaged with HTT to be offered to collaboratively develop a crisis plan [64]. Results included improvement from 22% of people having a crisis plan to 77% after the second PDSA cycle.

Opportunities: Poster presentation at the national AP network.

Challenges: It was important to acknowledge systemic pressures impacting on completion of crisis planning. Teamwork was essential, working together to identify adaptable ways to address challenges; one example was considering creative methods of crisis planning.

Key elements: Synthesise relevant research, evaluation and audit, using the results to develop practice; presentation of quality improvement via appropriate forums.

MPF pillars: 4.1–4.4, 4.6–4.8.

4. **Engage in research and promote further research: CAMHS Goes Wild**

    Scenario: A qualitative research project looking at the impact of specialist ecopsychology training with a cohort of CAMHS practitioners.

    APMH role: Involvement to assess feasibility of incorporating nature-based approaches.

    Opportunities: This has benefited the well-being of young people and practitioners and has contributed to cultural shifts within CAMHS. Additional developments include a children's participation group, nature-based staff away days and a community of practice for practitioners using nature-based approaches.

    Challenges: Changing practice within an established system; navigating risk assessment and infection control governance whilst influencing positive risk taking approaches has been challenging but is not insurmountable.

    Key elements: Critical engagement in research activity; developing evidence-based strategies; contribution of development of robust governance systems.

    MPF pillars: 4.1–4.8

5. **Appraise and synthesise research: Knowledge and Action**

    Scenario: Complex case team discussion QI project.

    APMH role: Synthesis of available literature and contextual factors resulting in a project led by the APMH supported by the team manager and clinical lead whereby complex case team discussions are held underpinned by an adaptation of the action consequences model [39, 40, 42, 45].

    What has this involved: The project proposal was presented by the APMH and team manager at the trust clinical quality and assurance group.

    The project will be evaluated through collation of anonymised staff feedback in relation to confidence when making complex risk decisions (compared to previous practice) and by collating patient and family feedback where appropriate.

    Opportunities: Capturing practitioner feedback enables involvement in onwards planning of this project, this appears to be positively influencing 'buy in' from the team, feedback suggestions can be implemented as part of subsequent PDSA cycles [64].

    Challenges: Once evaluated, consideration will be given to the transferability of this project to other clinical areas.

Key elements: Synthesise relevant research, evaluation and audit, using the results to develop practice; presentation of quality improvement via appropriate forums; contribution of development of robust governance systems.

MPF pillars: 4.1–4.4, 4.6–4.8

Reflection

How will you advocate for value of the research pillar to enhance AP? How could you contribute to research about the AP research pillar?

Tips

- Utilise the AP Research Pillar Toolkit [60].
- Link in with your local research team and your local clinical audit team.
- Consider involvement in local service accreditation processes.
- Sign up to relevant email newsletters.
- Consider relevant policy development opportunities.

CASE STUDY: INTEGRATING THE FOUR PILLARS OF ADVANCED PRACTICE INTO CLINICAL INTERVENTIONS

Presenting Information: Amy is 28 years old. She is engaged with the CMHT. Amy was referred to HTT following Mental Health Act assessment whilst under section 136; she came to police attention due to reckless driving with reported suicidal ideation.

Amy has a history of self-harm via cutting to varying degrees. She has made multiple previous attempts to end her life.

Her current medication is quetiapine 50 mg, taken twice daily as needed; which she finds calming. She has previously trialled various antidepressants with little effect.

Amy has two children (9 and 4 years old); they are subject to a Child in Need plan.

Amy has been assessed by HTT practitioners; the current plan is daily HTT review. Amy has had three previous unplanned admissions within the last year. HTT practitioners requested APMH consultation due to complexity and risk.

Before Advancing to the Next Part of the Case Study:

As part of APMH consultation, what models of assessment and formulation might you use, and why? How will collaborative working and shared decision-making feature?
Based on the information available, how might research and education pillars be relevant?

AP CONSULTATION

The APMH facilitated consultation using Trenoweth and Moone's biopsychosocial assessment model [65]; prior review of records helped to enable focus on the salient areas and avoid repetition of the recent HTT assessment. This model facilitates holistic understanding of what may have contributed to Amy's current crisis presentation. Collaborative use of the Five Ps formulation model with Amy supported her understanding of her current presentation and potential contributory factors [66]. Five Ps can be useful as part of crisis intervention when processing ability may be impacted due to acuity of presentation.

Amy briefly spoke about her childhood, enough to know she has experienced multiple event trauma. The APMH drew on research and education pillars to discuss adverse childhood events and the potential impact of this with Amy and her partner [67]. The APMH consultation drew to a natural conclusion; it was agreed for the APMH to return the following day.

> **Before Advancing to the Next Part of the Case Study:**
>
> What intervention planning models might you use with Amy? From the information available, is there possibility of complex ethical dilemmas? Where might advocacy and trauma informed approaches feature?

Follow-up AP Consultation

Amy was curious about potential diagnosis; it was discussed that being amid a crisis may complicate this and may not be an appropriate time to consider diagnosis. However, at time of the consultation, Amy was engaged and calm, effective history taking enabled careful consideration of potential working diagnoses.

The APMH utilised First's framework for differential diagnosis in conjunction with the ICD-11 [68, 69]. The differential diagnoses considered included complex post-traumatic stress disorder (CPTSD), post-traumatic stress disorder (PTSD), acute stress disorder, adjustment disorder, personality disorder, major depressive disorder and generalised anxiety disorder. Amy's working diagnosis was identified as CPTSD.

Broader consideration was given to potential primary or comorbid neurodiversity. However, accurate diagnosis in relation to neurodiversity is crucial and can be challenging within acute mental health services. Therefore, neurodiversity remained a potential differential diagnosis.

NICE guidelines were used to discuss complex PTSD in more detail [70].

The APMH used an adapted version of the Integrative Treatment Planning model (Figure 19.7) to explore intervention options and collaborative care planning with Amy [71].

The APMH explained to Amy that short-term HTT intervention would be beneficial to support her through her current crisis, and Amy agreed to this plan. Aligned with NICE guidelines, it was discussed with Amy that pharmacological intervention is unlikely to be a key component of her treatment plan but could be explored further if she wishes [70]; Amy declined this, explaining quetiapine helps and previous antidepressants have not been helpful for her.

Amy explained she would like increased support from Children's Social Care and consented to APMH liaison with them. Whilst there was no evidence of immediate safeguarding children concerns, liaison supports a 'think family' approach to ensuring appropriate support [72, 73].

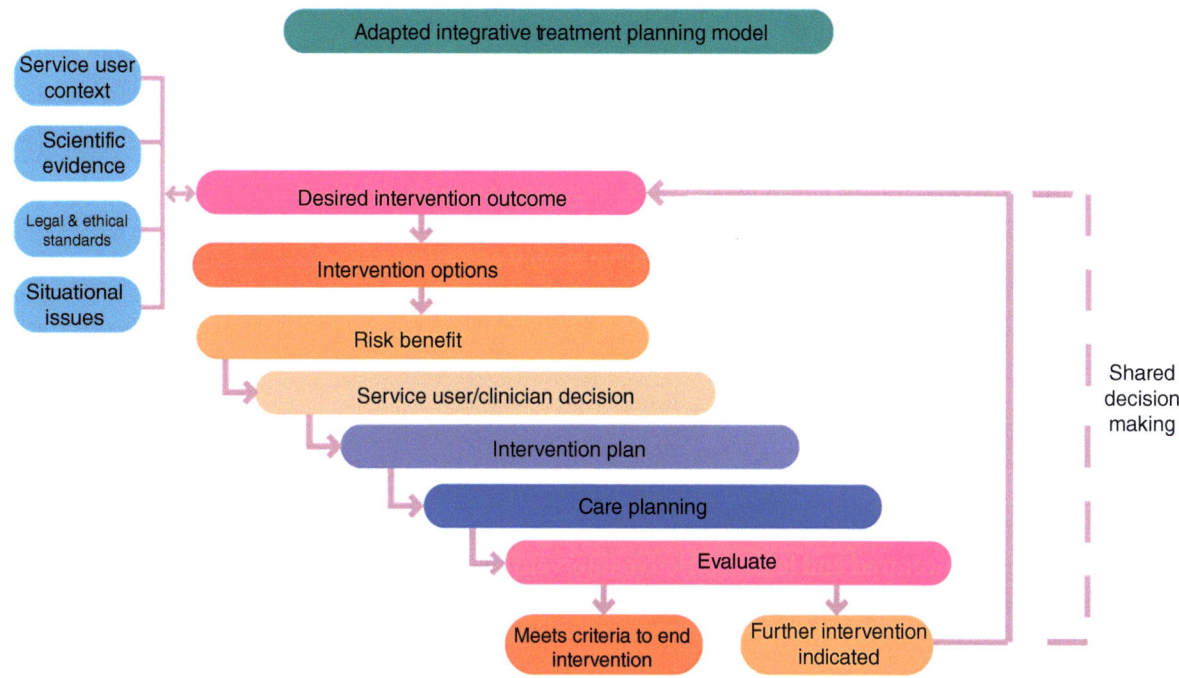

FIGURE 19.7 Adapted integrative treatment planning model. Source: [71] / with permission of Springer Nature.

AP ACTIONS

Telephone discussion with Children's Social Worker to facilitate effective communication [72]. The Social Worker held concerns about Amy's parenting ability; part of the APMH role was to advocate for Amy [14].

A letter outlining the APMH consultation was sent to Amy and copied to the CMHT, GP and Children's Social Worker.

A Few Days Later

During HTT practitioner review, Amy requested informal admission stating she will end her life if she remains in the community. HTT held concerns that admission may be unhelpful based on previous admissions which appeared to escalate Amy's risks to herself.

> **Before Advancing to the Next Part of the Case Study:**
>
> What approaches could you and the team take? What might your management plan include? What considerations would you have, across the four pillars?

AP INTERVENTION

Review of records, particularly in relation to Amy's levels of risk. Amy expressed thoughts to end her life if she remained in the community. Amy had not taken any further actions to harm or endanger herself.

Utilising leadership skills, the APMH facilitated a complex clinical meeting with HTT and the CMHT Key Worker using the Action Consequences model to weigh up the ethical complexities around Amy's risks and the potential decision to admit her to hospital [39, 40, 42, 45].

The team discussion lasted an hour and was documented using an adapted framework of the model. The team considered the potential action to admit Amy to hospital, and the benefits, dangers, short- and long-term implications of this, and how she may interpret decisions; additionally, the team considered the same concepts in relation to the possibility of continuing community support. On balance, it was considered that continued enhanced community intervention was indicated.

The documented team discussion was shared with Amy and her partner sensitively by a HTT practitioner who had previously met her. Amy reported feeling listened to and validated, and that she could understand the potential concerns. Amy agreed to continue to work with the HTT.

Outcome

Amy felt validated and listened to, as did her partner.
Collaborative, person-centred and least restrictive intervention planning.
Prevented potential escalation in presentation, distress and risks.
Short-term HTT intervention; joint working with the CMHT to enable a cohesive approach.
Avoided medical review.
Avoided admission to hospital.
Avoided further detentions under Section 136.

> **Mapping Amy's Case to the Pillars**
>
> **Clinical**: Complex clinical case; complex risk management; mental health legislation application; complex ethical decision-making; trauma-focused care.
>
> **Leadership and management**: Lead on complex case; facilitate complex clinical meeting; role model collaboration; consultancy across professional boundaries; patient advocacy.
>
> **Education**: Role model complex ethical decision-making with team; psychoeducation to patient, partner and to other services.
>
> **Research**: Use of relevant research; evidence-based practice; patient feedback collated to inform service design/developments.

CONCLUSION

APMHs are autonomous registered practitioners working across the four pillars of AP and the six domains of mental health AP [1, 3]. Deconstruction of AP highlights potential scope to adapt the 'pillars' to demonstrate their intersectionality and strengthen understanding of AP.

APMHs enhance capability within teams to increase clinical continuity and person-centred care. This chapter focused on outlining examples of the pillars in practice to both reassure existing APMH practice and inspire new directions, whilst exercising caution to avoid fuelling unhelpful comparison.

Limitations in the literature are clear with a requirement for focus on reviewing the AP in MH role, evaluating AHPs in AP roles and evaluating the AP role within non-clinical pillars to help understand and shape the future for the AP landscape.

APMH development enables exciting opportunities for mental health practitioner career progression. The future of AP in mental health is reliant on APMHs meeting, exceeding and pioneering in each of the pillars; this will advance care for people and their families, inspire and role model to peers, colleagues, teams and services and ultimately to justify the role of the APMH.

Reflection

- Which pillars resonate most with you?
- Where does your expert practice lie?
- Where are the opportunities within your practice to enhance fulfilment of all pillars?
- How will you advocate for the future of APMH?

REFERENCES

1. Health Education England (2017). Multi-professional framework for advanced clinical practice in England. London: HEE; 24 p. https://advanced-practice.hee.nhs.uk/multi-professional-framework-for-advanced-clinical-practice-in-england
2. Kristofersson, G.K., Higgins, A., and Kilkku, N. (2022). Role and competencies of advanced practice mental health nurses. In: *Advanced Practice in Mental Health Nursing: A European Perspective* (ed. A. Higgins, N. Kilkku, and G.K. Kristofersson), 19–42. Cham: Springer.
3. Health Education England (2022). Advanced practice in mental health curriculum and capabilities framework. London: HEE. 29 p. http://cc-private-storage-prod.s3.amazonaws.com/media/apps/heecapc2022/documents/51d5eaf591f5492593eb9cc21a77515e.pdf?response-content-disposition=inline%3B%20filename%3D%22advanced-practice-in-mental-health-curriculum-and-capabilities-framework.pdf%22%3B%20filename%2A%3DUTF-8%27%27advanced-practice-in-mental-health-curriculum-and-capabilities-framework.pdf&response-content-type=application%2Fpdf&X-Amz-Algorithm=AWS4-HMAC-SHA256&X-Amz-Credential=AKIAITK5SVR52HMXS5QQ%2F20240131%2Feu-central-1%2Fs3%2Faws4_request&X-Amz-Date=20240131T113011Z&X-Amz-Expires=30&X-Amz-SignedHeaders=host&X-Amz-Signature=139590896a903f9ffb697808ae7ed7f81096066d347c3937bdf06d4427f2c493
4. Evans, C., Poku, B., Pearce, R. et al. (2021). Characterising the outcomes, impacts and implementation challenges of advanced clinical practice roles in the UK: a scoping review. *BMJ Open* 11: e048171. https://doi.org/10.1136/bmjopen-2020-048171.
5. Fothergill, L.J., Al-Oraibi, A., Houdmont, J. et al. (2022). Nationwide evaluation of the advanced clinical practitioner role in England: a cross-sectional survey. *BMJ Open* 12: e055475. https://doi.org/10.1136/bmjopen-2021-055475.
6. Dean, S. (2023). Advanced clinical practitioners and the research pillar. *International Journal for Advancing Practice* 1 (1). https://www.internationaljournalforadvancingpractice.com/content/education/advanced-clinical-practitioners-and-the-research-pillar.
7. Stewart-Lord, A., Beanlands, C., Khine, R. et al. (2020). The role and development of advanced clinical practice within allied health professions: a mixed method study. *Journal of Multidisciplinary Healthcare* 25 (13): 1705–1715. https://doi.org/10.2147/JMDH.S267083.
8. Royal College of Nursing. RCN credentialing for advanced level nursing practice. London: RCN; 2023 www.rcn.org.uk/professional-development/professional-services/credentialing

9. Innes, E. and Harris, M. (2022). The importance of retaining professional identity within multidisciplinary advanced clinical practice [internet]. *BMJ Journals Evidence-Based Nursing Blog* https://blogs.bmj.com/ebn/2022/05/22/the-importance-of-retaining-professional-identity-within-multidisciplinary-advanced-clinical-practice/.
10. Mortimore, G., Reynolds, J., Forman, D. et al. (2021). From expert to advanced clinical practitioner and beyond. *British Journal of Nursing* 30 (11): 656–659. https://www-doi-org.plymouth.idm.oclc.org/10.12968/bjon.2021.30.11.656.
11. Kristofersson, G.K., Higgins, A., and Kilkku, N. (2022). Role and competencies of advanced practice mental health nurses. In: *Advanced Practice in Mental Health Nursing: A European Perspective* (ed. A. Higgins, N. Kilkku, and G.K. Kristofersson), 71–90. Cham: Springer.
12. Kristofferson, G.K. and Kaas, M.J. (2022). Integrative care planning. In: *Advanced Practice in Mental Health Nursing: A European Perspective* (ed. A. Higgins, N. Kilkku, and G.K. Kristofersson), 123–146. Cham: Springer.
13. Polhuis, D. and Grealish, A. (2022). Advanced mental health nursing assessment, formulation and decision-making. In: *Advanced Practice in Mental Health Nursing: A European Perspective* (ed. A. Higgins, N. Kilkku, and G.K. Kristofersson), 91–121. Cham: Springer.
14. NHS England (2023). Mental health nurse's handbook. London: NHSE; 30 p. [PR1011]. https://www.england.nhs.uk/wp-content/uploads/2022/10/B1011_Mental-Health-Nurses-Handbook_August-2023-v1.1-RCN-Endorsement.pdf
15. Health and Care Professions Council (2018). Standards of conduct, performance and ethics. London: HCPC. 14 p. https://www.hcpc-uk.org/globalassets/resources/standards/standards-of-conduct-performance-and-ethics.pdf
16. Nursing and Midwifery Council (2018). The Code: professional standards of practice and behaviour for nurses, midwives and nursing associates. London: NMC. 26 p. www.nmc.org.uk/globalassets/sitedocuments/nmc-publications/nmc-code.pdf
17. Murphy, R. and Higgins, A. (2022). Diversity and culturally responsive mental health practice. In: *Advanced Practice in Mental Health Nursing. A European Perspective* (ed. A. Higgins, N. Killku, and G.K. Kristofferson), 309–334. Cham: Springer.
18. Flanagan, S., Broholm, C., McClellan, L., and Yingling, C. (2022). LGBTQ+ issues: care of sexual and gender minority clients. In: *Advanced Practice Psychiatric Nursing*, 3rde (ed. K.R. Tusaie and J.J. Fitzpatrick), 625–644. New York: Springer Publishing.
19. Tusaie, K.R. (2023). Stages of treatment. In: *Advanced Practice Psychiatric Nursing*, 3rde (ed. K.R. Tusaie and J.J. Fitzpatrick), 116–127. New York: Springer Publishing.
20. Beauchamp, T.L. and Childress, J.F. (2021). *Principles of Biomedical Ethics*, 8the, 512. Oxford: Oxford University Press.
21. Benner, P. (1984). *From Novice to Expert, Excellence and Power in Clinical Nursing Practice*, 284. California: Addison-Wesley Publishing Company.
22. Mitchell, A. and Pearce, R. (2021). Prescribing practice: an overview of the principles. *British Journal of Nursing* 30(17). https://www.britishjournalofnursing.com/content/advanced-clinical-practice/prescribing-practice-an-overview-of-the-principles/.
23. Mann, C., Timmons, S., Evans, C. et al. (2023). Exploring the role of advanced clinical practitioners (ACPs) and their contribution to health services in England: A qualitative exploratory study. *Nurse Education in Practice* 67: 103546. https://doi.org/10.1016/j.nepr.2023.103546.
24. Mental Capacity Act (2005). (c 9) London, HMSO.

25. National Institute for health and care excellence (2020). Depression in children clinical knowledge summary. NICE. https://cks.nice.org.uk/topics/depression-in-children/
26. Montgomery v Lanarkshire Health Board (2015). United Kingdom Supreme Court, UKSC 1. Supreme Court. https://www.supremecourt.uk/cases/docs/uksc-2013-0136-judgment.pdf
27. Department of Health (2015). Mental health act 1983: code of practice. Norwich: the stationery office. 460 p. https://assets.publishing.service.gov.uk/media/5a80a774e5274a2e87dbb0f0/MHA_Code_of_Practice.PDF
28. McCulloch and others v Forth Valley Health Board (2023). United Kingdom Supreme Court, UKSC 26. Supreme Court. https://www.supremecourt.uk/cases/docs/uksc-2021-0149-judgment.pdf
29. Low M, Noblet T, Taylor J et al. (2024). Complex clinical reasoning. Elearning for Healthcare. https://www.e-lfh.org.uk/programmes/complex-clinical-reasoning/
30. Reed, L. and Carter, M. (2022). Leadership. In: *Hamric & Hanson's Advanced Practice Nursing: An Integrative Approach*, 7the (ed. M.F. Tracy, E.T. O'Grady, and S.J. Phillips), 279–314. Missouri: Elsevier.
31. Heinen, M., van Oostveen, C., Peters, J. et al. (2019). An integrative review of leadership competencies and attributes in advanced nursing practice. *Journal of Advanced Nursing* 75 (11): 2378–2392. https://doi.org/10.1111/jan.14092.
32. Wood, C. (2021). Leadership and management for nurses working at an advanced level. *British Journal of Nursing* 30 (5): 282–286. https://doi.org/10.12968/bjon.2021.30.5.282.
33. McGee, P. (2019). Leadership in advanced practice. In: *Advanced Practice in Health Care: Dynamic Developments in Nursing and Allied Health Professions*, 4the (ed. P. Mcgee and C. Inman), 251–264. West Sussex: Wiley Blackwell.
34. Royal College of Nursing (2023). Advanced level nursing practice: introduction. London: RCN; www.rcn.org.uk/professional-development/publications/PUB-006894
35. Johnson, J., Talley, M., and Watts, P. (2020). A quality and policy focus to academic Leadership. In: *Advanced Practice Nursing Leadership: A Global Perspective* (ed. S.B. Hassmiller and J. Pulcini), 185–204. Cham: Springer.
36. West, M. (2021). *Compassionate Leadership: Sustaining Wisdom, Humanity and Presence in Health and Social Care*, 340. UK: The Swirling Leaf Press.
37. Bailey S, West M (2022). What is compassionate leadership? www.kingsfund.org.uk/publications/what-is-compassionate-leadership
38. Fuggle, P., Talbot, L., Campbell, C. et al. (2023). *Adaptive Mentalisation-Based Integrative Treatment (AMBIT) for Working with Multiple Needs: Applications in Practise*, 384. Oxford: Oxford University Press.
39. Warrender, D. (2017). Borderline personality disorder and the ethics of risk management: the action/consequence model. *Nursing Ethics* 25 (7): 918–927. https://doi.org/10.1177/0969733016679467.
40. Warrender, D. (2023). The action/consequences model: a tool to prompt thinking and ethical decision making around risk. Poster presented at: British and Irish Group for the Study of Personality Disorder; Glasgow. https://www.researchgate.net/publication/371038224_The_ActionConsequences_Model_a_tool_to_prompt_thinking_and_ethical_decision_making_around_risk
41. Pearce, C. and Breen, B. (2018). Advanced clinical practice and nurse-led clinics: a time to progress. *British Journal of Nursing* 27 (8): 444–448. https://doi.org/10.12968/bjon.2018.27.8.444.
42. Hooks, C. and Walker, S. (2020). An exploration of the role of advanced clinical practitioners in the east of England. *British Journal of Nursing* 29 (15): 864–869. https://doi.org/10.12968/bjon.2020.29.15.864.
43. Health Education England (2022). Advanced practice workplace supervision: minimum Standards for supervision. London: HEE; 16 p. https://heeoe.hee.nhs.uk/sites/default/files/advanced_practice_workplace_supervision-_minimum_standards_for_supervision.pdf

44. Bloom, B.S. (1956). *Taxonomy of Educational Objectives: the Classification of Educational Goals*, 403. New York: Longmans, Green.
45. Anderson, L.W. and Krathwohl, D.R. (2001). *A Taxonomy for Learning, Teaching, and Assessing: A Revision of Bloom's Taxonomy of Educational Objectives*, 352. New York: Longman.
46. Mortimore, G., Forman, D., Brannigan, C., and Mitchell, K. (2021). From expert to advanced clinical practitioner and beyond. *Advanced Clinical Practice* 30 (11): 656–659. https://doi.org/10.12968/bjon.2021.30.11.656.
47. Howell, W.C. (1982). An overview of models, methods, and problems. In: *Human Performance and Productivity. Volume 2: Information Processing and Decision Making* (ed. W.C. Howell and E.A. Fleishman), 29–33. Hillsdale, NJ: Lawrence Erlbaum Associates, Incorporated.
48. Kolb, D.A. (2015). *Experiential Learning: experience as the Source of Learning and Development*, 2nde, 416. New Jersey: Pearson Education.
49. Gibbs, G. (1988). *Learning by Doing: A Guide to Teaching and Learning Methods*, 129. Oxford: Further Education Unit.
50. Driscoll, J. (2006). *Practicing Clinical Supervision: A Reflective Approach for Healthcare Professionals*, 2nde, 272. Edinburgh: Bailliere Tindall Elsevier.
51. Kirk, S. (2017). Waves of Reflection: seeing knowledges in academic writing. In: *EAP in a rapidly changing landscape: issues, challenges and solutions. Proceedings of the 2015 BALEAP Conference* (ed. J. Kemp), 109–118. Reading: Garnet Education.
52. The National Confidential Inquiry into Suicide and Safety in Mental Health (2018). The assessment of clinical risk in mental health services. The University of Manchester: 26 p. https://documents.manchester.ac.uk/display.aspx?DocID=38466
53. Littlewood, D.L., Quinlivan, L., Graney, J. et al. (2019). Learning from clinicians' views of good quality practice in mental healthcare services in the context of suicide prevention: a qualitative study. *BMC Psychiatry* 19: 346. https://doi.org/10.1186/s12888-019-2336-8.
54. The National Confidential Inquiry into Suicide and Safety in Mental Health (2023). Annual report: UK patient and general population data, 2010-2020. The University of Manchester: 44 p. https://documents.manchester.ac.uk/display.aspx?DocID=66829
55. Mukhalalati, B.A. and Taylor, A. (2019). Adult learning theories in context: a quick guide for healthcare professional educators. *Journal of Medical Education and Curricular Development* 6. https://doi-org.plymouth.idm.oclc.org/10.1177/2382120519840332.
56. Brown, J. (2020). Using learning theory to shape learning experiences in health care education: not scary at all! *Innovative Teaching and Learning in the Health Professions* 162: 81–89. https://doi-org.plymouth.idm.oclc.org/10.1002/tl.20393.
57. NHS England and NHS Improvement (2021). Making research matter chief nursing officer for england's strategic plan for research. London: NHSE/I; 32 p. https://www.england.nhs.uk/wp-content/uploads/2021/11/B0880-cno-for-englands-strategic-plan-fo-research.pdf
58. Health Education England (2022). Allied health professions' research and innovation strategy for England. London: HEE; 21 p. https://www.hee.nhs.uk/sites/default/files/documents/HEE%20Allied%20Health%20Professions%20Research%20and%20Innovation%20Strategy%20FINAL_0.pdf
59. Gaskin, K. (2023). Achieving the research pillar: a research toolkit for advanced practitioners. *BMJ Evidence-Based Nursing Blog* https://blogs.bmj.com/ebn/2023/06/11/achieving-the-research-pillar-a-research-toolkit-for-advanced-practitioners/.

60. Gaskin, K. (2023). Advanced practice research pillar toolkit. https://sway.cloud.microsoft/8hcpK9Gor8m2bVzT?ref=Link
61. National Mental Health Intelligence Network (2023). Premature mortality in adults with severe mental illness (SMI). https://www.gov.uk/government/publications/premature-mortality-in-adults-with-severe-mental-illness/premature-mortality-in-adults-with-severe-mental-illness-smi
62. National Institute for Health and Care Research (2023). Supporting the physical health of people with severe mental illness. https://evidence.nihr.ac.uk/collection/supporting-the-physical-health-of-people-with-severe-mental-illness/
63. Baugh, C, Singh, P, Talwar, K (2022). QN CRHTT standards for crisis resolution and home treatment teams 5th edition. London: Royal College of Psychiatrists; www.rcpsych.ac.uk/docs/default-source/improving-care/ccqi/quality-networks/htas/qn-crhtt-5th-edition-standards.pdf?sfvrsn=22cfa1dc_2
64. NHS England and NHS Improvement (2022). Online library of quality, service improvement and redesign tools: plan, do, study, act (PDSA) cycles and the model for improvement. London: NHSE/I; https://www.england.nhs.uk/wp-content/uploads/2022/01/qsir-pdsa-cycles-model-for-improvement.pdf
65. Trenoweth, S. and Moone, N. (2017). *Psychosocial Assessment in Mental Health*, 256. London: SAGE Publications Ltd.
66. Macneil CA, Hasty MK, Conus P, Berk M. Is diagnosis enough to guide interventions in mental health? Using case formulation in clinical practice. BMC Medicine. 2012 10(111). https://doi.org/10.1186/1741-7015-10.111
67. Felitti, V.J., Anda, R.F., Nordenberg, D. et al. (1998). Relationship of childhood abuse and household dysfunction to many of the leading causes of death in adults: the Adverse Childhood Experiences (ACE) study. *American Journal of Preventive Medicine* 14 (4): 245–258. https://doi.org/10.1016/S0749-3797(98)00017-8.
68. First, M. (2014). *DSM-5 Handbook of Differential Diagnosis*, 338. Washington: American Psychiatric Association.
69. World Health Organization (2022). ICD-11: international classification of diseases (11th revision). https://icd.who.int/
70. National Institute for Health and Care Excellence (2018). Post-traumatic stress disorder. London: NICE; 54 p. [NG116]. www.nice.org.uk/guidance/ng116/resources/posttraumatic-stress-disorder-pdf-66141601777861
71. Kristofferson, G.K. and Kaas, M.J. (2022). Integrative care planning. In: *Advanced Practice in Mental Health Nursing. A European Perspective* (ed. A. Higgins, N. Killku, and G.K. Kristofferson), 123–146. Cham: Springer.
72. Department for Education (2023). Working together to safeguard children: a guide to multi-agency working to help, protect and promote the welfare of children. London: DFE; 168 p. https://assets.publishing.service.gov.uk/media/65803fe31c0c2a000d18cf40/Working_together_to_safeguard_children_2023__statutory_guidance.pdf
73. Social Care Institute for Excellence (2009). Think child, think parent, think family: a guide to parental mental health and child welfare. London: SCIE 90 p. https://cypsp.hscni.net/wp-content/uploads/2014/02/SCIE-Guidance.pdf

CHAPTER 20

Advanced Practice in Mental Health: Personal and Professional Growth

Kayleigh Brown[1] and Stephanie Tempest[2]

[1] Mental Health Division, Humber teaching NHS Foundation Trust, Hull, UK
[2] Stephanie Tempest Consultancy Ltd., London, UK

Aim

This chapter aims to encourage readers to reflect on the relationship between the personal and professional aspects of self and to understand that each career development journey to working as an advanced practitioner in mental health is unique to the individual and their area of practice. Resources, tools and concepts are presented, alongside reflective questions, to empower clinicians to understand and take ownership of their professional growth.

LEARNING OUTCOMES

By the end of this chapter, the reader will be able to:

1. Reflect on the meaning and impact of personal growth for career development and the importance of being a reflective practitioner.
2. Critically evaluate the inter-relationship between personal and professional growth.
3. Critically consider the process of learning to advance career development.
4. Consider a range of multi-professional sources to support individual growth as an advanced practitioner in mental health, across the four pillars of practice.

Table 20.1 outlines how the content of this chapter maps to the mental health advanced practice area specific capability and curriculum framework [1].

The Advanced Practitioner in Mental Health, First Edition. Edited by Clare Allabyrne.
© 2026 John Wiley & Sons Ltd. All rights reserved, including rights for text and data mining and training of artificial intelligence technologies or similar technologies. Published 2026 by John Wiley & Sons Ltd.

TABLE 20.1 Mental health advanced practice area specific capability and curriculum framework.

Domain F: Leadership and Management, education and research

6.1 Exemplify leadership, resilience and determination; manage situations that are unfamiliar, uncertain, complex or unpredictable; and seek to build confidence in others.	6.6 Receive, lead and exemplify a culture of critically reflective clinical practice supervision.
6.2 Lead the development of effective relationships, fostering clarity of roles across teams.	6.7 Act as a professional role model and educator in understanding and practice, in accordance with evidence-based practice and statutory responsibilities, including legislation, guidance, standards and regulatory requirements.
6.5 Negotiate an individual scope of practice within legal, ethical, professional and organisational policies, governance and procedures, with a focus on mitigating risk and upholding safety.	6.8 Critically and strategically apply advanced clinical expertise across professional and service boundaries to enhance knowledge and understanding of mental health.

INTRODUCTION

There is a transitional period when you start working as an advanced practitioner in mental health. You may come to the role feeling like an expert in your clinical area and then arrive as an advanced practitioner in mental health with room to grow across the Four Pillars of Practice. This transition requires you to take an intentional approach to developing a set of skills that aligns with the required level of practice.

For example, think of a time in your adult life, but a few years back, where you were learning something new for the first time. It could be learning to drive, learning to be a parent for the first time or the early weeks in your first job as a qualified healthcare practitioner. Now think of your current level of performance, knowledge and skills doing the same role and how this has changed over time and with experience.

Let's take driving as an example. It is likely that a driver with years of experience no longer says 'Mirror, signal, manoeuvre' in their head when changing lanes. Their ability to reverse park may come from a tacit place which requires little cognitive processing. It's unlikely they hold the steering wheel at 'ten minutes to two' or check their blind spot as prescriptively as when they were learning. The point here is, that with experience, a driver learns how to drive the roads and perform the associated activities with less conscious thinking *after* they learn the prescriptive methods in which to pass their test. However, some bad habits might creep in too, and it could take a penalty notice or speed awareness course to act as a reminder of the need to refocus on their driving knowledge and skills. Alternatively, some drivers choose to take the advanced driving qualification to enhance their skills further.

The journey to becoming an advanced practitioner in mental health also develops over time. It is not a singular role in one setting, so it will take many forms, in part based on local service needs, which will be explored later in the chapter.

Throughout this chapter, the authors have drawn upon their own stories and experiences including a focus on one career story as an illustrative example. The story belongs to Kayleigh, a registered mental health nurse, an advanced practitioner in mental health and a clinical lead, who has chosen to share in the spirit of linking the theoretical concepts to a practical, real-world example. These sections are written in the first person and the career story represents Kayleigh's story alone.

PERSONAL GROWTH

Hello, my name is Kayleigh and I'm going to start my career story with an honest reflection of where it began. Twenty years or so on, I am now the Divisional Clinical Lead for a large Mental Health Trust responsible for the development and delivery of multi-professional services across a range of settings.

> ### Where I started
>
> As a person who didn't take a conventional education route, I never really knew what a career looked like. I knew about working and graft; I'd watched my whole family do that, but not necessarily about higher education and academia.
>
> When I got to about 16, I was introduced to people who had some higher education which broadened my horizons; my mum was also taking opportunities (as she had all my life) to develop her career in social care. I think watching her do this, and others, made me realise that if I wanted to enjoy a work life, I needed to explore options of what I might like.
>
> I remember heading into college at 16 and being told that I would have to do hairdressing with the qualifications I had (or lack of). I did as I was told and HATED it. I marched back into the college with my GNVQ and asked the question again – I want a childcare course – how do I make that happen? They relooked and low and behold, found a way for me to get on to a BTEC course.
>
> I didn't love it, but I saw it as a stepping stone, an opportunity. I then sat one night at the computer and looked at different jobs on the NHS jobs website. I read a few and nothing stuck, until I read about mental health nursing. It was one short paragraph and I knew, that's it, I'm going to be an RMN. First hurdle, it was a degree. I had zero GCSEs, nothing that aligned to any core curriculum like English or Maths, which we all know is a must. I took myself back in to college again and asked the question, what do I need to do to get in to university? Key skills from scratch and an access course. Off I went.

THE ROLE OF REFLECTION TO SUPPORT PERSONAL GROWTH

The best development often emerges from the most challenging circumstances, and Kayleigh's story illustrates that much of our best personal growth comes from being in and navigating our way through difficult places. Personal growth contributes to professional development [2], and reflection is key to supporting growth.

Role of Reflective Practice

Reflective practice allows us to make sense of a situation, understand how it has affected us and identify areas for learning and development to improve our everyday practice [3].

From a regulatory perspective, space to reflect helps registrants manage the challenge and pressure of working in health and care, to support safe and effective practice [4].

Reflective practice is a life practice and is not without its challenges, as explored by Kayleigh:

> Reflective spaces have not always shown up at the right time in the right places throughout my career; however, the more I did get to experience them, the more I learned of the value and sought them out in my development journey. Looking back now, this highlights that structures may not have been set up consistently to support clinicians to reflect in their roles or to embed an approach to structure reflective conversations in practice.

Safe and effective health and care delivery is enhanced through reflective practice, and there are three elements required to create a safety-based culture:

- Continuous learning and improvement of safety risks
- Supportive, psychologically safe teamwork
- Enabling and empowering speaking up by all [5]

Reflective practice provides a vehicle to develop these three elements because it requires us to discuss personal/professional learning and development, evaluation and improvement. This supports the creation of a culture of shared learning, which is pivotal to our development as practitioners and for service provision.

An exploration of various reflective models is beyond the scope of this chapter – and it is likely that readers have established preferences already. Wider reading is encouraged, including resources from the regulators and professional bodies for those wishing to refresh or enhance their knowledge, skills and practice further.

While reflective practice can be encouraged through formal processes, it is also important to view it as a habit, recognising that it is influenced by the culture we work in. As Kayleigh discusses:

> Supervision is one example of a structured, contracted and explicit way to support reflection, but it can also be an everyday process that, with practice and intentional structures, over time becomes a habit. This allows us to explore and accept our vulnerability in order to grow and build self-awareness. However, we have to be mindful that the systems in which we work are not always sophisticated enough to guarantee psychological safety, which is key to authentic and transparent growth and vulnerability. This stresses the importance of being an habitual reflective practitioner to manage the challenges at work, including establishing advanced practice within mental health.
>
> Experience has shown me that working in cultures where there is less emphasis on continuous learning, a lack of support for reflective practice and ineffective mechanisms to support speaking up and being heard, negatively impacts on me as an individual practitioner. A difficult workplace culture also negatively impacts on the team, service and the system and creates wider problems. Regardless of the workplace culture, we need to look after ourselves and this requires professional and personal self-awareness.

PROFESSIONAL AND PERSONAL SELF-AWARENESS

This section focuses on self-care, outlines the importance of understanding personal and professional values, explores a range of self-leadership skills and critically discusses the concept and impact of feeling like an imposter.

Self-Care

In mental health practice, service users are often encouraged to know and understand early warning signs or red flags, as early indications for struggle and challenge. As an act of self-care, practitioners also need to notice these, alongside the dysregulation in the systems and practices which can often reflect and impact on practitioner well-being.

It is important to notice when additional support is required and to access the mechanisms that meet your needs, e.g. to regulate or to self-soothe including but not limited to:

- Supervision
- Safe reflective spaces with colleagues
- Positive and transparent working relationships
- Coaching
- Formal learning opportunities
- Communities of practice and networks

As part of engaging in these mechanisms, practitioners may be invited to explore their own values and skill sets and some of these will be explored next.

Knowing Your Values and Skill Set

It is not uncommon for colleagues who advance their practice into leadership roles to report that they have 'found' themselves in the role, but do not feel they have been shown, or invested in, to develop their leadership skills and understanding. Readers may be able to relate to this from their own experience too.

However, reflective conversations on why people choose to hold specific responsibilities, e.g. leadership roles, will often be linked to personal and professional values that feel important to them as an individual. When moving into advanced practice roles or when there are any periods of rapid career development, it is important to reflect on personal and professional values to understand how they influence and drive individual career paths, including into leadership.

To inspire people to take action, effective leaders start by asking **why** do you do what you do and then seek to explore the **how** and **what** [6]. Identifying values can feel like quite a daunting task and if readers wish to explore some of this work, they are encouraged to search for reputable sources using the term 'identifying values' including the work undertaken by Dr. Brene Brown in her work Dare to Lead [7].

Leadership development opportunities are evolving and are now taught in some pre-registration programmes, as well as offered to practitioners at different career levels, including advanced practice. Tools which seek to identify individual strengths and developmental areas are increasingly being embedded into leadership programmes to promote self-awareness and to identify values, drivers and behaviours that feature in daily work. Readers are encouraged to explore the opportunities available within their setting, including via the Learning and Development Teams.

Leadership as a Set of Skills

Kayleigh reflects on what leadership means to her and offers these thoughts:

We need to view leadership as a set of skills which we can develop and hone including transferable elements from our existing roles. Advanced practitioners in mental health have clinical expertise which is based on the area in which they have gained enhanced and advanced skills. However, there is also a core set of leadership skills to support us to work at this level of practice. We can lift and shift these skills across teams and systems, ones which we may not be as attuned with, but allow us the skills to understand and navigate work areas to support teams and service delivery.

Indeed, in the broader world of work, there are eight key leadership skills that individuals are encouraged to develop [8], skills which are seen as transferable and these include:

- Relationship building
- Agility and adaptability
- Innovation and creativity
- Employee motivation
- Decision-making
- Conflict management
- Negotiation
- Critical thinking

REFLECTION QUESTION: Consider the eight leadership skills in the list and identify learning and experiences from across your career where you have learnt to develop these.

Imposter Syndrome/Phenomenon

One challenge to self-care and to advancing careers, which is receiving more attention, is the impact of imposter syndrome, including how this can negatively impact high-functioning, high-achieving individuals, especially those working within the context of health and care including clinical practice and academia. This section explores and challenges some of the existing narrative and evidence and readers are invited to consider the debate here in relation to their own beliefs and experiences.

Imposter syndrome has been defined as a behavioural health phenomenon comprising self-doubt of intellect, skills or accomplishments, among high-achieving individuals. Characteristics may include perfectionism, fear of failure, super-heroism, feeling like a fraud, denial of competence, over-preparedness and procrastination [9]. There appears to be a relationship between imposter syndrome, depression, anxiety and burnout [10].

In the academic literature, the topic is indexed primarily as 'imposter phenomenon' while the lay literature uses the term 'imposter syndrome' [11]. The latter potentially medicalises a set of emotions and feelings that occur as a response to experiences, and this may or may not be helpful. For example, there are many factors, including the workplace culture and societal attitudes, that impact on a person's level of super-heroism.

The first published synthesis of peer-reviewed evidence [11] concluded there is no consensus on the prevalence, diagnoses and treatment for imposter phenomenon. Indeed, the nature of it as a condition has been challenged – there is currently no widely agreed definition and it is not listed in the DSM-V criteria or the International Classification of Diseases (ICD-10). There is also debate, from a feminist perspective, to challenge and reframe the narrative around imposter syndrome including debating its existence [12].

That being said, the emotions and feelings that are evoked and are classed as features within the concept of imposter syndrome/phenomenon must not be undermined or invalidated. Feelings, such as the need to be perfect and the fear of failure, are real and can have significant negative consequences on individuals at home and in the workplace. It may be that the source comes from the expectations within the workplace rather than from the individual themselves.

As the debate continues as to the nature of imposter syndrome/phenomenon, it may be more effective to address directly the individual behavioural responses, through reflective practice, group supervision, mentoring, coaching and counselling, to enable individuals to challenge and build new internal strategies for managing a range of emotional responses to challenges at work. Labelling these responses as a syndrome carries the risk of being a barrier to supporting people to grow and advance in their careers.

PROFESSIONAL GROWTH

So far this chapter has focused on personal growth and development including becoming reflective, understanding personal values and drivers and the importance of self-care. This next section focuses on professional growth. It will briefly outline key concepts in the theories that support adults to learn and then explore the role of experience to aid learning and skill development so practitioners can grow and advance their careers within mental health. It will explore specific frameworks that can be used in practice so readers can consider some of the resources available to them.

Acquiring and Developing Skills – Theoretical Concepts

In order to define what professional growth looks like, it is important to understand the ways in which adults learn and develop knowledge and skills.

There are five main theory bases (see Table 20.2), and this section is intended as a starting point or brief reminder. They are not mutually exclusive and readers are encouraged to reflect on the extent to which they have preferences for elements of some or all of them. The role of reflection is a key element across the learning theories in order to support individuals to develop new knowledge and skills and to change behaviours. This was discussed in an earlier section when exploring personal growth which reinforces the inter-relationship between being a reflective person (for personal growth) and the development of the professional self too.

There are many theories that seek to define and conceptualise how people grow professionally in order to learn the knowledge and skills they need for the workplace, and it is beyond the scope of this chapter to explore them all in detail. Readers are encouraged to explore the wider literature for more details.

Learning theories are different from learning styles (e.g. visual, auditory etc) and while defining preferred ways of learning receives much attention and is widely promoted, there is a lack of evidence to show the effectiveness of aligning learning styles to teaching methods [14].

TABLE 20.2 A brief summary of learning theories.

Learning theory	Key points
Behaviour	Change in behaviour occurs through training, education and stimuli in the external environment, e.g. reinforcement after a behaviour (positive or negative reinforcement).
Cognitive	New knowledge is interpreted through cognitive (thinking) processes including from experience, e.g. skills in analysis, application, problem-solving, memory and perception.
Humanistic	Learning focuses on cognitive (thinking) aspects and also includes the role of emotions and feelings. Individuals learn (and respond to the learning) based on an interpretation of the knowledge and experiences in relation to their own values, thoughts and feelings.
Social	Learning happens through the interactions with others including in a social context, through communities of practice and from real-life action.
Constructivist	A learner constructs meaning and knowledge from experiences and from reflecting on those experiences. A new experience will be related to previous ones to either change a way of thinking or working or reject it.

Source: Adapted from Hayden [13].

Regardless of the theoretical basis, there are also models that propose the different stages through which individuals work, consciously or subconsciously, to acquire new knowledge and skills.

A five-stage model to conceptualise the mental activities and processes involved in acquiring and developing new skills was published in seminal work in 1980 [15]. The model was based on observational analyses of chess players and airline pilots and identifies five stages of skill acquisition:

1. Novice
2. Competence
3. Proficiency
4. Expertise
5. Mastery

This model proposes that experience alone accounts for higher levels of performance [15]. So, for example, Stage 2 (Competence) can only be achieved after considerable real-world experience as a novice. This links back to the example in the introduction of learning to drive before and after passing the test. The role of supervision is central as a process for supporting people to learn from experience and to enhance knowledge and skill acquisition.

Further work was undertaken to explore what these five stages look like when applied to clinical competence in healthcare, with a focus specifically on nursing practice (see Figure 20.1) [16]. Figure 20.1 reinforces that expertise in any field, such as mental health, must be viewed as a process that is learned over time.

The influences of these theories can be seen in contemporary resources used to conceptualise and support career development today. The novice to expert continuum is one such example, and it features widely in multi-professional and uni-professional resources.

Stage	Clinical competence level
1	Novice
2	Advanced Beginner
3	Competent
4	Proficient
5	Expert

FIGURE 20.1   Benner's stages of clinical competence [16].

The advantage of using the novice to expert continuum within the context of advanced practice is that people new to this level of practice can recognise there is room to grow within it, as they develop expertise through experience. It also enables experienced advanced practitioners to recognise where they sit too.

Significant work has been undertaken in the last decade to conceptualise the healthcare workforce. A Venn diagram approach has been proposed [17] to conceptualise different levels of practice within the health and care workforce, namely: supportive, assistive, novice, intermediate/foundation, enhanced, advanced and consultant. Individual professional growth can be plotted along the diagram appreciating that many people will choose to self-actualise at different levels – not everyone wants to become an advanced or consultant level practitioner. Equally, there are barriers that prevent some people from being recognised for working at specific levels, placed there by the system itself.

When reflecting on the underlying principles across the theories, models and the frameworks, there are several key message that emerge.

Advancing practice:

1. Is a process that requires experience to develop the necessary knowledge and skills.
2. Is a level of practice built upon from previous levels.
3. Requires a learning and development approach to support knowledge and skills acquisition which includes paying attention to the role of external environment, the learner's cognitive processes, emotions and feelings and the way in which people can learn together to draw on experiences to make sense of new learning.

Later in this chapter, the role of frameworks will be explored in more detail as mechanisms to support professional growth.

Professional Growth Is a Cognitive and Emotional Process

As already discussed, learning can be viewed as a cognitive, emotional and social process. As a previous educator within Higher Education, I (Steph – second author) lost count of the number of learners who told me that they were 'more practical and not really academic' and then I had the privilege of watching them graduate with bachelor's and master's qualifications – the mismatch between how I perceived their reality and their own belief always surprised me.

Individual beliefs are shaped in part by past experiences, including the impact of childhood schooling experiences and family attitudes to study. Internal, subconscious thought patterns exist and these impact the way that individuals approach learning – two will be briefly explored next as, left unchecked, they both have the potential to impact on professional growth.

Growth Mindset Theory

Growth-mindset theory proposes that people primarily approach their capacity to learn with one of two mindsets – a growth mindset or a fixed one [18] which shapes the brain's capacity to learn and solve problems.

A person with a fixed mindset believes their capacity to learn is fixed so, for example, they are academic, sporty, good at maths or they are not. A person with a growth-mindset believes they have capacity to make incremental changes in their ability. In reality, most people's mindset lies somewhere along the spectrum with fixed and growth at the extreme ends, and this may fluctuate depending on a range of factors including the learning environment and recent experiences.

Career advancement and professional growth can be positively influenced by adopting more of a growth-mindset approach, as it enables individuals to thrive when they feel challenged, to help them to expect to make mistakes as part of the growth process and to be more resilient to learn from them [19].

Further research on mindset theory is required, especially as the majority of the work has been conducted within the formal educational system and with children [20]. However, a scoping review [21] identified that the use of the growth mindset model has been applied within the health and care professions to develop critical thinking, enhance resilience and help practitioners to learn how to respond to mistakes.

> **REFLECTIVE QUESTIONS** based on [22]
>
> 1. Fixed mindset: To what extent do you avoid risk, struggle to admit mistakes or default to a defensive position when challenged after a setback? What other factors could be impacting on these behaviours beyond the mindset approach?
> 2. Growth mindset: To what extent are you comfortable to try different strategies when something does not work, to learn more and to work through obstacles? What other characteristics do you have that support you to grow?

The Dunning-Kruger Effect

In 1999, Justin Kruger and David Dunning published a paper with the title 'Unskilled and unaware of it: how difficulties in recognising one's own incompetence lead to inflated self-assessments'. [23]. Across four studies, the research found that college students with lower skills in specific tests tended to overestimate their abilities. This presented the students with a dual burden – they did not know what they did not know and they overestimated their capacity. Conversely, when the skills of the student participants improved, they were able to recognise the limitations of their abilities better, using newly developed metacognitive processes. This cognitive bias became known as the Dunning-Kruger effect or the Dunning-Kruger learning curve [23].

It is important to reinforce that when referring to unskilled or low skilled, this is not the same as perceived level of intelligence in general. It refers to all individuals starting out to learn a new skill. To highlight this point, Table 20.3 includes a real-world example of learning to drive a manual car as an illustrative example, alongside the four stages within the Dunning-Kruger effect/learning curve.

TABLE 20.3 The four stages within the Dunning-Kruger effect and an everyday example of learning to drive a manual car.

Stage	Description	Learning to drive a manual car
Unconscious incompetence	I don't know what I don't know.	I have no idea how to drive any type of car.
Conscious incompetence	I know what I don't know but I haven't learnt it yet.	I know there is one pedal to go faster, one to go slower and one to help change the gears. I know what the gear stick does too.
Conscious competence	I know what I don't know and I'm gaining knowledge about it.	I can use all three pedals and the gear stick but sometimes I stall the car when I pull away and sometimes I brake too hard.
Unconscious competence	I have mastered something.	I can use the three pedals and the gearstick in a responsive manner without having to think about it.

> **REFLECTIVE ACTIVITY:** think about a time in your professional career when you embarked on learning a new skill, e.g. the first time you worked with a student on placement as their educator. Apply the stages of the Dunning-Kruger learning curve to your example to reflect on how your performance developed and where it could go next.

Later in this chapter, the role of supervision and coaching for professional growth will be explored. Some of the techniques used in supervision and coaching seek to explore the different learning stages proposed in the work by Dunning and Kruger and to enact other theories that seek to increase metacognition and self-awareness.

Acquiring and Developing Skills – the Practical Use of Frameworks to Support Professional Growth

There are many frameworks to support professional growth and advancement that can be used within the context of advancing multi-professional careers in mental health. In my current role (ST), I have been involved in the development and implementation of many of them, including the mental health advanced practice area specific capability and curriculum framework [1]. There are also frameworks for specific professions and settings (see Table 20.4 for a summary).

Before exploring the practical use of different frameworks in more detail, it is important to recognise and acknowledge the concept of 'framework fatigue' – not an actual disorder, rather an emotional response to the proliferation of resources that are now available from multiple sources including NHS England, Royal Colleges, Professional Bodies, the Council of Deans and many more. In the realities of a busy work life, it is understandable that finding time to source and engage with the various frameworks may feel like a challenge and one task to many. And that is a valid response. However, I'd like to offer an alternative viewpoint to 'framework fatigue', expressed by a colleague in a podcast we recorded together [24], who reflected on the reality that we when we go into a library, we expect to find well-stocked shelves and a range of reference books from which we can select the ones that help to meet individual need. The key point is to ensure we browse the section that feels relevant to us and select the books/frameworks we want to read at that moment in time.

The dictionary definition for framework is 'a supporting structure or object comprising a set of rules, ideas or beliefs to help you decide what to do' [25]. With so many professions and so many exciting and rewarding places for healthcare practitioners to advance their careers (e.g. in clinical practice, education roles, leadership roles and research), there is no wonder there are so many frameworks to support individualised growth and career planning.

One common theme that runs across most of the resources is the Four Pillars of Practice, albeit named slightly differently for different audiences, i.e. clinical practice, leadership and management, education and research [1]. Individual professions have chosen to adapt the language, for example, occupational therapists and speech and language therapists use 'professional practice' instead of 'clinical practice' [26, 27] choosing to reflect the multiple settings where their members work including prisons, schools and leisure centres among others.

TABLE 20.4 A summary of some of the recent frameworks to support the advancement of practice in mental health across the Four Pillars of Practice.

Name of Framework
Multi-professional framework for advanced practice in England [28]
Mental health advanced practice area specific capability and curriculum framework [1]
Profession-specific frameworks to cover the career lifespan including advanced level, e.g. RCOT Career Development Framework [26], RCSLT Professional Development Framework [27]
AHP Educator Career Framework to support development of knowledge and skills in the **Education Pillar** [29].
Multi-professional practice-based research capabilities framework to support development of knowledge and skills in the **Research Pillar** [30]
NHS Healthcare Leadership Model to support development of knowledge and skills in **Leadership Pillar**

Each framework provides a structure for individuals to reflect on their current level of performance, knowledge and skills with key capabilities. The mental health advanced practice area specific capability and curriculum framework [1] is also used by higher education institutes, providers and commissioners to quality assure their courses. They provide a structure to recognise and articulate that each advanced level role in mental health will look different, depending on the needs of the service and the requirements of different roles. Most importantly, the frameworks support us to identify and celebrate our achievements and plan the next element in our continuing professional development.

Continuing professional development and lifelong learning are different concepts to the mandatory training that we all have to complete to function at work (although in practice, this is often not the perception). There are a range of definitions, including from different regulators, but the following definitions were agreed across a broad range of health and care professions including nurses, midwives, allied health professions and trade unions [31] and are cited here:

CPD is:

The way in which you continue to learn and develop throughout your career. CPD is essential. It adds to your skills, knowledge, professional identify and ways of thinking so that you stay up to date and practice safely and effectively, now and in the future.

Lifelong learning is:

Formal and informal learning opportunities that allow you to continuously develop and improve the knowledge and skills you need for employment and personal fulfilment.

The frameworks available to us help to guide the process of engaging in CPD and lifelong learning to support our personal and professional growth.

> **REFLECTIVE QUESTION:** Which frameworks do you feel you would like to explore in more detail? How can you use the frameworks, or sections within them, to support your own career growth? Which other frameworks would you like to use?

HUMAN SUPPORT FOR PROFESSIONAL GROWTH

From experience, frameworks have their place to support career growth and development, but their strength lies in the conversations they promote. This section focuses on sources of human support to promote growth. It will briefly explore coaching, mentoring and supervision, networks and communities of practice, alongside the need for health and well-being approaches for all health and care practitioners seeking to grow and advance their careers within mental health.

Throughout this section readers are encouraged to identify anchor points they already have or feel they need – sources that can act as scaffolding through career transitions and periods of growth, especially when those periods of growth are also causing growing pains.

Arguably the system has yet to fully embrace the potential and the range of advanced practice roles in mental health nor fully understand their contribution in practice. It is common for advanced practitioners in mental health to feel like they are trailblazing new ways of working which can be exhausting on top of the 'day job'. With this in mind, it important that advanced practitioners in mental health prioritise their own wellness as part of being able to deliver safe, compassionate and effective services to people who need them. Selecting the right scaffolding to build around ourselves is a priority.

Coaching, Mentoring, Supervision

There are many different definitions for coaching, mentoring and supervision, and Table 20.5 provides an overview adapted from [32]. The definitions show there are some similarities but also differences, and there may be occasions where individuals feel one form of support would be better than another. Additionally, there may be times, especially during transition between roles, where elements of all three feel appropriate.

TABLE 20.5 Defining coaching, mentoring and supervision.

Coaching	Traditionally is: • time-limited. • focused on improving performance in a particular skill set. • linked to individual or organisational goals. • based on solution-focused techniques. • a process that seeks to reframe challenges. • delivered by people with specific training.
Mentoring	Traditionally is: • based on a relationship between two people. • focused on the whole person and their future career plans. • delivered by someone beyond the immediate work team (who may traditionally be someone more senior/experienced, but in the case of 'reverse mentoring', it may be with someone earlier on in their career who is living the experience that the mentee wishes to learn more about).

TABLE 20.5	(Continued)
Supervision	Traditionally is: • a formal process of learning and professional development. • designed to promote optimal outcomes, safety and the well-being of people who access services. • designed to support practitioner well-being. • linked to the maintenance of professional and organisational standards.

Source: Martin et al. [32] / with Permission of Taylor & Francis.

Advanced practitioners within large organisations may be able to access coaching, mentoring or supervision support through formal channels including via their Learning and Development team, although local and regional policies vary. Readers are advised to seek clarification on the availability within their organisation and region, including local forums for peer support.

Recognising that supervision and assessment for and with advanced practitioners is essential to develop confidence and capabilities within the workforce, the Centre for Advancing Practice have published a range of supporting resources [33]. Led by Professor Deborah Harding, minimum standards of supervision are now available, alongside a set of supervisor capabilities and a collection of stories and podcasts. Also available are action plan templates and checklists for supervisor readiness and advanced practitioner readiness. These tools support individuals and organisations to develop the necessary infrastructure to enhance safe and effective advanced practice.

Networks and Communities of Practice

Healthcare practitioners are always learning and the type of learning extends way beyond mandatory training or 'the amount' required to satisfy the needs of the regulators.

Informal or formal networks, including communities of practice, play a valuable role in connecting people to learn and grow. They deliver learning opportunities that fit effectively with the cognitive, humanistic and social learning theories previously discussed. It was one such Network (Advanced Practice in Mental Health Network – APMHN) that led the two authors to meet, connect and learn from each other in the first place and now we're writing this book chapter together.

A community of practice is a group of people who share a common interest and passion for something they do and learn how to do it better through interacting with each other [34]. The community may be local, regional, national and international with the ability to form connections in the real and virtual worlds.

Returning to the APMHN – the first version of the network was funded as a pilot for 2 years until 2023. It provided a virtual space for people aspiring to be, studying to be or working as advanced practitioners in mental health to share their experiences across sectors and settings. Regular features at virtual events included: a 'Brag and Steal' item – where individual Network members shared something they have found useful within their context for other people to 'steal' should they wish. A 'Three minute thesis' section provided a space where colleagues could briefly and informally share the findings from their academic studies or practice-based audits and evaluations. Time was ring-fenced after the features for smaller groups to discuss what had been learnt and identify elements to take back into their own workplace. The APMHN members also contributed to the development of national resources to support advancing practice in mental health, including an implementation guide and a myth-busting resource [35, 36].

There are many benefits to actively participating in a Community of Practice. For example, the evaluation data from the APMHN showed that people valued a safe space to belong, to share information and experiences with each other and feel less isolated as they developed roles within their organisations.

Readers are encouraged to explore the availability of communities and networks to meet their learning and development needs. And if it is not possible to locate one, then consider setting one up. The APMHN started with 12 members (including Kayleigh) who came together and initially shared email addresses. Over the course of 2 years, it grew to over 1000 people!

Mental Health and Well-Being Especially During Transitions

Sometimes the type of support that individuals need within the workforce extends beyond what is provided by methods such as coaching, mentoring or supervision.

Trauma-informed approaches can help personal and professional well-being. For example, Talking Therapies can help with work-related anxiety, to make career choices and manage emotional distress, the impact of bullying and our own life events and health conditions [37]. The everyday experiences of working within healthcare may also impact on an individual's well-being, including, but not limited to the negative impact on mental and emotional well-being as the pandemic progressed [38].

Talking Therapies may support us as individuals to grow both personally and professionally for a range of inter-related reasons. Acknowledging that self-funding may be required, if this is something you wish to explore, a starting point is the BACP Directory, which is a searchable directory of private therapists who offer a range of services.

> **REFLECTIVE QUESTION:** Which human-based opportunities do you feel you would like to explore in more detail? How can you use them to support your own career growth?

CONCLUSION

The focus of this chapter has been on personal and professional growth to advance multi-professional careers in the mental health setting. It has explored different aspects of growth in separate sections but, in conclusion, the inter-relationship between personal and professional growth must not be overlooked.

The use of resources to support growth has been critically debated including the resources we have within ourselves (e.g. our mindsets, our approaches to learning and our ability to self-assess our level of performance), as well as resources available to us in the form of frameworks and human support (supervision, coaching, mentoring, etc).

The overall purpose of this chapter, coming at the end of the book, is to reinforce the need for individual practitioners to proactively own and drive their careers in advanced practice in mental health and maybe beyond that level of practice to consultant level or into other roles of interest. This needs care and intention, including to look after ourselves along the way, in order for us to best serve the people who access our services.

REFERENCES

1. NHS England (2022). Mental health advanced practice area specific capability and curriculum framework. https://advanced-practice.hee.nhs.uk/wp-content/uploads/sites/28/2025/01/Mental-health-advanced-practice-area-specific-capability-and-curriculum-framework-NHSE.pdf (accessed 11th June 2025).
2. Nutley, T (2023). The links between personal and professional development. UK College of Personal Development. https://ukcpd.co.uk/the-links-between-personal-and-professional-development (accessed 11th June 2025).

3. Nursing and Midwifery Council (2024). Guidance sheet – reflective practice. www.nmc.org.uk/global assets/sitedocuments/revalidation/reflective-practice-guidance.pdf (accessed 11th June 2025).
4. Health and Care Professions Council (2024). Recognise, reflect, resolve: the benefits of reflecting on your practice. https://www.hcpc-uk.org/standards/meeting-our-standards/reflective-practice (accessed 11th June 2025).
5. NHS England (2022). Safety culture: learning from best practice (webpage). https://www.england.nhs.uk/long-read/safety-culture-learning-from-best-practice (accessed 11th June 2025).
6. Sinek, S. (2011). Chapter 3: The golden circle. In: *Start with why: how Great Leaders Inspire Everyone to Take Action*. Great Britain: Portfolio Penguin.
7. Brown, B. (2020). Dare to lead list of values. https://brenebrown.com/resources/dare-to-lead-list-of-values (accessed 11th June 2025).
8. International Institute for Management Development (2024). The 8 key leadership skills you need to know in 2024. https://www.imd.org/reflections/leadership-skills (accessed 11th June 2025).
9. Huecker, M.R., Shreffler, J., McKeny, P.T., and Davis, D. (2023). Imposter Phenomenon. In: *StatPearls [Internet]*. Treasure Island: StatPearls Publishing. https://www.ncbi.nlm.nih.gov/books/NBK585058 (accessed 11th June 2025).
10. Thomas M, Bigatti S. (2020). Perfectionism, impostor phenomenon, and mental health in medicine: a literature review. *International Journal of Medical Education* 11:201–213. https://doi.org/10.5116/ijme.5f54.c8f8. https://www.ncbi.nlm.nih.gov/pmc/articles/PMC7882132 (accessed 11th June 2025).
11. Bravata, D.M., Watts, S.A., Keefer, A.L. et al. (2019). Prevalence, predictors, and treatment of impostor syndrome: a systematic review. *Journal of General Internal Medicine* 35 (4): 1252–1275. https://www.ncbi.nlm.nih.gov/pmc/articles/PMC7174434 (accessed 11th June 2025).
12. Saujani, R. (2023). Imposter syndrome is a scheme: Reshma Saujani's Smith college commencement address. https://www.youtube.com/watch?v=BoHDDgeQtlc (accessed 11th June 2025).
13. Hayden, D. (2023). Learning theories that impact on design. CIPD factsheet. https://www.cipd.org/en/knowledge/factsheets/learning-theories (accessed 11th June 2025).
14. Newton, P., Najabat-Lattif, H., Santiago, G., and Salvi, A. (2021). The learning styles neuromyth is still thriving in medical education. *Frontiers in Human Neuroscience* 15. https://doi.org/10.3389/fnhum.2021.708540 (accessed 11th June 2025).
15. Dreyfus, S. and Dreyfus, H. (1980). A five stage model of the mental activities involved in directed skill acquisition. California university Berkeley operations research center [monograph on the internet]. https://www.researchgate.net/publication/235125013_A_Five-Stage_Model_of_the_Mental_Activities_Involved_in_Directed_Skill_Acquisition (accessed 11th June 2025).
16. Benner, P. (1982). From novice to expert. *American Journal of Nursing* 82 (3): 402–407.
17. Leary, A. (2019). Enhanced Practice: a workforce modelling project for Health Education England. https://www.hee.nhs.uk/our-work/enhanced-practice-0 (Accessed 11th June 2025).
18. Dweck, C.S. (2017). *Mindset: Changing the Way you Think to Fulfil your Potential*, 6th. Robinson Publisher.
19. Dweck, C.S. and Yeager, D.S. (2019). Mindsets: a view from two eras. *Perspectives on Psychological Science* https://doi.org/10.1177/1745691618804166 14: 481–496.
20. Yeager, D.S. and Dweck, C.S. (2020). What can be learned from growth mindset controversies? *American Psychologist* 75 (9): 1269–1284. https://doi.org/10.1037/amp0000794.
21. Williams, C. and Lewis, L. (2021). Mindsets in health professions education: a scoping review. *Nurse Education Today* 100: 104863. https://doi.org/10.1016/j.nedt.2021.104863.
22. Dancza, K., Tempest, S., Baird, J., and Volkert, A. (2023). Chapter 2. Concepts that help us do supervision well. In: *Supervision for occupational therapy: practical guidance for supervisors and supervisees* (ed. K. Dancza, A. Volkert, and S. Tempest), 25–47. Routledge.

23. Kruger, J. and Dunning, D. (1999). Unskilled and unaware of it: how difficulties in recognising one's own incompetence lead to self-inflated self-assessments. *Journal of Personality and Social Psychology* 77 (6): 1121–1134. https://doi.org/10.1037/0022-3514.77.6.1121.
24. Royal College of Speech and Language Therapists (2023). Making Frameworks work for you and your team [podcast]. https://soundcloud.com/rcslt/making-frameworks-work-for-you-and-your-team?utm_source=clipboard&utm_medium=text&utm_campaign=social_sharing (accessed 11th June 2025).
25. Collins dictionary online (2024). Definition of 'framework'. https://www.collinsdictionary.com/dictionary/english/framework
26. Royal College of Occupational Therapists (2021). Career development framework: guiding principles for occupational therapists. RCOT www.rcot.co.uk/explore-resources/rcot-publications/career-development (accessed 11th June 2025).
27. Royal College of Speech and Language Therapists (2023). Professional development framework. https://www.rcslt.org/learning/professional-development-framework (accessed 11th June 2025)
28. NHS England (2025). Multi-professional framework for advanced practice in England 2025. https://advanced-practice.hee.nhs.uk/mpf2025 (accessed 11th June 2025).
29. Council of Deans for Health (2023). AHP educator career framework. www.councilofdeans.org.uk/wp-content/uploads/2023/04/Allied-Health-Professions-Educator-Framework.pdf (accessed 11th June 2025).
30. NHS England (2024). Multi-professional practice-based research capabilities framework. https://advanced-practice.hee.nhs.uk/our-work/research/multi-professional-practice-based-research-capabilities-framework (accessed 11th June 2025).
31. Broughton, W. and Harris, G. (2019). *on behalf of the Interprofessional CPD and Lifelong Learning UK Working Group. Principles for Continuing Professional Development and Lifelong Learning in Health and Social Care.* Bridgwater: College of Paramedics. https://collegeofparamedics.co.uk/COP/ProfessionalDevelopment/Principles_for_CPD.aspx (accessed 11th June 2025).
32. Martin, P., Dancza, K., Volkert, A., and Tempest, S. (2023). Chapter 1. Setting the stage for supervision. In: *Supervision for Occupational Therapy: practical Guidance for Supervisors and Supervisees* (ed. K. Dancza, A. Volkert, and S. Tempest). London: Routledge.
33. NHS England (2024). Supervision and assessment resources. https://advanced-practice.hee.nhs.uk/our-work/supervision/supervision-and-assessment-resources (accessed 11th June 2025).
34. Wenger-Trayner, E; Wenger-Trayner B. (2015). Introduction to communities of practice: a brief overview of the concepts and its uses. https://www.wenger-trayner.com/introduction-to-communities-of-practice (accessed 11th June 2025).
35. NHS England (2022). Mental health resources. https://advanced-practice.hee.nhs.uk/resources/mental-health-resources (accessed 11th June 2025).
36. NHS England (2020). Workplace supervision for advanced practice – An integrated multi-professional approach for practitioner development. https://advanced-practice.hee.nhs.uk/our-work/supervision (accessed 11th June 2025).
37. British Association of Counselling and Psychotherapy (2024). What therapy can help with. www.bacp.co.uk/about-therapy/what-therapy-can-help-with (accessed 11th June 2025).
38. British Medical Association (2023). Covid-19: The impact of the pandemic on the medical profession. www.bma.org.uk/advice-and-support/covid-19/what-the-bma-is-doing/covid-19-the-impact-of-the-pandemic-on-the-medical-profession (accessed 11th June 2025).

Index

A

abductive reasoning, 71t, 74–75
Accessible Information Standards, 293
adapted integrative treatment planning model, *373*
adaptive information processing (AIP) model, 120
advanced care planning, 170
advanced clinical practice, 201–202
Advanced Decision to Refuse Treatment (ADRT), 155
advanced practice in mental health, 12–13
    application of digital innovation, 188–193
    co-production and co-creation in, 206–207
    four pillars of, *13*
    importance of experts by experience in, 201–205
    logo for, *21*
Advanced Practice Mental Health Curriculum and Capabilities Framework, 20–21, *21*
advanced practitioner (AP)
    actions, 373
    clinical pillar, *355*, 355–358
    consultation, 372
    follow-up, 372
    intervention, 373–374
    role, 14–17, 288
Advanced Practitioners in Mental Health (APMH)
    case study, 371
    clinical pillar, 355–358
    definition, 4
    diagnostic overshadowing, 6
    education, 6, 362–368
    examples, 356–358
    history, 4–5
    human support for professional growth, 392–394
    leadership, 359–362
    management, 359–362
    parity of esteem, 5–6
    personal growth, 382–383
    positioning, 6–7
    professional and personal self-awareness, 383–386
    professional growth, 386–391
    research, 368–371
advanced risk assessment, 301–316
Adverse Childhood Experiences (ACEs), 109–111
adversity, 110
African Alliance for Maternal Mental Health (AAMMH), 224
All Party Parliamentary Group (APPG), 226
anchoring bias, 92–93
antipsychotics, 311, 313
anxiety, symptoms of, 290
Approved Clinician (AC), 15, 163
Approved Mental Health Professional (AMHP), 15, 162
artificial intelligence (AI), 186, 191–192, 256
Assist-Lite tool, 334
attention deficit hyperactivity disorder (ADHD), 117, 118t, 136, 250, 309
autism
    and gender identity, 287
    and mental illness, 286–287
Autism Act, 293
autism spectrum disorder (ASD), 117, 118t, 250, 310
autistic people, learning disabilities
    autism and gender identity, 287
    autism and mental illness, 286–287
    case study, 296–297
    clinical learning event 1, 295
    clinical learning event 2, 295–296
    introduction, 285
    learning disability, 287–288
    mental health assessment tools, 291
    mental ill health, 287–288
    pharmacology and, 291–292

B

Beck Youth Inventory (BYI), 255t
behaviour learning theory, 387t
Behavioural and Emotional Rating Scale (BERS-2), 255t

The Advanced Practitioner in Mental Health, First Edition. Edited by Clare Allabyrne.
© 2026 John Wiley & Sons Ltd. All rights reserved, including rights for text and data mining and training of artificial intelligence technologies or similar technologies. Published 2026 by John Wiley & Sons Ltd.

benzodiazepines, 312, 340
Berlin Wisdom Paradigm, 101
Best Use of Medicines in Pregnancy (BUMPs), 238
biopsychosocial model
   clinical guidance, 32
   definition, 28
   future, 33–34
   historical influences, 29–32, *30*
   integrative care, 40–41, *41*
   multi-professional consultant practice, 39–40, *40*
   psychology and technology, 34–35
   social determinants, 35–39
bipolar personality disorder (BPD), 109, 117
boundary seesaw model, 97, *98*
breastfeeding, 135–136, 142
Brief Parental Self-Efficacy Scale (BPSES), 255*t*

C

Care Act, 157, 293
Care (Education) and Treatment Review (CETR), 258
care planning theory, 168, 237
Care Quality Commission (CQC), 54, 58–59, 199, 307
Centre for Addiction and Mental Health (CAMH), 207
Child and Adolescent Mental Health Services (CAMHS), 176–177, 187, 212, 288, 356
   case studies, 259–260
   child development theories, 249–250, 249*t*
   historical context of, 246–248
   neurodivergence, 250–251
   outcome and experience measures, 255–256, 255*t*–256*t*
   physical health and, 252–255
   prescribing in, 251–252
   and psychopharmacology, 251–252
   roles in, 247
   safeguarding, 258–259
   societal cultural shifts and, 252
   specific risks in, 256–258
   systemic and multi-agency working, 248–249
   tiers, *246*
   types of medications, 251
child development theories, 249–250
Child in Need Plan (CIN), 232*t*
Child Outcome Rating Scale (CORS), 256*t*
Child Outcomes Research Consortium (CORC), 255
Child Protection Plan, 232*t*, 239
Children and Young People (CYP), 310–311
children with learning disabilities, 290
Children's Global Assessment Scale (CGAS), 255*t*
chronic kidney disease (CKD), 56, 57
chronic pain, 119, 119*t*
clinical competence, *388*
clinical leadership, 360–361, 362
clinical pillar
   development of, 355–356
   examples, 356–358
   professional perspectives, 356
clinical reasoning
   abductive reasoning, 71*t*, 74–75
   Bloom's cognitive taxonomy, 66, 67*t*
   clinical practice, 64–66
   complication, 80
   curriculum and capabilities framework, 64, 64*t*
   deductive reasoning, 70, 71*t*, 72–73, 75
   definitions, 66
   dual process theory, 66–68, 69*t*
   education, 65
   inductive reasoning, 71*t*, 73–75
   leadership and management, 65
   PTSD, 76–78, *79*
   research, 65–66
   role and place of formulation, 76
   System 1 thinking to System 2 thinking, 79–80
   System 2 thinking to System 1 thinking, 75
coaching, 392–393, *392t*–*393t*
co-creation, 206
cognitive awareness, 103
cognitive biases, 95*t*–97*t*, 95–98, *98*
cognitive load, 68
cognitive processing, 111
cognitive regulation, 103
cognitive theory, 387*t*
collaborative care planning
   advanced care planning, 170
   CAMHS, 176–177
   care planning theory, 168
   curriculum and capabilities framework, 167, 167*t*
   legal frameworks, 169–170
   legal implications, 171
   multidisciplinary team, 168–169, 174–176
   patient and family, 171–173
   shared decision-making, 169
   SMART objectives, 170
collaborative planning, 337, 357–358
collaborative risk assessment, 307
Community Mental Health Nurse (CMHN), 156–157
Community Mental Health Team (CMHT), 356
Community Treatment Order (CTO), 159
competence, stages of, 365
complexity
   definition, 80
   diagnostic formulation, *82*, 82–83
   external model, 81
   risk factors, 81
Comprehensive Health Assessment Tool (CHAT), 310
confidentiality, 308
confirmation bias, 93, 95*t*
constructivist theory, 387*t*
contemporary issues, 30–32
continuous professional development (CPD), 204

co-occurring mental health and drugs and
  alcohol (COMHAD)
  assessment and treatment, 331
  assessment of alcohol, 335
  case study, 343–344
  clinical practice, 328
  collaborative planning, 337
  considerations in, 329
  cultural competence, 330
  definition, 329
  education, 328
  education and research, 345
  formulation, 337
  harm minimisation, 342
  inequalities, 330–331
  intervention and evaluation, 337–338
  introduction, 329
  leadership, 328, 345
  legal issues and implications, 332t
  management, 328
  motivational interviewing, 343
  person-centred therapeutic alliance, 331
  physical investigations, 336
  relapse prevention, 343
  research, 328
  risk assessment, 336–337
  stigma, 330
  trauma-informed care, 343
coping, 111
co-production, 206
covert administration of medications, 161
C-Reps, 77
Critical Appraisal Skills Programme (CASP), 138, *138*
cultural competence, 330
Current Risk of Violence (CuRV), 310
CYP-IAPT strategy, 247
cytochrome P450 (CYP450) system, 133

D

DCB0129, 184–185
DCB0160, 184–185
deductive reasoning, 70, 71t, 72–73, 75
default-mode network (DMN), 66, 67
delirium, 276
depression, 35–38, 274, 277–278, 288
Deprivation of Liberty Safeguards (DoLS) Best Interests
  Assessor, 162–163
Derby model, 364, *365*
diabetes, 35–38
diagnostic overshadowing, 6, 289
Diagnostic Statistical Manual (DSM), 32
digital technology
  classification of, 182–184
  classification rules, 183t
  clinical practice, 189

clinical risk management standards, 184–185
  education, 189–190
  Embers the Dragon, 187–188
  experience-based co-design approaches, 186t
  introduction, 181–185
  leadership and management, 189
  management of care, 185–188
  and medical devices, 182–184
  patient's perspective, 186
  research, 190
  social media, 192–193
District Nursing (DN) team, 156–157
drug distribution, 133
dual process theory, 66–68, 69t
Dunning-Kruger effect, 91, 99, 389–390, 390t
Dynamic Risk Assessment and Management System
  (DRAMS), 310
Dynamic Support Register (DSR), 258

E

early life experiences, 109–110
EBE. *see* experts by experience
emergency department, 307
Equality Act, 152–153, 293
estimated date of delivery (EDD), 232t
ethical leadership, 362
European Conformity Marking (CE), 183, *184*
Experience of Service Questionnaire (ESQ), 256t
Experience-Based Co-Design (EBCD), 202–203
experts by experience (EBEs)
  co-creation, 206
  contributions of, 199–200
  co-production, 206
  definition of, 199
  education, 203–204
  emotional and psychological challenges, 208
  ethical and professional challenges, 208
  ethical framework for, *209*
  importance of, 201–205
  integration, 206–214
  involvement of, 202, *205*
  in leadership, 202–203
  overview, 198–199
  pharmacology in, 210t–211t
  practical and logistical challenges, 208–209
  professionals, 212–213
  research, 204–205
  systemic and organisational challenges, 209
  testimonials, 212–213
eye movement de-sensitisation and reprocessing
  (EMDR), 120

F

facilitating learning, 363
factual knowledge, 101

FivexMore, 229
forensic mental health, 301–316

G

General Pharmaceutical Council (GPhC), 201
gifted experience, 198
Global Alliance for Maternal Mental Health (GAMMH), 224
governance
    acknowledgement, 11–12
    advanced practice, 12–13, *13*
    advanced practice roles of, 16–17
    advanced practitioner role, 14–17
    curriculum and capabilities, 20–21, *21*
    history, 11
    scope of practice, 17–19, *19*
    training, 19
    workforce and service transformation, 14
Greater Manchester Mental Health Recovery Academy (UK), 206
Green Light Toolkit, 293–294
growth mindset theory, 389

H

harm minimisation, 342
Health and Care Professions Council (HCPC), 201
Health and Social Care Act, 185, 293
Health Education England Older Adults Mental Health (HEE OAMH), 268
health policy leadership, 360
health systems leadership, 361
Health-Based Place of Safety (HBPoS), 307–308
heuristics
    anchoring bias, 92–93
    cognitive biases and mitigation, 95*t*–97*t*, 95–98, *98*
    confirmation bias, 93
    definition, 90
    metacognition (*see* metacognition)
    representativeness, 93–94
High Dose Antipsychotic Therapy (HDAT), 312
holistic care. *see also* biopsychosocial model
    definition, 28
    historical influences, 29–32, *30*
Human Rights Act 1998, 151–152, *152*
humanistic theory, 387*t*
hyponatraemia, 276

I

iatrogenic harm, 112–113
inductive reasoning, 71*t*, 73–75
initial child protection conference (ICPC), 239
inpatient environment, 55–59
integrative care, 40–41, *41*. *see also* physical health
Interim Care Order (ICO), 239

J

Johari Window, 99, *99*

L

lack mental capacity, 155–156
last menstrual period (LMP), 232*t*
Lasting Powers of Attorney (LPAs), 154–155
learning disability (LD), 287–288, 310
    learning difficulties *vs.*, 250–251, 251*t*
    mortality, 292
learning, taxonomy of, 363
LeDeR report, 289
legal issues
    clinical and leadership, 151
    clinical investigation and examination, 158–159
    Equality Act 2010, 152–153
    Human Rights Act 1998, 151–152, *152*
    Mental Capacity Act 2005, 154–157
    Mental Health Act, 157
    Mental Health Units (Use of Force) Act, 157–158
    reasonable adjustments, 153–154
    social workers, nurses and occupational therapists, 162–163
    treatment, 159–161
local authority (LA), 232*t*
Lord Darzi report, 11

M

Maternal Mental Health Alliance (MMHA), 224
Medical Device Regulations, 182
medical devices
    categories of, 182*t*
    characteristic of, 184
    classes of, 183*t*
Medicines and Healthcare products Regulatory Agency (MHRA), 139, 183
Mental Capacity Act, 59, 154–157, 171, 293
mental health, 252
    experts by experience (EBEs), 198
    good practice in, 293–295
Mental Health Act (MHA), 102, 157, 159–161
mental health in older people
    assessment of mental health problems in, 271–272
    assessment tools, 272–273
    capacity assessment in, 278
    and care planning, 275
    case study, 271, 272, 274–275, 277
    clinical history, 272–273
    cognitive impairment, 277–278
    cognitive screening tests, 278
    depression, 274, 277–278
    formulation and collaborative treatment, 275
    frailty, 275–276
    introduction, 267–268

person-centred care and, 268–269
physical conditions and medications, 273t
physical health complexity, 275–276
prescribing in, 276
safety planning, 278
Mental Health Units (Use of Force) Act, 157–158
mentoring, 392–393, 392t–393t
metacognition
knowledge, 98–99
regulation, 101–103
role descriptors, 91, 91t–92t
self-awareness, 99–101, 101t
Mindfulness Based Cognitive Behaviour Therapy (MCBT), 191
mitigation, 95t–97t, 95–98, 98
mother and baby units (MBUs), 226
motivational interviewing, 343
multidisciplinary team (MDT), 168–169, 174–176
multimorbidity, 52–53
multi-professional consultant practice, 39–40, 40

N

National Development Team for Inclusion (NDTI), 293, 294
National Disability Strategy, 293
National Framework for Recovery, 207
National Institute of Clinical Excellence (NICE), 184
National Institute of Health Research (NIHR), 188
neurodivergence, 250–251
neurodiversity, 117–118, 118t
neurotransmitters, 136, 137t
Newton's third law, 77
NHS Long Term Plan, 7, 268
NHS Long Term Workforce Plan, 11, 14
Nursing and Midwifery Council (NMC), 50, 201

O

obsessive compulsive disorder (OCD), 139, 176–177, 289
older adults, 135
older people, mental health in
assessment of mental health problems in, 271–272
assessment tools, 272–273
capacity assessment in, 278
and care planning, 275
case study, 271, 272, 274–275, 277
clinical history, 272–273
cognitive impairment, 277–278
cognitive screening tests, 278
depression, 274, 277–278
formulation and collaborative treatment, 275
frailty, 275–276
introduction, 267–268
person-centred care and, 268–269

physical conditions and medications, **273**
physical health complexity, 275–276
prescribing in, 276
safety planning, 278
Older People's Mental Health (OPMH), 356, 361
Organisation for the Review of Care and Health Apps (ORCHA), 186
Outcome Rating Scale (ORS), 256t
owned experience, 198

P

parity, 232t
parity of esteem, 5–6
perinatal mental health
assessment in, 231–232
factors, 228t
four pillar capabilities, 224t
health inequalities, 229
introduction, 224–225
obstetric history, 232–233
pathways, 230
perinatal professional network, 226, 226
person-centred alliance, 231
policy context, 225–226
prevalence, 227
safeguarding, 239–240
specific assessment information, 232
suicidality and suicide in, 228
personal growth, 382–383
personality disorder (PD), 287
pharmacodynamics, 132–134
pharmacogenomics, 136–138, 137t, 138
pharmacokinetics, 132–134
pharmacology, 237–238
physical health
context of, 49–50
deteriorating patient, 54–55
inpatient environment, 55–59
law, 59
mental health problems, 59
serious mental illness, 50–53
physical health monitoring, 144
physiological response, 111
Plan, Do, Study, Act (PDSA) cycle, 190, 190
postnatal period, 237
post-traumatic stress disorder (PTSD), 70, 76–78, 79, 116, 117, 119, 119t
pregnancy
and breastfeeding, 135–136
management of acute agitation in, 238–239
or breastfeeding, 142
stages of, 136
prescribing rights, 16
procedural knowledge, 101

professional growth, 386–391
  human support for, 392–394
professional leadership, 361–362
Psychiatric-Mental Health Nurse Practitioners (PMHNPs), 4
psychological impact, 111
psychopharmacology
  children, 134–135
  curriculum and capabilities framework, 131t
  definition, 131
  history, 131–132
  older adults, 135
  pharmacodynamics, 132–134
  pharmacogenomics, 136–138, 137t, 138
  pharmacokinetics, 132–134
  pregnancy and breastfeeding, 135–136
  prescribing, 139, 142–144
  treatment, 139–142

Q
quality-adjusted life year (QALY), 144

R
randomised control trials (RCTs), 251
reasonable adjustments, 153–154
recidivism, 314
recognition, 102
Recovery Colleges Characterisation and Testing in England (RECOLLECT) program, 207
relapse prevention, 343
representativeness heuristics, 93–94
research
  development of, 369, 368
  examples, 369–371
resilience, 111
Responsible Clinician (RC), 15, 163
re-traumatisation risks, 112
Revised Children's Anxiety and Depression Scale (RCADS), 256t
risk
  assessment of, 304–306, 305t–306t
  confidentiality, 308
  demographic subgroups, 308
  five Ps, 306
  gender, 311
  learning disability, 310
  management, 314
  neurodiversity, 309–310
  older adults, 311
  pharmacological considerations, 311–313
  pharmacological interventions for, 313
  race, 308–309
  sexual orientation, 309
  therapeutic risk, 315–316
  types of, 303–304

S
safeguarding, 112, 239–240, 258–259
  child, 239
schizophrenia, 52, 68, 69t, 76, 102, 132, 139, 288, 289
Screening Tool of Older Persons Prescriptions (STOPP), 135
Screening Tool to Alert to Right Treatment (START), 135
seizures, 53
selective serotonin reuptake inhibitor (SSRI), 52, 276
self-awareness, 91, 99–101, 101t
serious mental illness (SMI), 6, 49–53
service transformation, 14
shared decision-making, 169
Short Dynamic Risk Scale (SDRS), 310
situationally accessible memories (SAMs), 77
social and environmental factors, 111
social theory, 387t
social workers, 162–163
South London and Maudsley (SLaM), 207
S-Reps, 77
statutory principles, 154
stigma, 330
Strengths and Difficulties Questionnaire (SDQ), 256t
structured clinical judgement, 257
structured professional judgement (SPJ), 304
Substance Abuse and Mental Health Services Administration (SAMHSA), 109, 113
substance misuse, 102
substance use
  capabilities in, 332t
  clinical assessment in, 333
  considerations in, 329
  pharmacological principles in, 338–339
  questions, 333
  screening tools, 334
supervision, 392–393, 392t–393t
Synthetic Cannabinoid Receptor Agonist (SCRA), 331

T
termination of pregnancy (TOP), 232t
termination of pregnancy for medical reasons (TFMR), 232t
Tourette's syndrome, 250
trauma-focused cognitive behavioural therapy (TF-CBT), 120
trauma-informed care (TIC), 343
  ACEs, 110–111
  assessment, 115–116
  curriculum and capabilities framework, 108t
  definition, 111
  diagnosis of, 116–117
  early life experiences and predisposing factors, 109–110
  EMDR, 120
  iatrogenic harm, 112–113

implementation, 113–114
neurodiversity, 117–118, 118*t*
pharmacology, 121
principles of, 112*t*
PTSD and chronic pain, 119, 119*t*
re-traumatisation risks, 112
risk management, 122
R's assumptions, 112*t*
safeguarding, 122–123
screening tools, 114–115, 115*t*
TF-CBT, 120
therapy, 119, 119*t*
warning signs, 121

U

UK Conformity Assessed (UKCA), 183, *184*
uncertainty, 52–53, 102

United Kingdom Teratology Information Service (UKTIS), 238

V

vaginal birth after caesarean section (VBAC), 232*t*
value relativism, 102
venous thromboembolism (VTE), 56
verbally accessible memories (VAMs), 77
virtual reality (VR), 191

W

Western Australia Recovery College, 207
WYSA study, 192

Y

young people, 143–144
Youth Offender Institutions (YOI), 310